Reconstructing Early Intervention after Trauma

Reconstructing Early Intervention after Trauma

Innovations in the Care of Survivors

Edited by

Roderick Ørner
Consultant Clinical Psychologist
Lincolnshire Partnership NHS Trust
UK

and

Ulrich Schnyder
Head, Psychiatric Department
University Hospital Zurich
Switzerland

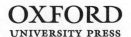

OXFORD
UNIVERSITY PRESS

BS

OXFORD
UNIVERSITY PRESS

Great Clarendon Street, Oxford OX2 6DP

Oxford University Press is a department of the University of Oxford.
It furthers the University's objective of excellence in research, scholarship,
and education by publishing worldwide in

Oxford   New York

Auckland Bangkok Buenos Aires Cape Town Chennai
Dar es Salaam Delhi Hong Kong Istanbul Karachi Kolkata
Kuala Lumpur Madrid Melbourne Mexico City Mumbai
Nairobi Sao Paulo Shanghai Taipei Tokyo Toronto

Oxford is a registered trade mark of Oxford University Press
in the UK and in certain other countries

Published in the United States
by Oxford University Press Inc., New York

A catalogue record for this title is available from the British Library

Library of Congress Cataloging in Publication Data
(Data available)

ISBN 0 19 850834 4 (Pbk)

10 9 8 7 6 5 4 3 2 1

Typeset by Cepha Imaging Pvt Ltd
Printed in Great Britain
on acid-free paper by Biddles Ltd, Guildford and King's Lynn

10/21/03

Dedication

With thanks to our families and friends, some of whom, at great personal risk, campaigned tirelessly for the human rights of free speech, unfettered writing and public debate that makes this book possible.

Preface

We are pleased and honoured to have edited the first book in a new series of publications jointly produced by the European Society for Traumatic Stress Studies and Oxford University Press. Most of all though, we are proud to be associated with the high quality contributions and the levels of passionate convictions expressed by all chapter authors. We do not necessarily agree with the positions taken, but it is to recognize their substantial contributions to shaping this book into what we, as editors, believe is a watershed publication in the continuing quest for promoting a professional commitment to evidence-based practice for early intervention after trauma and within psychotraumatology generally.

At a personal level, we are gratified to realize that, having come through the protracted stages involved in developing this book from an inspired idea first articulated in February 1999 to a material product published in 2003, readers will share with us a sense of being challenged by ideas, rationales and recommendations that underpin reconstructed early interventions after trauma. This is not to imply an expectation of consensus being forged between all parties with an interest in early intervention. Rather, it is a declaration of editorial intention to promote critical, but open-minded assessments and evaluations that inspire informed practices referenced to published evidence. Linked to the same, we hope future debates and service provision for survivors of recent traumas will take comprehensive account of the need to incorporate new knowledge and experience so as to establish a dynamically creative evidence base.

We have edited this book with an eye to the need for a truly informative reference source offering sensible guidance and advice. It should be of help to everyone with an interest in early intervention after trauma, irrespective of personal positions taken in the current debate about post-incident care and support. Particularly, we have sought to offer a broader perspective on early intervention than that which would be engendered by a focus on psychological debriefing alone. By setting out to reconstruct early intervention after trauma, chapters should be of equal interest to students, professionals in practice and training, students, faculty members in academic institutions, service planners, members of high risk professional groups in both military or civilian contexts, and possibly trauma survivors. We note with particular interest a recurrence of the theme of a window of opportunity that now presents itself for the latter two groups to exert a more decisive influence upon service provision. A new era, characterized by unprecedented user influence, is therefore heralded. Practitioners and 'experts' will, in future, have to give consideration to the possibility that trauma survivors are their pre-eminent information source and not vice versa. By implication, we believe this book marks the point where the field of psychotraumatology demonstrates the positive achievements that can be engendered through increased user involvement.

If only for these reasons, the timing of this book is apposite. Other considerations should be taken into account as well. For instance, the early part of the twenty-first century is generating more considered perspectives on both theory and practice in the field of early intervention. Because of this, we believe our respected friends and colleagues have contributed chapters evincing levels of sophistication previously attained only exceptionally in this branch of psychotraumatology. Their texts bear witness to impressive standards of expertise and an admirable capacity to integrate new knowledge into theory, as well as applied practice. By so doing, they demonstrate a too infrequently appreciated aspect of promoting evidence-based practice; namely, that evidence confers degrees of freedom of thought and opportunities for innovation that are far preferable to the trappings of doctrinaire orthodoxy and prescriptive practice.

For this and much else we are truly grateful to all chapter authors. The many hours spent editing draft manuscripts have been times of privileged access to some of the most distinguished experts who define the cutting edge of early intervention after trauma. It has been a time for learning and reflection for us both. Any editorial project is carried along by an expectation of defining new standards of knowledge and standards of practice. In both these respects, authors have delivered chapters of commendable quality. If any reader feels the book fails in respect to these aspirations, we, as editors, take full responsibility.

Our book is not only the product of contributions made by chapter authors. Thanks are due to many others whose generous help and support has been crucial for the completion of our assigned task. They are too many for all to be named in person. All the same, particular thanks are due to Dr Stuart Turner. As Chair of the Editorial Commissioning Subgroup of the Board of Directors of the European Society for Traumatic Stress Studies he took an inspired lead on this project, and has steered it with consummate skill and discretion. Richard Marley, Senior Commissioning Editor with Oxford University Press and his assistant Carol Maxwell succeeded in bringing clear guidance and advice to all involved in this project. The standards of professionalism shown augurs well for other books to be published in a collaborative venture between the European Society for Traumatic Stress Studies and Oxford University Press. Expert secretarial support provided by Pam Hare and Norma Carter has been unfailingly patient and, at times of uncertainty they oiled the wheels of this project by infusing reassuring notes of enthusiasm. To all the above we are truly grateful.

This book can be read from cover to cover or be used as a reference source. Its structure is intended to make explicit both theoretical and practical considerations incorporated in the process of reconstructing early intervention after trauma. In support of these aims, each section is preceded by a brief content summary. The first section of invited contributions starts with an overview of different historical, conceptual and theoretical perspectives on early intervention. To some extent these overlap, but taken together, a clearer impression is formed of the origins of early intervention. In turn, this leads to a consideration of what early intervention can realistically be expected to achieve in the light of published evidence and accumulated experience. In the next section, attention is focused on the nature of initial reactions to trauma plus theoretical perspectives that help foster a greater understanding of biological, psychological, cognitive and systemic processes engendered by traumatic experiences. It is from such theories that rationales for reconstructed early intervention can be formulated, but innovation should not be inspired by theory alone. Of equal importance is recently published evidence about early intervention and Section 3 furnishes a new knowledge base to which future provision should be referenced. Readers of the penultimate section will benefit from authors' accumulated experience of how to provide early intervention following a broad range of trauma. These are 'how to do' chapters, notable for their recurrent emphasis on routine service evaluation and research. In the first part of our concluding chapter we seek to draw together the theoretical and conceptual models described by chapter authors, and integrate these with emergent evidence about reconstructed early intervention. Thereafter, key principles informing evidence-based practice are explained before consideration is given to future directions for early intervention.

We are confident readers will learn as much from chapter authors as we have whilst editing this book. A bonus for all would be if some also feel inspired to further improve standards of help and support for survivors of recent trauma.

Roderick Ørner   February 2003
Ulrich Schnyder

Contents

Contributors

Ron Acierno, National Crime Victims Research and Treatment Center, 3rd Floor Bank Building, Medical University of South Carolina, 171 Ashley Avenue, Charleston SC 29451, USA

Dean Ajduković, Department of Psychology, Faculty of Philosophy, University of Zagreb, I. Lučića 3, 10 000 Zagreb, Croatia

Marina Ajduković, Marina Ajdukovic, Department of Social Work, Faculty of Law, University of Zagreb, Nazorova 51, 10 000 Zagreb, Croatia

Bernice Andrews, Department of Psychology, Royal Holloway, Egham, Surrey TW20 0EX, UK

Anna Avery, Department of Clinical Psychology, Lincolnshire Partnership NHS Trust, Baverstock House, St Anne's Road, Lincoln LN2 5RA, UK

Lionel Bailly, Department of Psychiatry and Behavioural Sciences, Royal Free & University College Medical School, Wolfson Building, 48 Riding House Street, London W1N 8AA, UK

Nancy Baron, Global Psychiatric and Psychosocial Initiatives (GPSI), P.O. Box 1360, The Sarit Center, 00606 Nairobi, Kenya

Jonathon Bisson, Department of Liaison Psychiatry, Room 222, Rawnsley Unit, Monmouth House, University Hospital of Wales, Heath Park, Cardiff CF14 4XW, UK

Chris R. Brewin, Subdepartment of Clinical Health Psychology, University College London, Gower Street, London WC1E 6BT, UK

Richard A. Bryant, School of Psychology, University of New South Wales, NSW 2052, Australia

Matthew J Cordova, Department of Psychiatry and Behavioral Sciences, Stanford University, Palo Alto, CA, USA

Chris Freeman, Rivers Centre for Trauma Stress, Royal Edinburgh Hospital, Morningside, Edinburgh, EH10 5HF, UK

Berthold P. R. Gersons, Academic Medical Center, Tafelbergweg 25, 1105 BC Amsterdam, The Netherlands

Søren Buus Jensen, Global Psychiatric and Psychosocial Initiatives (GPSI), P.O. Box 1360, The Sarit Center, 00606 Nairobi, Kenya

Kaz de Jong, Médecin sans Frontières, P.O. Box 10014, 1001 EA Amsterdam, The Netherlands

Stephen King, Department of Clinical Psychology, Lincolnshire Partnership NHS Trust, Baverstock House, St Anne's Road, Lincoln LN2 5RA, UK

Rolf Kleber, Professor of Psychotraumatology at Tilburg and Utrecht Universities, The Netherlands, and Head Research of the Institute for Psychotrauma

Lars Mehlum, Division of Disaster Psychiatry, University of Oslo, Sognsvannsveien 21, Bygning 20, N-0320 Oslo, Norway

Alexander McFarlane, University of Adelaide, Adelaide, Australia

Robin Minhinnett, National Crime Victims Research and Treatment Center, 3rd Floor Bank Building, Medical University of South Carolina, 171 Ashley Avenue, Charleston SC 29451, USA

Hanspeter Moergeli, Psychiatric Department, University Hospital, Culmannstrasse 8, CH-8091, Zurich, Switzerland

R. J. Ørner, Department of Clinical Psychology, Lincolnshire Partnership NHS Trust, Baverstock House, St Anne's Road, Lincoln LN2 5RA, UK

Sean Perrin, Department of Psychology, Kings College, Institute of Psychiatry, De Crespigny Park, Denmark Hill, London SE5 8AF, UK

Hazel Pilgrim, Duchess of Kent Hospital, Catterick Garrison, Catterick DL9 4DF, UK

Heidi Resnick, National Crime Victims Research and Treatment Center, 3rd Floor Bank Building, Medical University of South Carolina, 171 Ashley Avenue, Charleston SC 29451, USA

Suzanna Rose, West Berkshire Traumatic Stress Service, Berkshire Healthcare NHS Trust, 25 Erleigh Road, Reading, Berks RG1 5LR, UK

Josef I. Ruzek, National Center for Post-Traumatic Stress Disorder, Education and Clinical Laboratory Division, VA Palo Alto Health Care System, 795 Willow Road, Menlo Park, CA 94025 USA

Ulrich Schnyder, Psychiatric Department, University Hospital, Culmannstrasse 8, CH-8091, Zurich, Switzerland

Arieh Y. Shalev, Department of Psychiatry, Hadassah University Hospital, P.O. Box 12000, il-91120 Jerusalem, Israel

Patrick Smith, Department of Psychology, Kings College, Institute of Psychiatry, de Crespigny Park, Denmark Hill, London SE5 8AF, UK

Jane Stafford, National Crime Victims Research and Treatment Center, 3rd Floor Bank Building, Medical University of South Carolina, 171 Ashley Avenue, Charleston SC 29451, USA

Robert J. Ursano, Department of Psychiatry, Uniformed Services, University of the Health Sciences, Bethesda, Maryland, USA

Lars Weisæth, Division of Disaster Psychiatry, University of Oslo, Sognsvannsveien 21, Bygning 20, N-0320 Oslo, Norway

Simon Wesley, Academic Department of Psychological Medicine, Kings College Hospital, 103 Denmark Hill, London SE5 9RS, UK

William Yule, University of London Institute of Psychiatry, de Crespigny Park, London SE5 8AF, UK

Section 1 History and theory

In recent years the debate about early intervention after trauma has reached an impasse. Protagonists are taking increasingly doctrinaire positions inspired by personal conviction and anecdotal accounts of the impact of services provided. Any sense of engaging in constructive exchanges of ideas with some prospect of formulating a new consensus has largely been lost. The debate has become confused, media reports are contradictory and unprecedented levels of skepticism prevail about early intervention both in professional and public domains.

The process of reconstructing early intervention is unlikely to be served by perpetuating current levels of debate. As is often the case under such circumstances, a radical departure from orthodoxy is required. This book seeks to establish a new starting point for examining the complexities of early intervention. It does so initially by focusing on historical roots and critically assesses the veracity of some of the basic premises that inform practice. From such critical analyses emerge new foundations for championing evidence-based service innovations.

Readers are therefore invited to follow a staged process of reconstruction starting with the recognition that early intervention draws on a rich historical legacy originally driven by military expediencies. Symptom elimination is not made an explicit aim of help and support for soldiers with combat stress reactions. The imperative is to return service personnel to front line duties with their units. Considerations of symptom status and early intervention to monitor longer-term adjustment of war veterans are relatively recent innovations. So is the challenge to maintain operational readiness during peacekeeping missions, etc. This is described in the first chapter by Lars Weisæth, Professor of Disaster Psychiatry at the University of Oslo, Norway.

His observations reinforce the importance of being prepared to offer some form of psychosocial intervention after recent trauma. To do nothing is no longer a viable option for any survivor group. The prototype applied model, handed down from military psychiatry, recommends itself for its clarity of purpose, as do the principles of immediacy, proximity and expectancy. From these origins have emerged a number of developments both within and outside military settings; the focus of which have shifted away from an exclusive focus on restoring functionality in the short term to much broader considerations of human welfare.

Trauma, critical incidents and crises were never an exclusive domain of military organizations. They occur with great regularity in civilian settings too. Not surprisingly therefore, a parallel lineage of early intervention services can be traced through an examination of historical developments within psychiatry and psychology. These are discussed in the next chapter. Professor Berthold Gersons, from the Academic Department of Psychiatry at the University of Amsterdam, The Netherlands, describes highly nuanced conceptualizations that evolved from systematic observations of individuals and groups in crises. Natural inclinations to once again establish homeostasis inspired crisis theory from which are derived sensible practices within the specialist field of crisis intervention. Gersons points out how principles of service provision derived from crisis theory and social psychiatry were enthusiastically expropriated by recent champions of early intervention after trauma. In retrospect, this appears to have been ill advised, since in so doing they failed to take due account of differences between reactions associated with crises and those evoked in the early aftermath of trauma. Although often assumed to be identical they are not. Having failed to take account of significant theoretical or phenomenological differences between the two controversies have raged about how to deliver early intervention services and outcomes that might reasonably be expected from its provision. In years to come, reconstructed early intervention will be championed on the basis of crisis theory and crisis intervention being but two of the many important traditions that inform survivor care. Most usefully they advocate priority be given to practical measures that reduce victims' levels of psychophysiological arousal. More elaborate psychological interventions that involve developing trauma narratives with the explicit purpose of eliminating evoked symptoms should be contemplated during later phases of the recovery process.

Since the early 1980s early intervention after trauma appears to have been championed on theoretical and practical rationales presumed to be apposite when, in fact, they were not. With such inauspicious beginnings it comes as no surprise to find the field to be riddled with controversy. Most especially doubts prevail as to the types of outcomes that might reasonably be expected from early intervention. Uncertainties in this regard spring from a number of disparate studies with seemingly contradictory results. The next chapter authored by Suzanna Rose, Jonathan Bisson and Simon Wessely describes the process of conducting a systematic review of the most rigorous, symptom focused outcome studies of one off early interventions published to date. Their conclusions help clarify the extent to which risks accrue to survivors taken through early intervention protocols. As is also the intention of Cochrane Reviews, the investigation also recommends itself for raising standards of debate about past provisions for recent trauma survivors and clarifies what this form of early intervention can reasonably be expected to achieve. Given a lack of consistency of outcomes in studies selected for review these authors are right to conclude the evidence base is at best neutral. Their work also highlights problems inherent in comparing survivor populations whose demographic characteristics may differ as much as the types of traumas to which they have been exposed.

On a more positive note, the overall impression to emerge from all chapters in Section 1 is that reconstructed early intervention must be construed as comprising of more than one set formula or technique for offering help and support. This is because different trauma engender diverse configurations of changeable needs that vary according to the stage of post-exposure adaptation attained by each survivor. In keeping with the above, evaluations of outcomes to be achieved by reconstructed early intervention must document changes beyond the narrow focus of evoked symptoms that have preoccupied investigators to date.

1 Historical background of early intervention in military settings

Lars Weisæth

History deals with the past and is seen by some as a thing of the past. A contemporary military medical historian has, however, stated that doctors of the current PTSD generation are going through the same learning process, as did their colleagues during World War I (WWI) (Shepard, 2000). He points out an apparently recurrent cycle in respect of the war neuroses: 'At first denied, then exaggerated, then understood and finally forgotten'. This chapter sets out to delineate lessons that can be learned from past experiences by examining the changing conceptualizations of combat stress reaction (CSR) and how early intervention can help resolve these multifaceted reactions.

The German doctor Johannes Hofer termed CSR as Nostalgia in 1678 and ever since a range of different diagnostic terms have been used. Initial concerns about the psychological well being of soldiers were, however, not motivated by considerations of their value as individuals. Rather, it was realized that their mental state was crucial for the preservation of manpower and sustained combat effectiveness during battle.

Courage or cowardice

The forms of 'early intervention' offered to military personnel have been predicated by varying perceptions of the causes of observed incapacities to fight. Soldiers' own attitudes towards their symptoms and impairment have also played a decisive role.

Ever since the days of Herodotus and Socrates conflicts between fighting and fleeing are recurring topics in literature and science. By all accounts, the dividing line between fighting and fleeing is extremely thin. In a 4th century BC report on the battle of Thermopylae, Herodotus (1998) describes how a soldier named Aristodamus used illness (an eye infection) as an excuse to withdraw from battle and became the only survivor of the Spartan force. He met with abuse and disgrace from fellow citizens. Interestingly, during the Thermopylae battle another soldier also suffered an eye infection, but had fought on and was killed. Herodotus adds that had both soldiers withdrawn from battle they would not have been scorned because this illness would then have been considered an acceptable reason for not joining combat.

The soldier and his society: the individual and the collective

The Greek city states provided, for the first time in documented history, the stage for free and autonomous individuals to enter the world's stage. However, when society was threatened, individuals would submit to the needs of the larger group and be prepared to risk life for the pursuit of collective values. If killed in battle soldiers would be honoured and commemorated. During the 2000 years that followed soldiers were recruited as mercenaries whose pay comprised a concession to loot and pillage after victorious battle. This contractual arrangement meant that society owed them nothing. If killed they would be interred in anonymous mass graves and those injured had to fend for themselves.

Mass mobilization of free citizens as soldiers again became the rule at the time of the French revolution. Soldiers killed in action now had their names inscribed on war memorials so as never to be forgotten. Even 'The Unknown Soldier' was entitled to a memorial.

Definitions and constructions of combat stress reactions

Perusal of clinical texts reveals that definitions of combat stress reactions include not only descriptions of symptoms, but also imply, more or less explicitly, assumptions about cause–effect relationships. This aetiological approach is crucially important for conceptualizations of CSR, diagnosis and treatment. At one extreme, it has allowed the 'loss of nerve' to result in honourable discharge for those construed to have been courageous, whilst others in similar circumstances were executed for cowardice.

General George Patton, whose views on this subject are thought extreme, said 'Any man who says he has battle fatigue is avoiding danger'. The British Army echoed this perspective when it took the position that a psychiatric casualty is a soldier who becomes ineffective in battle as a direct result of his personality being unable to stand up to the stresses of combat. Similar views are still being advocated in textbooks in military psychiatry. For instance, Jones (1994) wrote 'The psychiatric casualty is a soldier whose instincts of self-preservation (or fears of death and being maimed) have temporarily overcome his loyalties to his fellow soldiers and his military mission'. Such definitions seek to prevent CSR and any apparent lack of compassion for incapacitated soldiers can be understood in relation to the goal of military medical corps, which is 'to preserve manpower'. However, if such priorities are applied indiscriminately for the planning and provision of early intervention, they can foster ruthless and cruel treatments. When such interventions were the subject of an Austrian Commission set up soon after World War I (WWI), Sigmund Freud stated that every war neurosis had a purpose and was a flight into illness by subconscious intentions. He also stated that war neuroses would disappear in the aftermath of the war (Eissler, 1986). History was to prove him wrong on all accounts.

In NATO terminology CSR is used to describe acute reactions of any severity and nature, which do not comprise a recognized mental disorder, manifested in military personnel exposed to exceptional physical or mental stress. As for PTSD diagnostic criteria, it is necessary to demonstrate that a severe stressor has evoked subsequent disabling symptoms. Combat stress reactions should therefore be seen as temporary and reversible reactions, the consequence of which is to reduce functional capability in a previously normal person who has become overwhelmed by severe stresses.

Measuring efficacy of early intervention for CSR

Some of the more powerful studies of the efficacy of early intervention come from wartime practices of 'forward psychiatry'. Its impact on CSR is measured by the number of affected soldiers who are able to return to their fighting units. A number of methodological objections may be raised in respect of the validity and reliability of these measures. Reflecting the imperatives of war, the overriding evaluation criterion is operational readiness, and not a presence or absence of symptoms as might be emphasized in civilian outcome studies. As a consequence, few figures exist that document the proportion of soldiers who could have utilized services or the balance of benefits and costs that accrue from their implementation.

The American Civil War

Cardiovascular symptoms reported by soldiers in armed conflict came to prominence during the American Civil War. This gave rise to a long-running tradition of diagnosis focusing on somatic aspect alone, and the condition became known as 'irritable heart', 'soldiers' heart' and 'Da Costa's syndrome' (Myers 1870; Da Costa 1871). Palpitations, cardiac pain, rapid pulse and respiratory problems were attributed to over-stimulation of special nerve centres at the base of the heart. Fairly high rates of return to battle were achieved if treated with a cocktail of drugs.

The medical model perspectives brought to the field by doctors have inspired this focus on somatization in the complex symptomatology of CSR. All the same, there has been a continuous struggle between those believing in a physical aetiology and those who have seen manifestations of trauma as primarily a psychological disorder. Amongst the latter, the syndrome of reactions are not construed as being indicative of an underlying medical disorder and, therefore, require early psychosocial interventions or therapy in preference to medication (Fischer-Homberger, 1975).

Before WWI

During its war with Japan, at the beginning of the twentieth century, the Russian army made the first experiments with providing treatment at the front. Initially, their services owed more to long evacuation lines than to an empirical understanding of what was best for traumatized soldiers or their units. However, their efforts were the forerunners to what is now known as 'forward psychiatry'. At about this time Hesnard (1914) conducted studies into the emotional changes that could follow in the aftermath of explosions. Advances in knowledge were integrated in the climate of ideas discussed during the period leading up to WWI. Thus, with the advent of the war itself, a fuller understanding of the mass occurrence of CSR was possible and contributed to a recognition of shell shock (Merskey, 1991).

World War I

Severe stresses inherent in the static trench warfare on the western front accrued through the use of high explosives and almost continuous artillery shelling. Every participating nation suffered numerous psychiatric losses from shell shock and it was soon recognized the new condition was caused by the way this war was fought.

However, nosological confusion prevailed during this period. For instance, the notion of 'soldier's heart' found continued expression in the frequently used diagnosis of 'neurocirculatory asthenia' or 'disorderly action of the heart'. It was the third most frequently quoted cause for discharge from the British army and, in 1917, was renamed 'Effort Syndrome' (Merskey, 1991). A clinical discovery of the period was that once a recruit had been told he had 'soldier's heart' it proved extremely difficult for doctors and carers to persuade him his heart could ever again become normal (Shepard, 2000).

The British psychiatrist Charles Samuel Myers (1915) introduced the term shell shock to the medical literature, and the early intervention programmes that followed from it involved evacuation away from front lines for hospital treatment and eventually discharge. However, Myers was also to play an important role in rejecting the connection between battle neurosis and 'organic molecular commotion' in the brain. He emphasized the similarities of this presentation to that of hysteria and later stated that emotional disturbance alone was sufficient to account for this condition (Myers, 1940). In time it was concluded from English, French and German studies that at least 80% of shell shock cases had an emotional aetiology.

By early 1916, Myers (1940) had decided that the diagnosis of shell shock was undesirable. It had apparently caught on like wildfire among the British forces and gave rise to a notion of shell shock being rapidly contagious. For reasons that are not too difficult to understand, soldiers had started to believe that such a diagnosis was synonymous with the occurrence of clinically significant changes in their central nervous systems. From July to December 1916, more than 16,000 cases of shell shock were recorded among British battle casualties and a disproportionate number had participated in the first battle of the Somme.

In France, England and Germany very different views prevailed about the aetiology of shell shock. A considerable body of opinion continued to accept an organic aetiology, even if it could not be demonstrated objectively. Ahrenfeldt (1958) attempted to explain why an organic interpretation of shell shock was held for so long. He lists the biased trends of 'modern' medical science of the time and the belief that British soldiers who were 'heroes' could not possibly show mental symptoms. Another contributing factor was that a condition construed as an injury with an organic basis offered a solution of sorts for all parties. The soldier stood to save his self-respect, and doctors did not have to diagnose personal failure or desertion. However, the diagnostic refinements that occurred during WWI only inspired more informed preventive and early intervention measures for the battle worn to a marginal degree.

Over time, some improved understanding was achieved about the relative roles played by individual vulnerability factors, battle stress factors and collective factors in the genesis of CSR. Whereas many previously stable men did break down, it was generally appreciated that those of vulnerable personality were strongly predisposed to develop shell shock. Nervous disposition, lack of experience, higher age and being amongst reserves brought forward to the front lines are amongst the risk factors linked to ease of developing CSR.

A further consideration was that a high proportion of shell shock cases often came from the same front line units. This pointed to the importance of collective factors in its generation, maintenance and resolution. The realization that combat breakdown was better predicted by collective factors than by individual vulnerability factors or characteristics of the combat situation was both an extremely important finding, from a theoretical and practical perspective. However, it is disappointing to note that during WWI the implications of this insight for selection, training and early intervention were only partly understood and implemented.

According to Shepard (2000), the notion that neurosis is a consequence of mental conflict arising from a sense of duty being matched by unconscious wishes to survive was first adapted to battle psychiatry by the Freudian psychoanalyst David Eder (1916), whilst working with soldiers evacuated from Gallipoli. 'Flight into illness' and 'illness gains' were the first psychoanalytic concepts accepted by the military psychiatric community. French clinicians appear to have been least willing to accept the idea of unconscious motives coming into play during battle. A prevalent view was that hysterical soldiers were indistinguishable from simulators and malingerers. So no expectations of evacuation to safety or war pension compensation should be engendered. To a significant extent this may help explain why their early intervention strategy involved offering front line treatments in accordance with the principles of 'forward psychiatry'. In 1916, the advanced posts of the French Army's Medical Service (*postes de chirurgie d'urgence*) and its neuropsychiatric department reported up to 90% of psychiatric casualties returning to fight at the front.

Early interventions for a military context

By the end of WWI it was understood that early evacuation to the rear imperilled soldiers' mental health by providing a primary gain of saving one's life. However, it reinforced soldiers' perceptions of personal failure, separated them from their peer group and effected a removal from the front, where mass-suggestion sustained men in the belief they were 'striving shoulder to shoulder'.

In August 1916 the British armies were ordered not to evacuate shell shock cases. Myers had created special centres near the front line that offered treatment based on promptness of action, maintaining a suitable environment and provision of appropriate psychotherapeutic interventions (Myers, 1940; War Office Committee 1922). In 1917, the American psychiatrist Thomas W. Salmon visited the Allied medical corps to be advised of the treatment principles applied to battlefront conditions. He had previously been in charge of psychiatric services for immigrants at Ellis Island, where up to 5000 individuals had to be assessed and processed in any one day. His observation on war neurosis was of it being an endless variation of the central themes of escape from a factually intolerable situation to one made bearable by the neurotic condition. Salmon recommended stricter selection of soldiers for combat duties and that treatment be provided by medical officers with special training in psychiatry, positioned as near the front as military exigency would permit. He took great care never to mention the word 'shell shock' since the risks of diagnostic labelling had been recognized. He put in place an organizational arrangement involving three tiers of psychiatric service: the division psychiatrist, the Advanced Neurological Hospital and, about 50 miles to the rear, a base hospital (Salmon, 1917). The principles that underlie forward psychiatry are, to this day, referred to as Salmon's principles in recognition of his important contributions to military psychiatry. American involvement in WWI was so brief that the efficacy of this approach to early intervention could not be systematically evaluated.

The advantages to early intervention achieved by retaining combat casualties near the front and in a military environment proved uncontroversial to senior officers. The same was true for the all-important creation of a proper atmosphere of cure, reassurance and rest. Also, the role of expectancy in helping soldiers back to active service was understood by all. Trials of clinical hypnosis sought to optimize the effects of persuasion and suggestibility. A fuller appreciation was shown for the ways the personality of the medical officer and the quality of the patient–doctor relationship influence outcomes. In fact, a form of ergotherapy (occupational therapy) had been introduced underpinned by the principle of 'cure by functioning' (Brock, 1918).

Controversies

The finding that shell shock was not an organic injury created a power vacuum, since the role of neurologists had been marginalized. A power struggle developed between those who saw shell shock as a 'disorder of will' that could be prevented and cured by disciplinary measures, and those who saw the need for more humane treatments in keeping with patient focused medicine. In seeking to serve both the interests of the individuals and the collective, military psychiatry had to confront difficult ethical dilemmas (Moran, 1945).

Although conceptual advances made during the first quarter of the twentith century could have set standards for care of recently traumatized war veterans, clinical practice remained in many instances primarily informed by prejudice and ill-advised opinion. As a result, brutal forms of electrical therapy were administered to soldiers from Great Britain, Germany and Austria. In part, these helped engender a sense of doctors being actively engaged in the war effort and met a need to be seen to be patriotic. After WWI, the prominent Viennese psychiatrist and subsequent

Nobel laureate Wagner-Jauregg was accused of having tortured patients in his clinic by administering brutal electrical treatments. Formal charges were eventually dismissed.

By and large, however, it seems that, by the end of WWI, a compromise had been reached between those who wished to pursue a moral, disciplinary treatment line and those whose treatment rationales drew on prevailing conflict models of war neurosis (War Office Committee, 1922). Psychiatry matured during WWI and demonstrated through clinical practice that early treatment of combat induced psychological reactions could be successful.

Early intervention between WWI and WWII

With the benefit of hindsight, it is interesting to note the extent to which cultural, social, historical and political forces have influenced the development of traumatic stress theory and clinical practice (Fischer-Homberger, 1975). During the inter-war years theories of traumatic neurosis developed in parallel with the spirit of the age and the focus of attention shifted from external characteristics of war stressors to an examination of their intra-psychic meanings of trauma. Thus, it came to be that CSR and the traumatic neurosis they often gave rise to were construed as neurotic disturbances and not as distinctive post-traumatic stress disorders.

Bonhoeffer (1926) and colleagues in Germany pioneered a school of thought that considered the traumatic neurosis a social illness that could only be cured by social remedies. The sociological perspective this gave rise to proposed that neurotic disorders can be understood if explanations incorporate social processes that are a feature of the daily lives of the general public. Accordingly, the cause of traumatic neurosis was construed to be the secondary personal and social gains associated with the disorder, which would therefore only arise in predisposed individuals (Jaspers, 1953).

Controversies continued to rage between those who saw traumatic neurosis as developing after exposure to real external trauma and those who construed internal or fantasy trauma as the most important etiological agents. Groundbreaking discoveries of the traumatic effect of severe external stressors had been published on several occasions, but in each instance they were followed by a surge of interest in and acceptance of the intra-psychic conflict such events might engender. This happened when Freud launched his theory of neurosis based upon sexual trauma. Unfortunately, this fascinating insight into internal psychic processes was accompanied by a reduced interest in the reality aspects of external trauma. This emphasis on unconscious conflicts to account for symptom generation helped create an impression of psychiatric disorders as 'irrational' and little credence was given to the notion they could be understood to be a function of actual developmentally disruptive experiences. Only a few new studies on the effects of traumatic life events were carried out during the 1920s and 1930s.

A notable exception was Rivers (1922), who drew upon his clinical work with traumatized soldiers to challenge Freud's theory of dreaming as a form of wish fulfilment. He proposed that dreams arise as an attempt to solve some of the persistently disturbing conflicts being experienced whilst awake.

World War II

Lessons learned during WWI about how to deliver early intervention during wartime had largely been set aside by the start of WWII and had to be resurrected. Thus, once again, faulty treatment procedures, such as evacuation away from front line areas, was practised at great prognostic cost for affected soldiers and resulting in severe loss of manpower for military forces (Stouffer *et al.*, 1949; Ahrenfeldt, 1958). As this realization dawned, steps were taken to improve understanding of combat stress reactions within implicated armed forces and early intervention was modelled on WWI policies.

BICEPS (brevity, immediacy, centrality, expectancy, proximity, simplicity) became the essential elements of forward psychiatry as practised amongst Allied nations. For the first time these treatment principles were also applied at the front line by personnel without a medical background. Distinctions were drawn between acute and chronic cases. For the latter, physical fatigue had often worn soldiers down and lowered their resistance to situational stresses. During battles in North Africa 30–70% would experience relief from CSR within 30 hours if given rest and assurance near front lines. Reports from other battlefronts also documented 30–70% return rates to the fighting unit within 3 days (Shepard, 2000). By April 1943 a decision was made that the initial diagnosis for all psychiatric casualties in the US Army would be 'combat exhaustion'.

It is interesting to note that early interventions involving re-experiencing of combat trauma alone had very disappointing results. Grinker and Spiegel (1943) reported a 2% return rate following 'narcosynthesis' and drug-induced abreaction. Of battle stress casualties evacuated to North Africa from Sicily, only 3% returned to their original units.

While stress-related gastric and intestinal disorders were frequently reported during WWII, true hysterical disorders presented less often than in WWI. The acceptance of fear as a natural response during combat that could be controlled may account for this change, but this may just reflect different diagnostic priorities. Merskey (1991) makes this point when stating 'If the military medical culture does not expect conversion symptoms—and expects anxiety ones, the former largely vanish'.

The German army reported very few cases of combat stress reactions during the first part of WWII. This contrasts with high levels of psychosomatic disturbances on the Allied side, but to make psychiatric diagnoses was practically forbidden in the Wehrmacht. Therefore, very little is known about CSR among German soldiers. Recent publications reveal severe psychiatric problems in the German Navy as losses of submarine crews grew dramatically during the U-boat war.

This said, few theoretical refinements were achieved during WWII. The main point of progress was a more considered view of what makes soldiers prepared to risk their lives. Marshall (1947) formulated this as 'Men do not fight for a cause but because they do not want to let their comrades down'. New and deeper understandings of group dynamics emerged from the accumulated experiences of psychiatrists who worked within the armed forces during WWII. In Britain, group therapy and milieu therapy grew directly from army experiences accrued by psychoanalysts (Main, 1989). In the USA, Colonel S.L.A. Marshall promoted group talks and a new research focus on protective factors, such as training, group cohesion, leadership, motivation and morale, helped develop military psychiatry (Arenfeldt, 1958).

Early interventions inspired by behaviour and learning theories received little recognition during WWII. However, Sargant and Shorvon (1945) incorporated these as adjuncts to eclectic treatments in the form of exposure training. How it came to be that traumatic stress syndromes were not systematically studied by behaviourists is hard to understand, since stressful war events offer laboratory-like experimental opportunities for research on stimulus-response relationships.

The Korean War

Like WWI, this campaign largely took the form of static trench warfare. Rotation from the front line after 9 months helped reduce psychiatric casualty rates, but the overall impression is that lessons learned during previous wars were, once again, set aside. However, as soon as evacuation rates reached levels that compromised operational readiness psychiatric expertise was called for once again. Help came from Colonel Albert Glass who had served as a WWII psychiatrist.

His contribution was to update and improve the Salmon principles for early intervention. Very tough BICEPS intervention programmes reduced psychiatric casualties to 37 per 1000 men (Glass, 1954).

Studies conducted during the Korean War again demonstrated that individual demographic or environmental factors accounted for only a moderate part of the risk of developing combat stress reactions. However, personality factors appeared to offer a credible explanation for how some soldiers did not show a positive response to early interventions.

The Vietnam War

Combat casualties in US troops during the early part of the Vietnam War reached an unprecedented low of 12 per 1000. Soldiers' morale was said to be high, although the quality of statistics used to support this conclusion have been questioned. These low rates were achieved in spite of having introduced less strict selection procedures that resulted in vulnerable individuals being recruited for active service and over-representation of ethnic minorities within the ranks. It is also possible that the 12-month rotation undermined unit cohesion.

Interestingly, once psychiatric disorders were acknowledged they took a form not typical of those observed during WWI, WWII or the Korean War. Behavioural and disciplinary problems were common and drug abuse was seen as a way of acting out frustrations. Surprisingly, no significant developments took place in respect of early intervention during this war. Given local conditions, it remains an open question whether any particular type of intervention could have significantly reduced the many problems that came to the public's attention during and after the war.

Extraneous social changes that took place in the Western world during the 1960s and 1970s had wide reaching implications for Vietnam War veterans. Not only did they make this war different because of tactical criticisms of the pursuit of this jungle guerrilla war, but observers also highlighted the lack of purpose and meaning of this military engagement.

A great difficulty that confronted US Vietnam War veterans upon returning stateside was how to readjust to a civilian life, the demands of which were entirely different from those faced by veterans of other wars. In spite of considerable efforts from military and civilian psychiatric services, little could be done to neutralize the effects of being rejected by one's own nation. This may highlight not only limitations inherent in early intervention under adverse social circumstances, but also help explain the complexities and chronicity of the 'Post-Vietnam Syndrome'.

Subsequent wars

It would appear British authorities made no special trauma services available to soldiers posted to Northern Ireland in the early 1970s and only two Royal Navy psychiatrists were sent with the task force that sailed to fight the Falklands war. Both served on board ships and were not assigned duties ashore. Upon returning to the UK all veterans were granted 6 weeks leave. According to one of the serving psychiatrist this was an ill-considered early intervention during a critical time of readjustment, because it removed soldiers from their units for several weeks. Given that Falklands war veterans and those who served in Northern Ireland have, since the mid-1980s, been reporting problems similar to those experienced by Vietnam war veterans (Abraham, 1982; Ørner, 1992), it is reasonable to speculate whether better informed early interventions could have lowered the prevalence rates of adjustment difficulties.

The first well-controlled study to document the efficacy of early return to combat units was conducted during the 1982 war in Lebanon. Israeli CSR casualties who had been given early intervention in line with the Salmon principles were found to be more likely to regain long-term health than fellow sufferers kept away from the front line (Solomon and Benbeniskti, 1986).

When the separate effects of the various elements of the PIE-principles (proximity, immediacy and expectancy) were compared, the latter was found to be most strongly associated with a return to front line units and good post-war adjustment.

Present doctrine in respect of early intervention for soldiers serving within NATO forces is detailed in the chapter by Mehlum in this book and will therefore not be considered further at this stage.

The Gulf War

The nations that participated in the Gulf War had made comprehensive preparations for early intervention of psychiatric casualties. For example, the British force had field psychiatric teams and battle shock recovery units at strategic locations. The principles of forward psychiatry were practised and appear to have worked well in preventing PTSD.

However, a post-conflict 'Gulf War Syndrome' has developed in nearly 20% of British veterans. Along with other post-war syndromes, this most recent version is a function of the character of the war that was fought. The nature of this ill-defined syndrome is still not fully described or understood. Current impressions are that it may relate more closely to other unexplained environmental syndromes, such as chronic fatigue syndrome or multiple chemical sensitivity than to disorders within the post-traumatic stress spectrum (Wessely, 2001). Combat stress and other psychological stressors on the battlefield are only some of many possible causal factors that have to be considered.

Amongst the most important lesson learned from the Gulf War is that early intervention should in future include a focus on gathering medical intelligence. This is an important development for reconstructed early intervention, which at least in some instances should embrace considerations of environmental health factors that can degrade the health and effectiveness of fighting forces. This should include information about industrial toxin and radiation accidents, environmental warfare of terrorism and hazardous waste. However, having made this point those involved in planning and delivering early psychological interventions should also keep in mind the fact that somatization disorders are amongst the most frequently reported sequelae of trauma.

Peacekeeping soldiers

Peacekeeping service has produced higher rates of stress casualties than predicted by the orthodox formula that calculates prevalence from the figure of number of soldiers killed and wounded. A particular type of post-traumatic stress response has been described and named 'the UN-soldiers stress syndrome'. It is characterized by dominant symptoms of anxiety evoked by fears of soldiers' own anger. Intense impulses may have resulted from duty related provocations, threats or exposures to dangers in situations where military personnel cannot fight back because operational orders prohibit such actions.

Any early indication that the required degree of control is compromised by stress reaction may make evacuation an imperative. This is contrary to the principles that guide early intervention for CSR and it is interesting to note that evacuation of soldiers who struggle with self-control is associated with relatively high morbidity (Weisæth and Sund, 1982; Weisæth et al. 1993).

Summary

The high number of shell shock cases reported during WWI marks a convenient starting point for following the development of early intervention for CSR. The theoretical models invoked to account for these reactions have varied from the purely organic to the moral, social and psychological. Each has engendered its own sets of early intervention techniques, and has tended to go through cyclical phases of widespread acceptance, neglect and eventual rehabilitation. The driving force for these recurrent developments appears to be the realization that high psychiatric casualty rates significantly impair the operational readiness of military forces. Steps been taken have in recent years to standardize early interventions for soldiers traumatized by battle conditions along the principles of proximity, immediacy and expectancy. These are known to be associated with encouraging outcomes and expectancy to remain in the soldier role with allocated units appears to exert marked positive benefits. However, with such consensus having been achieved, it is interesting to note that recent military engagements in the Gulf War have highlighted the necessity for early intervention to extend its remit to considerations of environmental health. UN peacekeeping missions also seem to require special forms of early intervention protocols due to the distinct and unconventional circumstances under which they take place. It may be that these nuances of understanding and their different implications for early intervention, may herald a period of greater appreciation of the broad range of psychiatric needs presented by soldiers in active service, and the flexible early interventions that may be called for to optimize combat or operational readiness.

References

Abraham, P. (1982) Training for battle shock. *Journal of the Royal Army Medical Corps* **128**, 118–27.

Ahrenfeldt, R.H. (1958) *Psychiatry in the British army in the Second World War*. New York: Columbia University Press.

Bonhoeffer, K. (1926) Beurteilung, Begutachtung und Rechtsprechung bei den sogenannten Unfallsneurosen. *Deutch Med Wochensch* **l.52**, 179–82.

Brock, A.J. (1918) The re-education of the adult: the neurasthenic in war and peace. *Sociolog Rev* **10**, 25–40.

Da Costa, J.M. (1871) On irritable heart: a clinical study of a form of functional cardiac disorder and its consequences. *Am J Med Sci* **61**, 17–52.

Eder, D. (1916) The psychopathology of the war neurosis. *Lancet*, **ii**, 264–8.

Eissler, K.R. (1986) *Freud as an Expert Witness: the discussion of war neuroses between Freud and Wagner-Jauregg*. Madison: International University Press.

Fischer-Homberger, E. (1975) *Die traumatische Neurose, von somatischen zum sozialen Leiden*. Bern: Verlag Hans Huber.

Glass, A.J. (1954) Psychotherapy in the Combat Zone. *Am J Psychiat* **110**, 727.

Grinker, R.R. and Spiegel, J.P. (1943) *War Neurosis in North Africa: the Tunisian Campaign January–May 1943*. New York.

Herodotus. (1998) *The Histories*. Book 7, paragraph 230. Book 9, paragraph 71. Oxford: Oxford University Press.

Hesuard, A. (1914) Les troubles nerveux et psychiques causēcutifs aux catastrophes navales. *Revue de Psychiartie* **18**, 139–51.

Jaspers, K. (1953) *Allegemeine Psychopathologie*. Berlin: Springer:-Verlag.

Jones, F.D. (1994) From combat to community psychiatry. In Zajtchuk, R. (eds), *Textbook of Military Medicine, Military Psychiatry: preparing in peace for war*, Part 1, pp. 227–237. Washington DC: Department of the Army.

Main, T. (1989) *The Ailment and Other Psychoanalytic Essays*. London: Free Association Press.

Marshall, S.L.A. (1978) *Men Against Fire: the problem of battle command in future war*. Gloucester: Peter Smith.

Merskey, H. (1991) Shell shock. In Berrios, G.E. and Freeman, H.L. (eds), *150 years of British Psychiatry 1841–1991*, pp. 245–267. London: Royal College of Psychiatrists.

Moran, C.M.W., Lord (1945) *The Anatomy of Courage*. London: Constable.

Myers, A.B.R. (1870) *On the Etiology and Prevalence of Disease of the Heart Among Soldiers*. London: Churchill.

Myers, C.S. (1915) A contribution to the study of shell shock. *Lancet*, 316–320.

Myers, C.S. (1940) *Shell Shock in France 1914–18*. Cambridge: University Press.

Ørner, R.J. (1992) Post-traumatic stress disorders and European war veterans. *Br J Clin Psychol* **31**, 387–403.

Plato (1993) *The Apology of Socrates*. Connecticut: Harvard Classics, Easton Press.

Rivers, W.H.R. (1922) *Conflict and Dream*. London: Harcourt, Brace and Co.

Salmon, T.W. (1917) The care and treatment of mental diseases and war neuroses ('shell shock') in the British army. *Ment Hyg* **1**, 509–47.

Sargant, W. and Shorvon, H.J. (1945) Acute war neurosis. *Arch Neurol Psychiat* **54**, 231–40.

Shepard, B. (2000) *A War of Nerves: soldiers and psychiatrists*. London: Jonathan Cape.

Solomon, Z. and Benbenishti, R. (1986) The role of proximity, immediacy and expectancy in frontline treatment of combat stress reaction among Israeli CSR casualties. *Am J Psychiat* **143**, 613–17.

Stouffer, S.A., *et al.* (1949) The American soldier. Vol. 2: combat and its aftermath. In *Social Science Research Council. U.S. Studies in social psychology in World War II*, Princeton: Princeton University Press.

War Office Committee of Enquiry into Shell Shock (1922) *Report of the Committee*, Cmd 1737. London: HMSO.

Weisæth, L. and Sund (1982) Psychiatric problems. *Int Rev Army, Navy Air Force Med Serv* **55**, 109–16.

Weisæth, L., Aarhaug, P. and Mehlour, L. (1993) *The UNIFIL Study. Report-Part 1. Research and recommendations*. Headquarter Defence Command, Norway. The Joint Medical Service, Oslo, Norway.

Wessely, S. (2001) Psychological injury. Fact and fiction. In Braidwood, A. (eds) *Psychological Injury. Understanding and Supporting*, pp 33–44. London: Department of Social Security, Stationary Office.

2 Historical background: social psychiatry and crisis theory

Berthold P. R. Gersons

The ideology of social and preventive psychiatry

Tracing back the steps our predecessors went through in order to develop improved perspectives on mental health for mankind helps us better appreciate how we have arrived at our present levels of understanding. Sometimes such an historical perspective is used to serve the notion of how wrong our predecessors were and how right we seem to be now. A book that exemplifies this latter approach is 'A history of Psychiatry' by Edward Shorter (1997). No mention of crisis theory or its pioneers can be found in this publication. The main message is that psychoanalytic theory has been a source of delay for the coming into existence of the jewels of biological psychiatry. Such historians of psychiatry are inclined to forget about the oscillating pictures one gets from looking into the history of science. In contrast, a very different approach is exemplified in *Madness and Civilization* by Michel Foucault (1965). Foucault, who is a philosopher, describes every major step in the history of psychiatry in terms of what we lost and what we gained by it. For the purpose of this chapter, the points made by him will be briefly summarized because they describe so well the progressive developmental steps that have helped us reach improved conceptualizations of mental health.

The history of mental illness focuses mainly on disordered behaviour and how society has sought to make sense of what was observed. In the Middle Ages medicine was preoccupied with infectious diseases like leprosy and pestilence. Disordered behaviour was not identified as a separate and distinct issue. For instance, there was no formal distinction between criminal and other deviant behaviour. Witches were singled out for persecution, and from contemporaneous descriptions clinicians now recognize 'hysterical states' in women who were burned or drowned because of their behaviour. During the Renaissance those with disordered behaviour were isolated in Doll houses. No formal psychiatric diagnoses were made and these houses served the single aim of separating the disordered from the rest of 'normal' society. Within the institutions disordered behaviours were accepted and no systematic attempts were made to effect change. During the French revolution Pinel was the first psychiatrist to make a distinction between a range of abnormal behaviour patterns observed in some individuals and those who could genuinely be said to be suffering from mental disorders. This was the starting point for setting up asylums that not only housed the insane who were 'unchained' by Pinel, but also offered treatment. In these institutions the notion of *moral treatment* was the first systematic attempt to provide some form of intervention with a view to returning individuals back to the community. According to Foucault the introduction of techniques to improve disordered behaviour amongst the insane had the effect that recipients accept a new assigned role and the label of 'mental patients'. Thus, insanity and disordered behaviour became a field of medicine. At this same stage psychiatrists like Janet, Charcot and Freud started to unravel the complexities of disordered psychological states. This development resulted in an interest not only in disordered behaviour, but also in socially unacceptable thinking and feeling. Foucault also points out how introducing new psychological therapies, such as psychoanalysis and psychotherapy, engendered a fuller appreciation of the general pervasiveness of 'non-typical' modes of psychological functioning. By implication, a shift occurred that meant that medical attention was brought to bear not only on the insane and those with other diagnosable disorders, but also individuals identified as presenting with 'abnormal' thoughts and feelings. It was at this juncture that the ambition of the mental health sciences extended to encompass not only the lives of the insane, but also the general well being of everyone.

In the twentieth century this ambition became known as the 'mental health movement'. The work of Adolf Meyer (1952), an American psychiatrist, exemplifies this approach as evidenced by his proposal to replace the police by mental health agencies. The World Federation of Mental Health was founded in 1930 as an optimistic and ambitious movement heavily inspired and influenced by two emergent realizations. The first was an apparent increase in the prevalence of psychiatric disorders that Durkheim (1951) had linked to population displacements away from the countryside to the cities. These changes had been brought about by the demands of increasingly industrialized societies and resulted in the experience of loneliness and anonymity for large numbers of people. Social factors became identified as causes for becoming mentally ill and to effect planned changes to social circumstance became a tool of preventive psychiatry. The second formative realization was engendered by World Wars I and II, during which soldiers as well as civilian populations became targets for mass scale killing, wounding and destruction (Sidel *et al.*, 1995). This coincided with the progressive development of psychoanalysis that highlighted the presence of conflicts at the level of the individual's psyche and its consequences for personal adjustment. The aim of therapy and treatment was formulated in terms of setting the individual free from the destructive consequences of seemingly irreconcilable conflicting processes.

Social psychiatry developed in response to increased understandings of the relationship between social factors and mental illness. So it was logical that pioneering social psychiatrists like Querido (1958) should focus on improving living conditions of the mentally ill. They started the de-institutionalization movement, which has as its aim to resettle those who have mental disorders in sheltered accommodation in the community. Also, day-treatment (Schene and Gersons, 1985) instead of institutionalization became an important aspect of social psychiatry provision. After the World War II (WWII) this movement developed further, especially in Italy, to become 'democratic psychiatry' at a time that corresponded to a wider socialist aspiration to improve society and eliminate its dehumanizing excesses (Bennett, 1985). In Italy, the UK and USA the number of available inpatient psychiatric beds reduced significantly with a maximum recorded being in the region of 80% (Bachrach, 1976). As a result, a whole range of new community care provision had to be put in place to 'open the back doors of the asylums'. Further developments within social psychiatry can best be described as an effort 'to close the entrance to the asylums'. It was Querido (1935), who first offered 'outreach emergency psychiatry', which sought specifically to prevent hospital admissions. This service innovation became the precursor of crisis intervention.

Crisis theory: concepts and practice

In 1932 the Harvard physiologist Walter Cannon published his book *Wisdom of the Body*, which coined the term homeostasis and applied it to the automatic systems that balance bodily functions, such as temperature, breathing, blood sugar, etc. Central to his considerations is the concept that such functions are usually kept in equilibrium dependent upon the different 'outside' circumstances to which an individual is exposed. This gave recognition to the body's capacity, within limits, to maintain its life-saving equilibrium under ever changing environmental conditions. Cannon argued that because of this homeostatic mechanism a person is free to move, act and think. However, when homeostasis processes fail to maintain a sustainable and dynamic balance illness will become manifest. Selye (1956) improved this concept by introducing the term heterostasis for any situation that effectively endangers a state of homeostasis. He invoked the term *stress* to describe such a situation and postulated that his model applies not only for psychic and somatic equilibrium, but also in respect of social processes.

Cannon and Selye laid the foundations for crisis theory as conceptualized by Gerald Caplan's definition of a crisis as 'an upset of a steady state' (1964, 1981). Querido was similarly influenced by Cannon in whose laboratory he had, as a young student, completed his dissertation. The then not generally recognized implication of the definition used for crisis is that everyone, in principle, can develop some form of mental disorder. It was the American psychoanalyst Karl Menninger who established this principle in *'The Vital Balance'* (1964). To a significant extent his hypothesis was influenced by clinical observations of the psychological and psychiatric sequels arising from two world wars. For instance film footage from the period documents soldiers presenting with catatonic like states that resemble those observed in some schizophrenic patients. As a result the distinctions that had previously existed between severe mental illness manifested, for instance, as psychotic states and other mental disorders became less clear.

At this juncture it is useful to reconsider developments that took place in the psychoanalytic theory and practice of the time. Menninger described a relationship between an individual's personality strength and the burdens of life, such as negative life events, that can be sustained. Similarly, Freud's psychoanalytic theory (1918) proposed an internal balance between conscious and unconscious drives and motives. So, the neuroses were postulated to be the result of struggles between sexual and aggressive drives expressed at the level of the Id, and the conflicting norms and values of society represented as the Superego (Freud, 1925). Crucial to personal development and subsequent adjustment are the ways individuals learn to balance these seemingly antagonistic forces. The manner of doing so gives rise to the Ego, the strength of which is seen as important for resolving and overcoming all sorts of negative circumstances in life. It was proposed that the technique of choice for promoting a better-balanced Ego was psychoanalysis and later this was extended to include psychodynamic psychotherapy. Making conscious previously repressed information stored in the unconscious can help a person in therapy. The resulting insights into important formative influences that shape individual development, from childhood to the present and promote better balanced functioning characterized by an acceptance of emotions, ambitions and frustrations. This is deemed essential for further maturing and strengthening of personality. These developments in psychoanalytic and psychodynamic theory were largely a product of observations made in clinical practice. They helped highlight the importance of standards of parenting to which an adult had been subjected during childhood and the quality of other formative relationships. In turn, this led to a more general recognition of the importance of help, which seeks to materially improve the quality of our significant relationships and our interactions with others. It is in this way that psychoanalysts have tried to transport the insights from consulting rooms into the public arena. The knowledge and experience accrued has been applied in child-guidance clinics, where the relationship between children and their parents is central to assessment and therapy that seeks to prevent later life psychiatric disorders.

Inspired by a similar insight two Harvard psychiatrists named Erich Lindemann (1944) and Gerald Caplan (1964) became pioneers of crisis theory and preventive psychiatry. Lindemann had aroused great professional interest by his article on the *'Symptomatology and management of acute grief'* (1944). The publication drew on his experiences with survivors of the Coconut Grove nightclub fire that had occurred about 12 months previously. More than 500 persons celebrating the annual regatta between Harvard and Yale had perished. This event had a massive impact on those most directly involved, but also a large proportion of the general population living in Boston, Massachusetts, and the surrounding areas. Lindemann's ideas, largely derived from impressions formed in his consulting room, were tested against observations made in the broader community. The disaster was like an '*in vivo* experiment' of psychological homeostasis and 'acute grief' was described as follows:

1. Acute grief is a definite syndrome with psychological and somatic symptomatology.
2. This syndrome may appear immediately after a crisis or may be delayed. It may be exaggerated or apparently absent.
3. In place of the typical syndrome distorted presentations may appear each of which represents one special aspect of the grief syndrome.
4. By appropriate techniques these distorted pictures can be successfully transformed into a normal grief reaction with resolution.

The techniques advocated by Lindemann comprised brief cathartic sessions. Their purpose was to promote psychological processing of emotional grief reactions. This treatment recommendation was inspired by Freud's account of cathartic treatment given to his patient Anna O (Freud and Breuer 1893). Freud and Lindemann thus provided the first two reported instances of how intense repressed emotions evoked by traumatic experiences can distort cognitions of that event. Furthermore, they demonstrated the treatment principle, whereby stimulating these emotions into conscious awareness can bring an end to these distortions. Nowadays, we realize how much psychotherapy is used as a tool to 'unfreeze' a neurotic state to bring patients into a 'healing' crisis through which healthy resolutions can be achieved.

The importance of Lindemann's observations derive from changing interest away from static diagnostic observations to a focus on process observations promoting resolution of grief and crises. Together with Klein, Lindemann outlined the principles of crisis intervention (1961):

1. Crisis is a temporary experience, a time-limited process lasting days or weeks.
2. Crisis develops within a network of committed persons.
3. Help and support will be delivered by involved persons from the immediate network.
4. Psychiatric symptoms present during a state of crisis are mostly of a temporary nature and relate directly to the crisis.
5. A minimum of help and support is sufficient to achieve maximum effect.

In retrospect, it is of interest to note that these propositions derived from subjective observations that, with time, were developed and tested through more systematic qualitative studies. Pre-eminent in this regard was Gerald Caplan's (Caplan and Killilea, 1976) emphasis of the healing power of mutual aid engendered within committed groups. He had seen and reported on this phenomenon as manifested in self-help groups for bereaved widows. Implicit in this perspective is a widening of the role of the mental health professional from treatment in the consulting room to preventive actions in the community.

Another important pioneer of crisis-theory was the Canadian psychiatrist Tyhurst (1957). His observations focused on individuals who had lived through a range of 'upsetting circumstances like fire, shipwreck or moving to a new house'. He distinguished three phases in the crisis response evoked by such incidents:

1. The *impact* phase, which is the period of danger or threat.
2. The *recoil* phase, which is the period immediately after danger has stopped.
3. The *post-traumatic* phase, which is the route back to the steady state of normal life.

In the impact phase the individual typically reacts adaptively to the situation without undue disruption caused by strong emotions. Cognitive orientation in time is powerfully focused on the immediate 'here and now'. Tyhurst described these characteristic responses as 'instrumental reaction'. Observations and self-report indicate these reactions serve the end of reaching safety or to fight danger without undue interference by strong emotions. When recalled, at a later stage, memories of what happened during this phase are usually strikingly precise and sharp. However, if no actions are taken, the person will stay in a sometimes dangerous state of disbelief and denial, a condition described as 'psychogenic death'.

The recoil phase is characterized by dramatic changes. There is no need for anyone to take immediate action, since at this stage catharsis of emotions is the paramount process. Denial, or outrage and crying may be prominent. A sense of utter exhaustion may also be felt. Cognitive orientation is now focused on the immediate past and there is typically no interest in the future or the more distant past. Usually, memories of this phase are not at all precise. Later in the post-traumatic phase the person tries to integrate the recent distressing experience within the register of life events that comprise his or her life history. This can help give personal meaning to what has happened. Tyhurst has called these different phases 'transitional' states within the crisis process.

Tyhurst also attracted our interest to a seldom-mentioned aspect of crises. Namely, the changes of roles that tend to occur during at such times. A role is defined as all the behavioural expectations a person may have about self and others in a given situation. Examples include those that pertain to friends, parents and children, people at work, teachers, etc. The importance of this role concept is that in unexpected and suddenly emergent situations it is possible to predict behaviour of someone else. For instance, parents are not expected to behave as children or vice versa. Working roles are different from the roles of being friends. This is how role behaviour and role expectation serve the purpose of making interactions more predictable. A crisis such as a life threatening fire may provoke sudden changes of role amongst those involved resulting in losses of previously held expectations of what constituted role-appropriate behaviour. For instance, a person who is registered as a guest in a hotel where a fire starts has to switch role into that of a survivor or victim, and possibly also a patient if hospitalized. Conceivably, too, the person may, in the long term, have to accept the role of a being functionally impaired and unable to work. Such adjustments are referred to as a sequence of role changes that have the effect of upsetting the steady state and producing stress (Caplan, 1981).

Based on the work of these pioneers Lindemann developed the field further by describing crisis intervention in terms of forces and equilibria. Actions can be assumed to be helpful to the extent they:

1. Alter the balance of forces within a group of people,
2. Restore a reasonable healthy equilibrium in a social orbit,
3. Redistribute role relationships within a group,
4. Repopulate the social space.

With the passing of time, these rather abstract formulations have gained prominence as powerful rationales for crisis therapy interventions. Most particularly so with families, but also other situations where patients present with more severe and enduring psychiatric disorders. For instance, a change of the 'balance of forces' can be recognized in crisis family therapy if one member is being blamed for harbouring 'all evil' within the group. Through crisis therapy, other members of the group may be asked to review their standpoint and to take some personal ownership of at least part of the overall burden of 'badness'. Furthermore, the notion of changing role-relations promotes a focus for therapy that involves changing and strengthening new roles to be assumed by the individuals involved. For instance, roles may be changed so as to redefine who is a 'victim' and who is an 'offender'. If the sought after role changes prove insufficient or are not attainable less stressful surroundings can be created through 'repopulation'. This involves asking those identified as being a burden to the person in crisis to leave the situation with a view to bringing in those who are more trusted and supportive. When such crisis therapy is offered with due care and consideration it can be an alternative to psychiatric hospitalization. Crisis theory has laid the basis for the setting up worldwide of crisis centers and mobile crisis-intervention services. These centres serve the goal of immediate intervention to prevent further psychiatric hospitalization (Katschnich and Cooper, 1991).

As will be appreciated from the above, crisis theory derives from a number of different and distinct roots that share a common and unifying element in being a search for a new equilibrium. However, the definition of crisis as an upset of a steady state has inadvertently engendered a misapprehension that after a crisis a person will once again re-establish the state of equilibrium that existed before disruptions occurred. This can occur, but is probably exceptional. More typically, crises engender outcomes that differ from previous steady states. In some instances, outcomes may be disadvantageous to the individuals concerned, but it is also possible for improved adjustments to follow in the wake of crises. When this happens the circumstances may be conducive to 'posttraumatic growth' (Tedeschi and Calhoun, 1996).

Life events and psychotrauma

Much interest appends to the development of crisis theory and crisis intervention because their aim is to prevent or change the course of psychiatric disorders. This has stimulated research into the extent to which disturbing circumstances can evoke such disorders. Foremost in this regard is the role that (dis)stressing life events can have in disrupting the steady state and influence the onset of depression. Erikson (1968) has made an interesting distinction between events that constitute a developmental crisis and those that are accidental. The former comprises situations that can be expected to occur during the natural course of the lives of most people. Examples are the death of parents, the birth of children, leaving home during adolescence and after marriage. Such events can effect very marked changes in the life situation of those involved. However, such events are expected and form part of normal life. With each there are associated transitional rituals that ease the passage from one situation to another. A further consideration is that the emotions involved are well accepted and their evocation is even encouraged by rituals.

In contrast, accidental events are characterized by not being expected and no transitional rituals are readily available to assist in the progression through the phased reactions that follow in their aftermath. Examples of such events are fires, wars, robberies, violence, rape, natural disasters, traffic incidents, etc. Although almost everyone is aware of the possibility such incidents may occur most people do not expect such accidents to feature in their lives and tend to deny the likelihood they themselves may become victims. When such accidental events do occur it stands to reason they are experienced as a source of great personal distress.

An interesting aspect of the life events lists published by Holmes and Rahe (1964), as well as Paykel (1969) is that they encompass both negative and positive events. Negative life events are sickness in the family, financial problems, being imprisoned and to loose one's job. Positive events in the lists are pregnancy or getting a better job. With this in mind, it is not unreasonable to presume life-event effects will depend on their frequency in a given time span, the social support available and possible vulnerability for specific psychiatric disturbances such as depression. In keeping with the above, Dohrenwend (Dohrenwend and Dohrenwend, 1981) has described different relationships between *stressful life events* and *adverse health changes* depending on their accompanying psycho-physiological reactions, and the social and personal dispositions of those involved.

The multifactorial nature of stressors, of which the event is only one aspect, is therefore important for the practice of crisis intervention (see Shalev, Chapter 11).

The different versions of the Diagnostic and Statistical Manual (DSM) of the American Psychiatric Association (APA) published before 1980 give expression to different and changing views about how the concept of crisis differs from that of trauma. Publications of DSMs before the 1980 version (DSM-III) only mentioned a reactive state in connection with stressful events, however serious these may be. This conceptualization was rooted in the then dominant perspective offered by psychoanalytic theory. In consequence, no specific distinction was made between a crisis (negative life-event) and a psychotrauma. However, studies of the long-term sequelae of the Holocaust combined with the devastating effects of early child abuse and high profile publicity given to the plight of many Vietnam veterans culminated in a new and distinct classification of posttraumatic stress disorder (PTSD) in DSM-III (APA, 1980).

Looking back it can now be appreciated how important the recognition of PTSD as a separate, and for some a chronic disorder, has been for promoting an understanding that trauma can be an entirely different entity from crisis. The first APA definition of a traumatic event presumed its distinguishing feature to be that is an event 'outside the usual range of human experiences'. By implication a crisis is construed as being within the range of normal events and traumas fall outside that range. It may therefore be argued that crisis intervention is not a sufficiently elaborate strategy for addressing the early sequelae of trauma related disorders. The event criterion used in DSM-III also resulted in the idea that traumas are infrequent and exceptional events the occurrence of which would, by implication and necessity, result in PTSD. These early notions were challenged by epidemiological studies that documented traumatic events to occur far more frequently than was first assumed (Kessler *et al.*, 1995; Breslau *et al.*, 1998). The many and varied ways in which trauma endanger the mental health of many people was also described.

A further realization fostered by these studies was that only approximately 20% of traumatic events, as defined in DSM-III, result in PTSD. This fact has profoundly changed the focus for how trauma is defined. According to the scheme proposed by Dohrenwend (Dohrenwend and Dohrenwend, 1981) the model changed from a linear victimization hypothesis to a stress-strain hypothesis. In this model, the effect of a trauma is mediated by the psycho-physiological responses they evoke. Therefore, trauma is now defined not only by its nature as an uncommon extreme event, but also by its accompanying psycho-physiological effects. The trauma concept had moved from being a crisis that can be evoked by a generally distressing event to a much more specific pathogenic event.

Limitations and perspectives on early intervention

Crisis intervention is now recognized as the early intervention technique of choice when seeking to prevent mental disorders. In the case of those recently exposed to traumatic experiences it is still not clear if it achieves the outcome of preventing PTSD. The primary prevention of PTSD is a task that should by addressed by society as a whole. For instance, psychotraumatology and victimology have a duty to confront society with the sometimes evil effects of traumatic events (Kleber *et al.*, 1995). In the aftermath of traumas it can be difficult to know which messages to prioritize for either victims or the general public. In our experience with large-scale disasters we have come to appreciate the value of informing members of the public that evoked reactions are 'normal reactions to an abnormal event' (Gersons and Carlier, 1993). Such a message seeks to foster acceptance of and reassurance about what is for most a temporary disturbance. This notion seems also to find ready acceptance amongst those recently exposed to trauma, particularly at a time when their sense of having been victimized may predominate. It also recommends itself for being a message of optimism and hope. Based on crisis theory, the message also predicts long-term resolution as the natural outcome to be expected for most of those involved. As stated above, this is generally true for the majority of recently traumatized persons who, although deeply distressed are, as a group, unlikely to develop chronic PTSD.

However, it also has to be recognized that for some this message will prove to be incorrect. A proportion may in the longer run be diagnosed with PTSD and other trauma-related disorders such as depression, addiction and anxiety disorders. The perspective offered by those who advocate a formal recognition of complex PTSD as an axis II disorder (van der Kolk, 1996) further complicates our conceptualizations of possible long-term effects of traumatization. A public message emphasizing the normality of reactions will prove to be an incorrect one in the case of those who develop longer-term disorders. This contradiction has given rise to a dilemma that, for the time being, we have to accept.

In the light of these developments it is reasonable to speculate about what may have been lost by distinguishing between crisis and trauma. In part, this may be answered by having a closer look at evidence engendered by studies of Critical Incident Stress Debriefing (CISD; Mitchell, 1983) and Psychological Debriefing (PD). A case in point is one of our own studies, which revealed striking and paradoxical outcomes (Carlier et al., 1998). Rescue officers who attended CISD meetings after a disaster were, at the time, extremely satisfied by the service offered. However, these same officers were also the ones to show more symptoms in the long run when compared to colleagues who had not attended CISD meetings. The paradox was further amplified by the latter group of police officers telling us they regretted not being participants in the debriefings. So how may it be explained that they favoured debriefing? We do not have a full set of facts to substantiate possible answers to this question, but a number of options come to mind. For instance, Beverly Raphael (1986) calls the first phase after a disaster the 'honeymoon' phase. Although this term may seem incongruous given that death and destruction may have occurred, the notion of a 'honeymoon phase' does seem to accurately describe some of the earliest reactions observed in some survivors of recent trauma. An example is the way survivors speak of how feeling much more connected to others implicated the incident. Role relationships are described in terms that emphasize friendship, whilst formality and hierarchy seems to vanish temporarily. Amongst survivors of some traumatic events everyone is equal and loyal. This is understandable if account is taken of the life-threatening characteristics of most traumatic events. The 'honeymoon phase' may be defined as a survival attachment that is functional to the extent that it serves a natural psychobiological survival reaction. Survivors are in particular need of support from one another in the early aftermath of being exposed to trauma. For some, hyper-activation experienced after trauma also engenders powerful feelings in which life seems more intense and emotional compared to the 'dull' routines of daily life.

The 'honeymoon' phenomenon serves to stress the importance of social support. This is reflected in guidelines, first offered by Salmon (1919) at the time of the World War I (WWI), to keep the traumatized together. The group gives mutual aid, warmth and emotional support along the same lines as postulated by the rules of crisis intervention. Taken together these considerations may account for the high acceptability ratings initially given for early intervention even if such subjective assessments have no absolute predictive power in respect of eventual outcome. A further speculation arising from our CISD study is that early intervention carried out by helping professionals may, in the longer term, militate against positive outcomes. Through their involvement it may be that inadvertent use is made of psychotherapeutic techniques that stimulate emotions as if in preparation for catharsis. To do so as part of any early intervention provision is likely to be inappropriate and may compromise processes that promote positive long-term adjustment.

It is in respect of this important point that a key lesson from crisis intervention appears to have been forgotten. Namely, that if a crisis is defined as an upset of a steady state it follows that priority should be given to early interventions that re-establish a steady state, which is promoted by regaining control over one's own life and especially the initial emotions engendered by a traumatic event. In this regard, it is useful to consider that theories about the function of emotions propose they serve as a vehicle for transitions towards regaining a state of control. This is as experienced in the observance of rituals commonly associated with trauma (Gersons, 1988). However, if early intervention engenders further stimulation and emotional arousal in the aftermath of trauma it will further deregulate the state of a person into an even more uncontrollable condition. Based on this realization crisis intervention has long recognized the importance of reaching a new and stable equilibrium as soon as possible. Only when psychological and social homeostasis is re-established should consideration be given to introducing further therapeutic methods. There is strong reason to believe that to the extent early intervention strategies incorporate the principles that underpin crisis intervention, and heeds other lessons learned from decades of providing such services, it may be possible to effect some secondary preventive interventions in respect of the development of PTSD. In order to establish if this is, in fact, possible and, more specifically, for whom early intervention may be indicated, it will be essential to conduct further research.

References

American Psychiatric Association (1980) *Diagnostic and Statistical Manual of Mental Disorders*, 3rd edn (DSM-III). Washington DC: APA.

Bachrach, L.J. (1976) *Deinstitutionalization: an analytical review and sociological perspective.* Rockville: National Institute of Mental Health.

Bennett, D.H. (1985) The changing pattern of health care in Trieste. *Int J Ment Hlth* 14: 70–92.

Breslau, N., Kessler, R.C., Chilcoat, H.D., Schultz, L.R., Davis, G.C. and Andreski, P. (1998) Trauma and post-traumatic stress disorder in the community; the 1996 Detroit area survey of trauma. *Arch Gen Psychiat* **55**, 626–32.

Cannon, W.B. (1932) *The Wisdom of the Body*. New York: Norton.

Caplan, G. (1964) *Principles of Preventive Psychiatry*. New York: Basic Books.

Caplan, G. (1981) Mastery of stress: psychosocial aspects. *Am J Psychiat* **138**, 413–20.

Caplan, G. and Killilea, M. (1976) *Support Systems and Mutual Help; Multidisciplinary Exploitations.* New York: Grune and Stratton.

Carlier, I.V.E., Lamberts, R.D., van Uchelen, A.J. and Gersons, B.P.R. (1998) Disaster-related post-traumatic stress in police officers: a field study of the impact of debriefing. *Stress Med* **14**, 143–8.

Dohrenwend, B.S. and Dohrenwend, B.P. (1981) *Stressful Life Events and their Contexts.* New Brunswick: Rutgers University Press.

Durkheim, E. (1951) *Suicide*. New York: Free Press.

Erikson, E. (1968) *Identity, Youth and Crisis*. New York: Norton.

Foucault, M. (1965) *Madness and Civilization*. New York: Random House.

Freud, S. (1918) *Introduction to Psychoanalysis and the War Neuroses*, standard edn, Vol. 17. London: Hogarth Press.

Freud, S. (1925) *Inhibitions, Symptoms and Anxiety*, standard edn, Vol. 20. London: Hogarth Press.

Freud, S. and Breuer, J. (1893) *On the Psychical Mechanism of Hysterical Phenomena: preliminary communication*, standard edn, Vol. 2. London: Hogarth Press.

Gersons, B.P.R. (1988) Adaptive defense mechanisms in post-traumatic stress disorders and leave-taking rituals. In: van der Hart, O. (ed.) *Coping with Loss*. New York: Irvington.

Gersons, B.P.R. and Carlier, I.V.E. (1993) Plane crash crisis intervention: a preliminary report from the Bijlmermeer Amsterdam. *J Crisis Intervention Suicide Prevent* **14**, 109–16.

Holmes, T.H. and Rahe, R.H. (1964) The social readjustment rating scale. *Am J Psychiat* **121**, 141–8.

Katschnich, H. and Cooper, Y. (1991) Psychiatric emergency and crisis intervention centers. In: Bennet, D.H. and Freeman, H.L. (eds), *Community Psychiatry*, pp. 517–542. Edinburgh: Churchill Livingstone.

Kessler, R.C., Sonnega, A., Bromet, E. and Nelson, C.B. (1995) Post-traumatic stress disorder in the National comorbidity survey. *Arch Gen Psychiat* **52**, 1058–60.

Kleber, R., Figley, C. and Gersons, B.P.R. (1995) *Beyond Trauma; cultural and societal dynamics*. New York: Plenum.

Klein, D.C. and Lindemann, E. (1961) Preventive intervention in individual and family crisis situations. In: Caplan, G. (ed.) *Prevention of Mental Disorder in Children*. New York: Basic Books.

Kolk van der, B.A. (1996) The complexity of adaptation to trauma; self-regulation, stimulus discrimination, and characterological development. In Kolk van der., B.A., McFarlane, A.C. and Weisaeth, L. (eds), *Traumatic Stress: the effects of overwhelming experience on mind, body and society*, pp. 182–213. New York: Guilford Press.

Lindemann, E. (1944) Symptomatology and management of acute grief. *Am J Psychiat* **101**, 141–8.

Menninger, K. (1964) *The Vital Balance*. New York: Viking Press.

Meyer, A. (1952) *Collected Papers of Adolf Meyer 1948–1952*, 4 vols. Baltimore: John Hopkins University Press.

Mitchell, J. (1983) When disaster strikes: the critical incident stress debriefing process. *J Emerg Med Serv* **8**, 36–9.

Paykel, E.S. (1969) Life events and depression: a controlled study. *Arch Gen Psychiat* **21**, 753–60.

Querido, A. (1935) Community mental hygiene in the city of Amsterdam. *Ment Hyg* **19**, 177–95.

Querido, A. (1958) Multiple equilibria. Folia Psychiatrica, Neurologica et Neurochirurgica Neerlandica, mei.

Raphael, B. (1986) *When Disaster Strikes; a Handbook for the Caring Professionals*. Boston: Unwin Hyman.

Salmon, T.W. (1919) The war neuroses and their lesson. *NY State J Med* **51**, 993–4.

Selye, H. (1956) *The Stress of Life*. London: Longmans Green.

Schene, A.H. and Gersons, B.P.R. (1985) Effectiveness and application of partial hospitalisation. *Acta Psychiat Scand* **74**, 335–40.

Shorter, E. (1997) *A History of Psychiatry*. New York: Wiley.

Sidel, V.W., Gersons, B.P.R. and Weerts, J.M.P. (1995) Primary prevention of traumatic stress caused by war. In Kleber, R., Figley, C. and Gersons, B.P.R. (eds), *Beyond Trauma; Cultural and Societal Dynamics*, pp. 277–98. New York: Plenum.

Tedeschi, R.G. and Calhoun, L.G. (1996) The post-traumatic growth inventory measuring the positive legacy of trauma. *J Traumatic Stress*, **9**, 455–71.

Tyhurst, J.S. (1957) The role of transition states—including disasters—in mental illness. In *Symposium on Preventive and Social Psychiatry*, Washington DC: Walter Reed Institute.

3 A systematic review of single psychological interventions ('debriefing') following trauma. Updating the Cochrane review and implications for good practice

Suzanna Rose, Jonathan Bisson, and Simon Wessely

Introduction

We live in an age of accountability and clinicians are increasingly being asked (particularly in public-funded services) to justify the interventions they use. In many countries, there is a move towards evidence-based practice (EBP) and systematic reviews form an important element of such an approach. In a nutshell, 'The underpinning of evidence based practice is that when we intervene in the lives of others we should do so on the basis of the best evidence available regarding the likely consequences of that intervention' (Macdonald, 1998). This chapter highlights the increasing importance of using an evidence based approach when considering early intervention after trauma and highlights findings of an updated Cochrane Collaboration Review of 'debriefing' (Rose *et al.* 2001).

What is evidence-based practice?

The bedrock of evidence based practice rests largely, but not exclusively, on formal evaluation. This is itself a process involving several well-recognized and distinct phases (Roth and Fonagy, 1996) that starts with comparing a new treatment with a well-established one (or comparing it with a no treatment control group). When enough studies have been undertaken a systematic review is performed so that systematic and meaningful comparisons can be made between the outcomes of these studies. Eventually, this important information affects treatment guidelines, public service purchasing policy, improved client care and fuels further research. Given the real and continuing demands on public-funded services, the system of EBP offers some way of providing systematic practice backed by evidence, but issues about the quality of that evidence remain crucial.

A systematic process for evaluating the quality of published evidenced is encapsulated in the Cochrane Collaboration, which was launched in 1992 as a non-profit making organization. Its origins lie in broad health care settings where practitioners from many backgrounds are facing pressure to justify the interventions they advocate. It is now an international multidisciplinary movement that works to prepare, maintain and disseminate systematic reviews of the effectiveness of health care interventions (http://www.cochrane.co.uk). For instance, British centres for EBP have been established or are planned in child health, nursing, social work, adult medicine and general practice. Evidence-based practice journals have also been successfully launched.

What is a systematic review?

The systematic review plays a pivotal role in the development of the EBP approach. It is a standardized process of performing literature searches on computerized databases and other information sources to identify randomized controlled trials. Through critical exploration, evaluation and synthesis, the systematic review separates the insignificant, unsound or redundant deadwood from the salient and critical studies that are worthy of reflection (Morgan, 1985). Ideally, the minimum criteria for a methodologically rigorous evaluation are that it reports clearly defined outcomes based on valid measures with explicit criteria for including and excluding participants, and random allocation to experimental and control groups.

We now move our consideration from general points about systematic reviews to its specific application for psychological debriefing. Since the mid-1980s, this form of early intervention after trauma has been advocated as an intervention of choice and has enjoyed considerable popularity. The background is that crisis intervention (Caplan, 1964) gained acceptance during the 1970s and, in 1983, Mitchell described Critical Incident Stress Debriefing as a semi-structured group intervention with emergency services personnel. Others (Dyregrov, 1989) have described the process as 'psychological debriefing' (PD) and the terms have been used interchangeably. Although there are some differences in the interventions (Rose, 1997), the term PD will be used in this chapter to refer to either and similar approaches. For instance, in more recent years other workers have adapted the Mitchell and Dyregrov models to debrief individuals (Lee et al., 1996; Hobbs et al., 1996).

During PDs participants are encouraged to give full narrative accounts of trauma. These encompass facts, sensory impressions, cognitions and feelings. Evoked emotional reactions are considered in some detail with an emphasis on normalization. That is, participants are reassured their responses are normal when seen in the light of abnormal events and are told to anticipate further emotional reactions. Finally, facilitators offer advice on how to deal with reactions and how to find further support if necessary. It is anticipated that this type of early intervention will achieve a number of outcomes including the prevention of PTSD.

Despite its widespread use there is a noticeable dearth of empirical evidence that PD achieves these declared outcomes and three reviews have called for further rigorous research in this area (Bisson and Deahl, 1994; Raphael et al., 1995; Rick et al., 1998). A first systematic review was published in 1998 (Rose and Bisson, 1998) and material from this formed the basis for a protocol, and subsequent Cochrane Collaboration Review of 'debriefing' (Wessely et al., 1998). The overall objective of the original systematic review (Rose and Bisson, 1998) and this most recent update is to examine the effectiveness of PD in preventing psychological sequelae following traumatic events.

Criteria for selecting studies for this review

Criteria used for inclusion of a study into this review were as follows: clear criteria for the inclusion and exclusion of study participants, random assignment to experimental and control groups, clearly defined outcomes including the use of standardized and valid measures, and delivery of the intervention within 28 days of the trauma. Selected studies involved participants aged 16 years or more, and the early intervention programme had incorporated a structured or semi-structured protocol that reviewed the traumatic event, discussed cognitions and emotions, normalized reactions and discussed future coping strategies. Therefore, all selected studies contain key components of Critical Incident Stress Debriefing (CISD) and psychological debriefing (PD) as described by Mitchell and Dyregrov. However, they do not necessarily adhere totally to their methods. Additionally, participants had to fulfil criterion A for post-traumatic stress disorder as listed in [DSM-III-R; American Psychiatric Association (APA), 1987]. This states:

> The person has experienced an event that is outside the range of usual normal human experience and that would be markedly distressing to almost anyone, e.g. serious threat to one's life or physical integrity; serious threat to one's life or harm to one's children, spouse, or other close relatives and friends; sudden destruction of one's home or community; or seeing another person who has recently been, or is being, seriously injured or killed as the result of an accident or physical violence.

Search strategy for the identification of studies

The search strategy used for this review is based on the method recommended by Chalmers and Altman (1995). In 1998 the following six steps were followed: first, electronic searches were made of the following databases EMBASE (1985–1996, issue 27), MEDLINE (1970–1995), PsycLIT (1974–June 1996), SOCIOFILE (Jan 1974–Dec 1995), BIOSIS PREVIEWS (1985–1996/June W4), OCC. SAFETY & HEALTH (1973–1996/April Q1) and PASCAL (1973–1996/JUNE). Later, when undertaking the update for the current review the following electronic searches were made: CCTR (Cochrane Collaboration Trial Register; Issue 2, 2000 April 00), CINAHL (Cumulative Nursing and Allied Health Literature; Update code 20000201 Feb-00), EMBASE (Update code 0018 Jun-00), LILACS (Nov. 1999 Nov-99), MEDLINE (Update code 2000073 Jul-00), NRR (Issue 2, 1999), PSYCINFO (Update code 20000401 Jun-00), PSYNDEX (Oct. 1999 Oct-99) and SIGLE (A database of 'grey' literature; 1999). The Cochrane Collaboration Anxiety and Neurosis Group Trials Register Facilitator facilitated this updated database search.

Within each database the following headings were used: Evaluation, Trial, Study, Studies, with subheadings psychological, debriefing, psychological debriefing, stress, debriefing, stress debriefing, crisis, intervention, crisis intervention, early, psychological, intervention, early psychological intervention, preventive, psychological, intervention, preventive psychological intervention. We also communicated with known experts in the field and S. Rose completed a hand search of the *Journal of Traumatic Stress* [Vols 1(1)–13(2)]. Additional information was requested via the electronic Trauma Forum based at Oregon University, USA. (mailto:traumatic-stress@freud.apa.org) and references within identified studies were also inspected for further publications. Finally, relevant conference papers were examined.

Methods following identification of a study

All studies identified as being potentially eligible were inspected by the reviewers to ensure they did fulfil the inclusion criteria outlined for both the original systematic review and this update. Each study was also examined for its year of publication, country of origin, funding and source of paper discovery, stated study objectives, type of traumatic event, demographics, description of the type of early intervention that was used, the settings where the interventions took place, subjective evidence of effectiveness and cost analysis.

After some thought it was decided to continue to use criterion A of the DSM-III-R (APA, 1987) for inclusion in this review. This earlier criterion does not require the additional response of intense fear, helplessness or horror introduced for criterion A2 in DSM-IV (APA, 1994). This detail could not be reliably elicited from many of the selected papers.

Studies examined, but not eligible for inclusion in this review

Studies that on initial examination were thought to fit the selection criteria for this review, but were later revealed not to do so are listed below in Table 3.1.

Results

The extensive search undertaken for this update realized six further studies that could be included in the review. Therefore, the review now encompasses a total of eleven systematic peer reviewed outcome evaluations (see Appendix A for characteristics of included studies). The publications in question are Mayou *et al.* (2000), which is a follow-up from an earlier study, and Hobbs and Adshead (1996) describe two relevant, but separate studies referred to as Stevens and Adshead (1993) and

Table 3.1 Studies examined but excluded from this study

Study	Reason for exclusion
Amir *et al.*, 1998	Non-randomized, group intervention
Andre *et al.*, 1997	Not single session, CBT
Brom *et al.*, 1993	Multiple sessions, intervention >1 month
Bryant *et al.*, 1998a	Sample selected on the basis of acute stress. Disorder–not a randomized sample of victims. Intervention 4 sessions
Carlier *et al.*, 1998	Non-randomized
Chemtob *et al.*, 1997	Non-randomized, intervention >1 month
Deahl *et al.*, 2000	Non-randomized
Deahl *et al.*, 1994	Non-randomized
Doctor *et al.*, 1994	Intervention not related to a traumatic event. Intervention not PD, 12 sessions of group counselling
Foa *et al.*, 1995	Non-randomized
Hytten and Hasle, 1989	Non-randomized
Kenardy *et al.*, 1996a	Non-randomized
Mathews, 1998	Non-randomized
McFarlane, 1988	Non-randomized
Polak *et al.*, 1975	Crisis intervention, not PD
Robinson and Mitchell, 1993	Non-randomized
Saari *et al.*, 1996	Non-randomized
Tadmor *et al.*, 1997	Pre-trauma intervention
Viney *et al.*, 1985	Not PD

Hobbs *et al.* (1993). For the purposes of this updated review, the studies in question are referred to as two separate studies authored by Stevens and Adshead (1993), and Hobbs *et al.* (1993), but listed jointly (as published) in the references. In addition, a brief report by Hobbs *et al.* (1996) was published separately. All the new studies were of interventions carried out with individuals with the exception of Bisson *et al.* (1997) who reported on PD with both individuals and couples. The studies evaluated single early interventions following a variety of traumatic events experienced by adults although specific age parameters were not given in all the studies.

Of the five more recent studies Dolan *et al.* (submitted), Lavender and Walkinshaw (1998), Rose *et al.* (1999), Conlon *et al.* (1999) and Small *et al.* (2000), three were carried out in an hospital environment. Exceptions to this were Lee *et al.* (1996), Rose *et al.* (1999) and Dolan *et al.* (submitted), where PD was carried out in the participants' homes. The 3-year follow-up by Mayou *et al.* (2000) extends the original study reported by Hobbs *et al.* in 1996 as a postal follow-up. Three studies (Small *et al.*, 2000; Bunn and Clarke, 1979; Bordow and Porritt, 1979) were carried out in Australia, one originated in Ireland (Conlon *et al.*, 1999) and the remaining eight were conducted in the United Kingdom.

Randomization/use of a control group

In all these studies, except one, participants were randomly allocated either to an early single intervention or no intervention. The exception is Bordow and Porritt (1979), which incorporated an additional intervention other than PD in the form of assistance from social workers for a 3-month period.

Clearly defined outcomes, the use of valid measures and follow-up

In two of the studies and (Lavender and Walkinshaw, 1998; Small *et al.*, 2000) no pre-intervention measures were taken. These obstetric studies utilized the Edinburgh Postnatal Depression Scale (Cox *et al.*, 1987) or the Hospital Anxiety and Depression Scale (HADS; Zigmond and Snaith, 1983), rather than the Impact of Events Scale (IES; Horowitz *et al.*, 1979) as outcome measures, since the overall aim in these studies was to prevent the onset of post-natal depression.

Other studies included in this review used pre- and post-intervention instruments that are of sound design, as well as further measures as listed in Appendix A. The follow-up periods varied in length, ranging from 1 month to 3 years. Bunn and Clarke (1979) considered outcome immediately post-intervention with no follow-up. Bisson *et al.* (1997) considered outcomes at both 3 and 13 months post-trauma, while Mayou *et al.* (2000) reported a 3-year follow-up.

Criteria for inclusion and exclusion of participants

All the studies reviewed mentioned inclusion and exclusion criteria for participants to be offered PD although the level of information given was variable. For example, in the two recent studies of PD following childbirth, Small *et al.* (2000) included women who had given birth by caesarean section, forceps or vacuum extraction. They excluded mothers who had not had operative births, had stillbirths or babies weighing less than 1500 g. Also excluded were those who were ill, had babies who were ill at the time and those whose obstetrician refused permission to participate. In Lavender and Walkinshaw's (1998) obstetric study participants in the evaluation comprised primagravidas with singleton pregnancies and cephalic presentations who were in spontaneous labour at term and proceeded to have normal vaginal deliveries of a healthy baby. Excluded from this study were mothers with a third degree perineal tear, those whose babies required special or high dependency care, or manual removal of the placenta. Hobbs *et al.* (1996) cite inclusion criteria as consecutive admissions to an Emergency and Accident Ward, but excluded those who had no memory of the road traffic accident (RTA) and those who had been discharged before the researchers could make contact. Conlon *et al.* (1999) included ambulant trauma clinic attenders with minor road traffic injuries, such as soft tissue injury, but excluded those with head injury. Rose *et al.* (1999) included victims of violent crime in the from of actual or attempted physical or sexual assault or a bag snatch, but excluded those who had been assaulted by someone from their own household. Dolan *et al.* (submitted) included patients presenting at an Accident and Emergency Department in a large Scottish Hospital following a life-threatening or near life-threatening event. These consisted of RTAs, assault, house-fires or industrial accidents. Excluded from this study were those who had incurred a serious head injury, were too unwell to co-operate, or patients injured through sports, self-harm, home repairs and maintenance, fights or those who were heavily intoxicated when the incident occurred.

Such wide and differing exclusion criteria reduce the generalizability of results. However, with successful randomization this does not necessarily affect the validity of reported findings. See Appendix A for further details of the studies included in this review.

Timing of interventions

Timing of early interventions varied greatly between studies. In some cases they took place very soon after the traumatic event. For instance, in the study by Bunn and Clarke (1979), it took place immediately following admission of the seriously injured or ill relative. Hobbs *et al.* (1996) provided PD between 24–48 hours after road traffic accidents or when patients' physical state allowed this to take place. Lavender and Walkinshaw (1998) and Small *et al.* (2000) allowed 2 days post-partum. In Bordow and Porritt's study (1979) participants were seen during the first week of hospital admission. Other investigations report time passed between trauma and early intervention to vary between 6 and 12 days. In Dolan *et al.* (submitted) it was 3–14 days post-accident (with a mean of 7 days), in Conlon *et al.* (1999) 2–19 days (with a mean of 6.3 days) after admission to a regional burns unit (Bisson *et al.*, 1997) and within 24 hours of attendance at a hospital casualty department (Stevens and Adshead, 1996). The studies in which PD took place at a later stage were Lee *et al.* (1996) and Rose *et al.* (1999). Here intervention took place at approximately two weeks post-miscarriage and 9–31 days post crime. In the latter study, the mean delay was 21 days, with a standard deviation of 5.6 days.

Description of early interventions after trauma

Descriptions of the intervention used in each of the most recent studies and the method used for rating its application (when given) are listed in Table 3.2.

For similar information on the earlier studies, e.g. Stevens and Adshead (1996), Bunn and Clarke (1979), Bordow and Porritt (1979), Bisson *et al.* (1997), Hobbs *et al.* (1996) and Lee *et al.* (1996) see Appendix A.

Methodological quality of the studies

Methodological quality of studies incorporated in this review was assessed by the chapter authors using three separate assessment ratings methods. Quality ratings were first made in accordance

Table 3.2 New studies incorporated in the Cochrane Review New studies incorporated in updated review

Study	Description of intervention/ method of rating
Lavender and Walkinshaw (1998)	'Interactive interview using as much time as necessary discussing their labour and exploring their feelings'. Respondent led. No method of rating stated.
Small et al. (2000)	'Provided women with the opportunity to discuss their labour ... content of the discussion was determined by each women's experiences.' No method of rating given.
Conlon et al. (1999)	'Standard protocol that encouraged expression of emotional and cognitive effects of the RTA experience and provided educational material'. No method of rating given.
Dolan et al. (submitted)	Using Mitchell/Dyregrov model adapted for individual use. Ten per cent of the interventions were audiotaped to confirm adherence.
Rose et al. (1999)	Using Mitchell model adapted for individuals. All PD interventions audiotaped and rated by two others to confirm adherence.

with the methods recommended in the Cochrane Collaboration Handbook. This examines the quality of the trial and, in particular, the quality of randomization. Four trials, namely those of Bisson et al. (1997), Lavender et al. (1998), Rose et al. (1999) and Small et al. (2000) had adequate allocation concealment using computer-generated random numbers, opening consecutively numbered sealed opaque envelopes or centralized telephone randomization. Two studies had intermediate levels of concealed allocation using opaque envelopes (Stevens and Adshead, 1996) or a sealed envelope method (Dolan et al. submitted). For the remainder, allocation concealment was either unsatisfactory or unclear.

The second quality rating took the form of each author using ratings devised and advocated by Churchill (1996) for studies of psychiatric interventions. The maximum obtainable score is 37 based on stated ratings of the objectives of each trial, sample size, length of follow-up, statistical power, randomization, standardization of treatment, blinding, source of population, recruitment procedures, exclusion criteria, demographic descriptions, blinded assessments, reasons for withdrawal, outcome measures, intention to treat, presentation of results, types of data presented, statistical analysis and control for baseline differences. Lastly, a quality measure developed specifically for studies of debriefing was used (Kenardy and Carr, 1996). This examines the population that will receive the intervention, delineation of the goals of debriefing, randomization, use of self-report and objective measures, descriptions of the debriefing procedures used including the stated goals, personnel conducting the intervention, manualization, amount of exposure to PD and use of outcome measures by raters blind to intervention conditions. Different rating results derived from using these three quality measures were discussed and resolved through group consensus. Discrepancies between the general Churchill and the specific Kenardy scales reflected the fact that the Churchill scale emphasizes general methodological issues relevant to all clinical and especially pharmacological trials. The Kenardy scale gives more weight to specific methodological challenges relevant to assessment of PD and, in particular, the content of debriefing protocols. Overall though, methodological quality of studies included in this review was variable. In part this was partly due to incomplete data recording. On occasions authors had to be asked for additional information and this was readily given. Most gave reasonable information on 'a priori' objectives and sources of samples studied. Only the Mayou et al. (2000) follow-up of the original study by Hobbs et al. (1996) used a true intention to treat analysis.

Subjective assessment of the early interventions after trauma

Subjective reports of effectiveness were assessed in six studies. Bisson *et al.* (1997) stated that 52% of the respondents found PD 'definitely useful'. In Lee *et al.* (1996) study of women who had miscarried 71% felt they had been given an opportunity to talk about how they felt. However, amongst those allocated to the non-PD control group the level of positive endorsement was 29% ($P<0.05$). In this study patients who received PD were asked to rate its helpfulness on a 100-mm scale spanning from 'extremely unhelpful' (0) to 'extremely helpful' (100). The mean score was 74, indicating the women in the early intervention group showed a tendency towards being satisfied with this aspect of their care. At 78% significantly more participants in the non-intervention control group had tried, by their own accord, to obtain additional information about their miscarriage. In the PD group the proportion having done so was only 29% ($P<0.05$). Stevens and Adshead (1996) stated that 66% of those counselled found the session useful, while 33% said they did not. Reasons given by the latter included feeling the early intervention had been offered too early or that they had not needed it. Rose *et al.* (1999) recorded subjective assessment of the intervention at 6 month follow-up by asking participants to rate the helpfulness of the original interview on a scale of 1–10 (0=unhelpful, 5=neutral, 10=helpful). Overall, the mean score of 138 participants to this question was 7 with a standard deviation of 2.1. Only six rated helpfulness as less than five. No statistically significant difference was found in respect of perceived helpfulness of PD reported by the intervention and non-intervention groups. In the recent obstetric studies Lavender and Walkinshaw (1998) reported a positive subjective assessment of early intervention expressed as 'more satisfaction recorded with the amount of information received'. Small *et al.* (2000) reported very positive views of PD with only 26 participants (5.6%), out of a total sample of 463 rating the session as unhelpful. Two-hundred (43.2%) rated it as 'very helpful' and 237 (51.2%) gave a rating of 'helpful'.

Main findings of the studies

Overall results of the 11 trials included in this review revealed three to have a positive outcome. The ones in question are Bunn and Clarke (1979), Bordow and Porritt (1979), and Lavender and Walkinshaw (1998). Six studies report neutral outcomes; namely Stevens and Adshead (1997), Lee *et al.* (1996), Conlon *et al.* (1999), Rose *et al.* (1999), Dolan *et al.* (submitted) and Small *et al.* (2000). Two studies report poor outcomes Bisson *et al.* (1997) and Mayou *et al.* (2000). The latter is a 3-year follow-up of the Hobbs *et al.* (1996) study. As in our earlier Cochrane Review we continue to take the view that in respect of a distinctive therapeutic effect attributable to PD the strength of evidence is still to be considered neutral.

It is worth noting that of the three studies with positive outcomes two were completed as long ago as in the late 1970s before PD protocols were described (Bunn and Clarke, 1979; Bordow and Porritt, 1979). These investigations probably utilized the most heterogeneous samples. The more recent positive study by Lavender and Walkinshaw (1998) evaluated PD with a very different and selective sample of women receiving obstetric care.

As regards evaluating the impact of PD specifically on post-traumatic stress disorder, only three studies by Bisson *et al.* (1997), Rose *et al.* (1999) and Conlon *et al.* (1999) incorporate a categorical diagnosis of PTSD in their methodologies. The longest follow-up studies by Bisson *et al.* (1997) and Mayou *et al.* (2000) showed an adverse intervention effect on PTSD symptomatology when the Impact of Event Scale (IES; Horowitz *et al.*, 1979) was used as an outcome criterion. This self-report questionnaire is one of the most commonly cited instruments for examining trauma-related symptoms and is used in all the most recently published studies incorporated in this review. It is reported as a continuous, rather than categorical outcome measure in these trials except for the Stevens and Adshead (1996) study, where the IES was not given to the treatment group. In all studies the variance of IES scores is considerable and only Lee *et al.* (1996) reported results in which the mean was more than 1.6 times the standardized deviation.

Methodological quality findings

All 11 studies were ranked for quality using the three separate assessments schemes referred to above. Overall the Bisson *et al.* (1997) and Rose *et al.* (1999) trials scored highly, Dolan *et al.* (submitted), Conlon *et al.* (1999), Lee *et al.* (1996) and Hobbs *et al.* (1996) was rated intermediate, and the remaining are of low standard. However, we decided to use the Kenardy ratings for the final ranking since this was specifically designed for trials of debriefing. The final rankings, from highest to lowest quality, were therefore Bisson *et al.* (1997), Rose *et al.* (1999), Dolan (submitted), Conlon *et al.* (1999), Lee *et al.* (1996), Hobbs *et al.* (1996), Stevens and Adshead (1996), joint eighth–Bordow and Porritt (1979) and Small *et al.* (2000), followed by Lavender and Walkenshaw (1998) and, lastly, Bunn and Clarke (1979).

Discussion

The 11 papers identified for this review continue to highlight the current paucity of published randomized controlled trials (RCTs) of PD, as well as a total absence of RCTs of group debriefings. As acknowledged above the studies featured in our Cochrane Review have some methodological shortcomings. These include raters not being blind to original treatment conditions at follow-up, small sample sizes which compromises the power of statistical tests and variations in the early intervention techniques used. Given the popularity and continued use of PD this updated review again shows how an intervention technique or protocol can come into common usage without consistent evidence demonstrating its capacity to deliver prophesied outcomes. At current levels of knowledge it is therefore imprudent for anyone to claim there is anything but scant evidence that early psychological interventions, as defined in this review, consistently and effectively prevent PTSD psychopathology following trauma.

At best, the evidence base provided by the collective of studies referred in this chapter is neutral, but it should not go unnoticed that some negative outcomes following single early psychological interventions have been reported by Bisson *et al.* (1997) and Mayou *et al.* (2000). These are also the studies that feature the longest follow-up periods. One of the seeming contradictions brought into focus by this review of PD is the disparity between subjective and objective findings over time. Subjective impressions of early interventions were usually positive when asked for, but this result is at variance with objective outcome measures.

At this juncture it is instructive to consider why these studies failed to show a consistent positive effect. For instance, might it be the case that the early interventions were too short? This is unlikely, since this proposition would not explain why only some of the studies report PD having an adverse effect, whilst others do not. It may also be postulated that in the reviewed studies interventions may have led to an increase in psychological distress by re-exposing participants to the traumatic events without allowing sufficient time for habituation. This raises the spectre of early interventions, under certain circumstances, inadvertently perpetrating a secondary traumatization.

A further argument frequently heard is that inexperienced debriefers carried out interventions. This is also difficult to sustain. One of the studies (Rose *et al.*, 1999) audiotaped the PD for rating by external assessors on two separate occasions to ensure adherence to the protocol that had been transcribed from the original training manuals. A general point to make is that, whilst it is not unreasonable to expect technical guidance for protocol driven early interventions to be sufficiently robust to be readily transferable between practitioners it is difficult to see how standards of practice can by systematically monitored in day-to-day practice.

However, is it possible that follow-up periods were too short and outcomes improve with time? This seems most unlikely since the two studies that used the longest follow-up (Bisson *et al.*, 1997; Mayou *et al.*, 2000) showed PD to be an intervention with sufficiently marked negative consequences to engender statistically significant group differences between those debriefed and those who were not.

Having documented adverse effects of single early interventions, it is instructive to ask how this may have come about. A number of possibilities warrant consideration. Already mentioned is the possibility of early interventions causing secondary traumatization. By its very nature, PD involves intense imaginal re-exposure to traumatic incidents within a short time of its occurrence. It may be that, for some individuals, this becomes a further trauma that exacerbates symptoms without assisting in emotional processing. Another possible adverse reaction to PD could be mediated by shame when this is experienced following certain traumatic events (e.g. assault, rape). In detail, group discussions of what happened may increase the felt sense of shame with possible adverse effects on coping and adjustment.

Another explanation for negative outcomes is that PD may 'medicalize' normal distress. It may also increase an expectancy of developing psychological symptoms amongst survivors who might otherwise not have done so. It is a constant finding that, no matter how severe the trauma, not everyone develops debilitating symptoms and only a minority report long-term diagnosable disorders. By increasing awareness of psychological distress PD may induce the distress felt or increase its intensity. There is also the danger that PD may be seen as a substitute for traditional forms of support provided naturally by friends and family. In general, the value of early practical support from friends, families and colleagues has not been fully recognized or evaluated, whilst rather more attention has focused on the presumed, but still unproven, benefits of professionally delivered early interventions.

The theory that has informed PD seems also to assume there is a uniform and to a certain extent predictable pattern of reactions to trauma the resolution of which will be promoted if the precipitating event is talked about in great detail. At the heart of PD resides the concept that discussing trauma is therapeutic. To deny its occurrence is presumed always to be unhelpful. This is based on a time-honoured tradition of psychological thought. However, this is not necessarily true in every case. Recalling and developing a narrative of such events may prove to be a 'secondary trauma', and attempts to forget or distance oneself from events may be adaptive. PD may therefore interfere with such adaptive defence mechanisms.

Taken as a whole we consider the implications of this review to be that the principle of offering psychological and social support to survivors in the aftermath of trauma is a sensible and humane way to show concern for others. However, the time has now come to bring an end to practices derived from uncritically applied protocol prescriptions for early interventions after trauma. Instead, priority considerations should be given to ensuring early practical and flexible support for all those affected. This support could prioritize improving survivors' safety, providing food and shelter, assistance to return home to be with family members, help to speak to relatives, allowing time off work, and participate in appropriate rituals and ceremonies. It should not be prescriptive but designed for each individual situation and thus practised selectively (Freeman *et al.*, 2001). Those involved need to be consulted about what they would find helpful. Paradoxically, by practising a more selective and arguably sensitive range of interventions may require wider and higher level of skills. However, it also makes more sense to target those who appear to be at greatest risk of developing PTSD and offering these survivors intensive therapeutic help along lines suggested by Andre *et al.* (1997) and Bryant *et al.* (1998a). In this context it is important to be aware of the predictive power of acute stress disorder (APA, 1994) for later chronic post-traumatic stress disorder (Bryant *et al.*, 1998a,b; Brewin *et al.*, 1999). Recently completed research by Brewin *et al.* (1999; see also this volume) has developed a relatively simple checklist to predict later onset of PTSD if no help is provided. These developments could eventually lead to a screening and brief focused treatment programmes for survivors 'highlighted' as being at risk at 1 month post-trauma. Such programmes would not be offered as 'one off' interventions. Clearly, while this method of working recommends itself for having great face validity and offers important preventive potential it will need rigorous evaluation. A Cochrane protocol was recently registered to systematically review studies carried out along these lines to date.

Conclusions

This updated review has again highlighted the relative paucity of evidence surrounding the use of PD. At a time of commitment to evidence-based practice it is a point of professional concern whenever PD, with its very weak evidence base, it is recommended as an early intervention of choice following trauma. It should be noted that no comment is made as to the use of PD with children since the systematic review highlighted does not address this important group. We also draw the conclusion that all concerned with early intervention after trauma should give consideration to offering a broad spectrum of psychosocial interventions and decide on which option to pursue after consultation with those for whom services are intended. This is especially important given that early interventions will become more intimately linked with clearly established needs in survivor groups, will have high face validity and, if flexibly delivered, can take account of emergent post trauma scenarios. Whilst all of these are important there will, in the final instance, be no substitute for evidence in respect of what early intervention after trauma can and cannot achieve.

References

American Psychiatric Association (1987) *Diagnostic and Statistical Manual of Mental Disorders DSM-IIIR*, 3rd edn. Washington DC: APA, pp. 247–251.

American Psychiatric Association (1994) *Diagnostic and Statistical Manual of Mental Disorders DSM-IV*, 4th edn. Washington DC: APA, pp. 427–428.

Amir, M., Weil, G., Kapin, Z., Tocker, T. and Witztum, E. (1998) Debriefing with brief group psychotherapy in a homogenous group on non-injured victims of a terrorist attack: a prospective study. *Psych Scand* **1009**, 237–42.

Andre, C., Lelord, F., Legeron, P., Reignier, A. and Delattre, A. (1997) Etude controlle sur l'efficacite a 6 mois d'une prise en charge precoce de 132 conducteurs d'authobus victimes de'agression. *L'encephale*, **23**, 65–71.

Bisson, J. and Deahl, M. (1994) Psychological debriefing and prevention of post-traumatic stress—more research is needed. *Br J Psychiat* **165**, 717–20.

Bisson, J., Jenkins, P., Alexander, J. and Bannister, C. (1997) A randomised controlled trial of psychological debriefing for victims of acute burn trauma. *Br J Psychiat* **171**, 78–81.

Bordow, S. and Porritt, D. (1979) An experimental evaluation of crisis intervention. *Soc Sci Med* **13a**, 251–6.

Brewin, C.R., Amdrews, A., Rose, S. and Kirk, M. (1999) Acute stress disorder and post-traumatic stress disorder in victims of violent crime. *Am J Psychiat* **156**, 360–5.

Brom, D., Kleber, R. and Hofman, M. (1993) Victims of traffic accidents: incidence and prevention of post-traumatic stress disorder. *J Clin Psychol* **49**, 131–40.

Bryant, R., Harvey, A., Dang, S., Sackville, T. and Basten, C. (1998a) Treatment of acute stress disorder: a comparison of cognitive behavior therapy and supportive counselling. *J Consult Clin Psychol* **66**, 862–6.

Bryant, R., Harvey, A., Dang, S. and Sackville, T. (1998b) Assessing acute stress disorder: psychometric properties of a structured clinical interview. *Psycholog Assess* **10**, 215–20.

Bunn. T. and Clarke, A. (1979) Crisis intervention: an experimental study of the effects of a brief period of counselling on the anxiety of relatives of seriously injured or ill hospital patients. *Br J Med Psychol* **52**, 191–5.

Carlier, I., Lamberts, R., Van Uchelen, A. and Gersons, B. (1998) Disaster related post-traumatic stress in police officers: a field study of the impact of debriefing. *Stress Med* **14**, 143–8.

Caplan, G. (1964) *Principles of Preventive Psychiatry*, London: Tavistock.

Chalmers, I. and Altman, D.G. (eds) (1995) Systematic Reviews. *British Medical Journal Publishing Group*.

Chemtob, C., Tomas, S., Law, W. and Cremniter, D. (1997) A field study of the impact of psychological debriefing on post-hurricane psychological distress. *Am J Psychiat* **154**, 415–17.

Churchill, R. (1996) *A systematic review and meta analysis of the effects of pharmacotherapy and psychotherapy for the treatment of depression in primary care*, MSc Thesis, London School of Hygiene and Tropical Medicine.

Conlon, L., Fahy, T.J. and Conroy, R. (1999) PTSD in ambulant RTA victims: a randomized controlled trial of debriefing. *J Psychosom Res* **46**, 37–44.

Cox, J.L., Holden, J.M. and Sagovsky, R. (1987) Detection of postnatal depression: development of the 10 item Edinburgh Postnatal Depression Scale. *Br J Psychiat* **150**, 782–6.

Deahl, M., Gillham, A.B., Thomas, J., Seale, M. and Scrinivasan, M. (1994) Psychological Sequelae Following the Gulf War. Factors Associated with Subsequent Morbidity and the Effectiveness of Psychological Debriefing. *Br J Psychiat* **165**, 60–5.

Deahl, M., Scrinivasan, M., Jones, M., Thomas, J., Neblett, C. and Jolly, A. (2000) Preventing psychological trauma in soldiers: the role of operational stress training and psychological debriefing. *Br J Med Psychol* **73**, 77–85.

Doctor, R., Curtis, D. and Isaacs, G. (1994) Psychiatric morbidity in policemen and the effect of brief psychotherapeutic intervention: a pilot study. *Stress Med* **10**, 151–7.

Dolan, B., Bowyer, D., Freeman, C. and Little, K. (submitted) Critical incident stress debriefing after trauma: is it effective?

Dyregrov, A. (1989) Caring for helpers in disaster situations: psychological debriefing. *Disaster Manag* **2**, 25–30.

Foa, E.B., Heart-Ikeda, D. and Perry, K.J. (1995) Evaluation of a brief cognitive-behavioural program for the prevention of chronic PTSD in recent assault victims. *J Consult Clin Psychol* **63**, 948–55.

Freeman, C., Flitcroft, A. and Weeple, P. (2001) *Psychological First Aid: a replacement for psychological debriefing*. Edinburgh: Lothian Primary Care NHS Trust, The Rivers Centre.

Hobbs, M. and Adshead, G. (1996) Preventive psychological intervention for road crash survivors. In Mitchell, M. (ed.) *The Aftermath of Road Accidents: psychological, social and legal perspectives*. London: Routledge, 159–71.

Hobbs, M., Mayou, R., Harrison, B. and Warlock, P. (1996) A randomised trial of psychological debriefing for victims of road traffic accidents. *Br Med J* **313**, 1438–9.

Horowitz, M., Wilner, N. and Alvarez, W. (1979) Impact of events scale: a measure of subjective stress. *Psychosom Med* **41**, 209–18.

Hytten, K. and Hasle, A. (1989) Firefighters: a study of stress and coping. *Acta Psychiat Scand* **80**, (Suppl. 355), 50–5.

Kenardy, J. and Carr, V. (1996) Imbalance in the debriefing debate: what we don't know far outweighs what we do. *Bull Aust Psycholog Soc* Feb 4–6.

Kenardy, J., Webster, R., Lewin, T., Carr, V., Hazell, P. and Carter, G. (1996) Stress debriefing and patterns of recovery following a natural disaster. *J Traumatic Stress* **9**, 37–49.

Lavender, T. and Walkinshaw, S.A. (1998) Can midwives reduce postpartum psychological morbidity? A randomized trial birth **25**, 215–19.

Lee, C., Slade, P. and Lygo, V. (1996) The Influence of psychological debriefing on emotional adaption in women following early miscarriage: a preliminary study. *Br J Med Psychol* **69**, 47–58.

Macdonald, G. (1998) Promoting evidence-based practice in child protection. *Clin Child Psychol Psychiat* **3**, 71–85.

Mathews, L. (1998) Effect of staff debriefing on post-traumatic stress symptoms after assaults by community housing residents. *Psychiat Serv* **49**, 207–12.

Mayou, R.A., Ehlers, A. and Hobbs, M. (2000) A three year follow-up of a randomised controlled trial of psychological debriefing for road traffic accident victims. *Br J Psychiat* **176**, 589–93.

McFarlane, A.C. (1988) The aetiology of post-traumatic stress disorders following a natural disaster. *Br J Psychiat* **152**, 116–21.

Mitchell, J.T. (1983) When disaster strikes. *J Emerg Med Serv* **8**, 36–9.

Morgan, P.P. (1985) The literature jungle. *Canad Med Ass J* **134**, 98–9.

Polak, P., Egan, D., Vandebergh, R. and Williams, W. (1975) Prevention in mental health: a control study. *Am J Psychiat* **132**, 146–9.

Raphael, B., Meldrum, L. and McFarlane, A.C. (1995) Does debriefing after psychological trauma work? *Br Med J* **310**, 1479–80.

Rick, J., Perryman, S., Young, K., Guppy, A. and Hillage, J. (1998) *Workplace Trauma and Its Management Review of the Literature*. London: Institute of Employment Studies.

Robinson, R. and Mitchell, J.T. (1993) Evaluation of psychological debriefings. *J Traumatic Stress* **6**, 367–82.

Rose, S. (1997) Psychological debriefing: history and methods. *Counselling—J Br Ass Counselling* **8**, 48–51.

Rose, S. and Bisson, J. (1998) Brief early psychological interventions following trauma: a systematic review of the literature. *J Traumatic Stress* **11**, 697–710.

Rose, S., Brewin, C.R. Andrews, B. and Kirk, M. (1999) A randomised controlled trial of individual psychological debriefing for victims of violent crime. *Psycholog Med* **29**, 793–9.

Rose, S., Bisson, J. and Wessely, S. (2001) A systematic review of brief psychological interventions ('debriefing') for the treatment of immediate trauma related symptoms and the prevention of post-traumatic stress disorder (Cochrane Review) update. *Cochrane Library* **3**. Update Software.

Roth, A. and Fonagy, P. (1996) *What Works for Whom? A Critical Review of Psychotherapy Research*. New York: Guilford Press.

Saari, S., Lindeman, M., Verkasalo, M. and Prytz, H. (1996) The Estonia disaster: a description of the crisis intervention in Finland. *Eur Psychol* **1**, 135–9.

Small, R., Lumley, J., Donohue, L., Potter, A. and Walderstrom, U. (2000) Midwife-led debriefing to reduce maternal depression following operative birth: a randomised controlled trial. *Br Med J* **321**, 1043–7.

Tadmor, C., Brandes, J. and Hofman, J. (1987) Preventive intervention for a caesarian birth population. *Br J Prevent Psychol* **3**, 343–64.

Viney, L., Clarke, A., Bunn, T. and Benjamin, Y. (1985) An evaluation of three crisis intervention programmes for general hospital patients. *Br J Med Psychol* **58**, 75–86.

Wessely, S., Rose, S. and Bisson, J. (1998) A systematic review of brief psychological intervention ('debriefing') for the treatment of immediate trauma related symptoms and the prevention of posttraumatic stress disorder (Cochrane Review). **In The Cochrane Library**, Issue 2, Oxford: Update Software: 1998. Updated quarterly.

Zigmond, A.S. and Snaith, R.P. (1983) The Hospital Anxiety and Depression Score. *Acta Psychiat Scand* **67**, 361–70.

Appendix A: characteristics of included studies

Study	Trauma	Subjects (total n)	Time post-trauma	Intervention (min)	Control condition	Setting	Facilitator	Main outcome measures	Follow-up period	Outcome	Comment
1. Bisson et al. (1997)	Acute burn trauma	130	2–19 days	IPD or couple PD (30–120)	Standard care	Hospital	Psychiatrist or nurse	HADS, IES, CAPS	3 & 13 months	Intervention group fared worse on all measures (P<0.05 at 13 months)	Initial distress far more predictive of outcome than PD
2. Bunn & Clarke (1979)	Relatives of seriously ill/injured	30	<12 hours	Ind Couns (20 min)	Standard care	Hospital	Medical practitioner (Psychology Undergrad*)	Anxiety content analysis scales	Immed post-couns	Intervention group less anxious (P<0.05)	No follow-up period
3. Bordow & Porritt (1979)	MVA victims	70	<1 week	'Immed Review' (60)	Standard care or 3 months SW input	Hospital	Social worker	8 Scales include Anxiety & Affect	3–4 months	Immediate Review fared better than no intervention but worse than extended input	
4. Conlon et al. (1999)	RTA victims	40	3–14 days (M=7 days)	IPD (30)	Standard care	Hospital	?	IES, CAPS-II.			
5. Dolan et al. (submitted)	Attendees A & E department	100	6–12 days	IPD 45 min to 2 hours	Standard care	Participants home or university dept	Nurse therapist	HADS, IES, GHQ.	1 month & 6 months	No significant differences between groups.	
6. Hobbs et al. (1996)	MVA victims	106	24–48 hours	IPD (60)	Standard care	Hospital	?	BSI, IES interview	4 months	Intervention group fared worse (P<0.05 on some measures)	Unclear if higher injury severity score in PD group controlled for.
Mayou et al. (2000)		61	3 year	Postal				BSI, IES travel anxiety, questions or	3 years		
3-year follow-up		61	Follow-up						3 years	Negative effects of the intervention	At 3 year follow-up it appeared that

Continued

Appendix A: characteristics of included studies (continued)

Study	Trauma	Subjects (total n)	Time post-trauma	Intervention (min)	Control condition	Setting	Facilitator	Main outcome measures	Follow-up period	Outcome	Comment
								longer-term effects of RTA		on patients with high initial IES scores at 4 months were maintained at 3 year follow-up.	overall the intervention may have made some patients worse. For those with a low IES score at 4 months the intervention appeared to make no difference but for those with a higher IES score at 3 months (>24) it appeared to make them significantly worse if they received the intervention.
7. Lavender & Walkinshaw (1998)	Normal cephalic birth at term	114	2 days post-partum	IPD (intervention did not include in-depth questioning) 30–120 mins.	All respondents were given the opportunity to discuss their birth experience when the study was completed.	Postnatal ward	Research midwife	HADS at 3 weeks: (no baseline measures)		Women in the PD group were significantly less likely to have high anxiety (P<0.00001) and depression (P<0.0001) 3 weeks following delivery.	Women in the control group had extremely high levels of depression HADS>11 = 31 from a sample of 56.
8. Lee et al. (1996)	Miscarriage	60	14 days	IPD (60)	Standard care	Home	Psychologist	HADS, IES	4 months	No difference between groups	

Study	Population	N	Timing	Intervention	Control	Setting	Provider	Measures	Follow-up	Results	
9. Rose et al. (1999)	Victims of violent crime	157	21 days	IPD 60 min	One group received standard care, while one group received education only	Home	Nurse therapist or research social worker	PSS, IES, BDI	6 months and 11 months	No difference between groups.	
10. Small et al. (2000)	Operative birth	908	2 days post-partum	IPD 'up to 1 hour'	Standard care	Maternity hospital	Research midwife	EPDS Overall maternal health status measures	6 months	No baseline measures taken. Utilizing the recommended cut-off of 13 for the EPDS the women who underwent PD were not less likely to be depressed at 6 months.	Odds for depression in the PD group were raised although not significantly. The mean EPDS scale scores did not differ significantly between the groups ($t=1.17$, $P=0.24$).
11. Stevens & Adshead (1996)	MVA, Assault or Dog Bite	63	<24 hours	Ind Couns (60)	Standard care	Hospital	Counsellor	IES, BDI, SEQ	1 week, 1 & 3 months	No difference between groups overall. High trait anxiety and BDI on entry in intervention group fared sig better	Unusually distressed during counselling excluded

IPD=Individual Psychological Debriefing
Couns. = Counselling
MVA=Motor Vehicle Accident
RTA=Road Traffic Accident
HADS=Hospital Anxiety and Depression Scale
IES=Impact of Event Scale
CAPS=Clinician Administered PTSD Scale
BSI=Brief Symptom Inventory
PSS=Post-traumatic Symptom Scale
BDI=Beck's Depression Inventory
SEQ=Spielberger Self Evaluation Questionnaire
EPDS=Edinburgh Postnatal Depression Score
*The Medical Practitioner was also a Psychology Undergraduate.

Section 2 Current theories and conceptualizations of early reactions to trauma

Section A of this book seeks to foster a recognition reconstructed early intervention after trauma cannot be premised by a doctrinaire notion of 'one technique fits all'. The era of confident assertions about routine prescriptions for post-incident care has come to an end. In its place has dawned a realization survivors' needs are probably as diverse as they are changeable. Even the notion of a narrow range of protocol prescriptions being sufficient to respond to all eventualities seems ill advised.

These conclusions may engender confusion on the part of readers who seek practical guidance on what to do to help trauma survivors. Indeed, such uncertainties are inconvenient under prevailing circumstances, but their implication is clear. In order to reconstruct early intervention it is necessary to go back to basics and start from fresh beginnings. One way of doing so is to temporarily suspend preoccupations with the practicalities of 'what to do'. In their place, effort may be expended more fruitfully by examining theories and conceptualizations of early reactions to trauma plus the factors that determine their development over time. This is a first step towards identifying appropriate rationales for interventions that are indicated in the aftermath of trauma. It should also help ensure provision remains rooted in theories that engender criteria for formulating informed opinions about the veracity of practice.

Section 2 sets out to lay solid theoretical and conceptual foundations for reconstructed early intervention. It does so by examining a range of informed opinions and facts pertinent to improved understanding of the nature of early reactions to trauma. By rooting practice in theories that are supported by empirical evidence reconstruction can proceed.

Professor Alexander McFarlane of Adelaide University, Australia examines the evolution of diagnostic terms used to describe early reactions to trauma. Nosological rigor is a desirable aspiration, since it promotes informed debate about the nature of reactions observed in trauma survivors. Crucial in this regard is the dynamic relationship between terminology and quality of research. He concludes the search for precise diagnosis is continuing under difficult circumstances. To a large measure this is because some of the main premises for appropriate use of medical diagnosis do not apply during the early aftermath of trauma. For instance, classification is rendered difficult by the diversity of observed reactions and their propensity for rapid change over relatively short periods of time. Readers should also note the suggestion diagnosis may be ill advised if evoked responses are primarily adaptive expressions of human distress at a time of personal crisis and not symptoms of a disorder. The point is also made that to impose seemingly arbitrary diagnostic criteria runs a risk of limiting systematic investigations to a restricted and unrepresentative range of evoked responses. Highlighting these difficulties is in no way meant to imply trauma survivors are not in need of prompt help or support. Undeniably, some do need very practical assistance, but decisions about what to do should not be premised by considerations of diagnosis alone.

Professor Arik Shalev from the Department of Psychiatry at Hadassah University Hospital in Jerusalem, Israel presents another vantage point for reconstructing early intervention. He traces sequences of psychobiological and neurochemical responses evoked by trauma. A convincing argument is put forward for viewing expressed reactions as phased and functional. That is, they can be adaptive in so far they increase chances of survival. Initially, this is achieved by eliciting primitive caring responses from those in a position to help. Thereafter, reactions can engender powerful processes of group cohesion and only at a later stage will more sophisticated psychological processing of events take place. Suggestions are offered for how reconstructed early intervention should aspire to be synchronized with the phasic nature of evoked reactions.

However, having explained the biological substrates that underpin survivors' prototype reactions Shalev acknowledges the course and development of evoked responses over time rarely conforms to a textbook 'ideal'. Rather, they are subject to marked individual variations that engender idiosyncratic presentations. Paramount amongst these are considerations of the general physical state of survivors at time of trauma, the meaning of the event to the person concerned, cognitive processing in the aftermath of actual experience and levels of social support. In this regard there is no simple cause-effect relationship between stimulus and response.

All the same Dr Sean Perrin from the Department of Psychology in the Institute of Psychiatry in London, UK delineates the value of learning theory perspectives for understanding some early behavioural and emotional reactions to trauma. Most particularly, the ways in which classical and operant conditioning paradigms account for high levels of psychophysiological arousal and persistent anxiety. He offers detailed advice about how selected behaviour therapy techniques can be adapted and incorporated within reconstructed early intervention. Of particular value is the way learning theory reinforces the imperative of lowering survivors' high levels of psychophysiological arousal. Only when this has been achieved should consideration be given to interventions requiring more sophisticated cognitive appraisal of what has happened.

Dr Hazel Pilgrim comprehensively reviews the importance of cognitive processes in the early aftermath of trauma. Her points are elaborated further in a number of other chapters. Survivors' immediate appraisals exert a crucial influence on the course and development of human reactions to trauma. For instance, if a given event is deemed to be life threatening, evoked reactions are likely to differ from those of survivors whose cognitive processes engender a sense of control and mastery.

Beyond the reflexive, behavioural and cognitive reactions evoked by trauma, language is the pre-eminent means by which survivors express subtle nuances of personal experience and subjective meaning. Consequently, many forms of reconstructed early intervention rely heavily on language. However, difficulties inherent in doing so should not be under-estimated. Dr Lionel Bailly, previously a project consultant for Médecins Sans Frontières, in Paris, France, but currently Honorary Consultant in Child and Adolescent Psychiatry at the Royal Free and University College London Medical School in London, UK, brings psychoanalytic theory to bear on this aspect of early intervention. He also describes some of the practical ramifications of this theoretical framework for systematic approaches to early intervention pursued in France.

Much merit derives from the theoretical perspective reviewed above. However, they are limited by being reductionist and person-centred. A comprehensive overview of theories that inform our understanding of early reactions to trauma and interventions indicated in their aftermath will be incomplete if no account is taken of the broader social context within which they occur.

Professor Dean and Dr Marina Ajducović from the Department of Psychology at Zagreb University, Zagreb, Croatia, extend the foundations for reconstructed early intervention into the realms of systemic theory. They make explicit the importance of mobilizing social, community and family networks in support of survivor care. In situations of mass violence or population displacement these networks are typically disrupted and a priority for reconstructed early intervention might be to systematically foster their regeneration.

Authors contributing to this book section have succeeded in engendering an appreciation of the many theoretical perspectives that are relevant to the process of reconstructing early intervention. Such diversity is no impediment to developing a clarity of purpose. Rather, it encourages not only recognition of survivors' complex and changing needs, but also that each of these can be systematically addressed with clear rationales for each intervention.

4 Early reactions to traumatic events. The diversity of diagnostic formulations

Alexander C. McFarlane

Historically, the traditions of medical nosology have, in many regards, had little to offer to the typology of acute reactions to traumatic stressors. Very few psychiatrists or psychologists would, in the course of normal practice, see patients in the immediate aftermath of such events. The theoretical frameworks that have underpinned psychiatric diagnosis are derived largely from sub-classifications of psychosis, and the various typologies used to separate pathological anxiety and depression into specific disorders. In most clinical settings the few cases that have provided opportunities for observation of the acute reactions to life events have generally been patients presenting with severe reactions such as psychotic episodes or suicide attempts. The lens for clinical observation and diagnosis has therefore been highly blinkered by the orthodox concepts applied to help categorizing and understanding patients' reactions in the face of adversity.

A legacy of the above is that until the 1990s no questionnaires had been designed for the observation of these reactions, especially those that are independent of symptoms associated with established psychiatric disorders. As a consequence, there is a poverty of systematic observations about these phenomena (Solomon *et al.*, 1996). Furthermore, in the vast majority of cases, those who develop psychiatric disorders in the context of adversity tend not to present to clinicians for weeks or months after the event. Patients who are seen soon after critical events are a small and atypical minority who may bias any generalizations derived from their reports. Recently designed instruments that have allowed systematic observation of acute symptoms have been influenced considerably by *DSM IV* formulations of acute stress disorder [American Psychiatric Association (APA), 1994].

Implicit in all endeavours to determine pathological reactions to trauma is a presumption of baseline knowledge about the nature of normal reactions to such events. However, the character and phenomenology of normal human distress has received remarkably little attention in psychiatric research. Even the word distress is seldom defined in psychiatric texts. So, it would appear that phenomenologists have concentrated on defining what is abnormal in relation to traumatic events without due consideration to the range or intensity of normal affective responses they may evoke.

Important theoretical biases have hampered research into the nature of emotions and their modulation. In particular, the growth of behaviourism and the dominant role this paradigm has played in the development of psychological theory in the twentieth century has hampered the development of more sophisticated typologies of emotion. Behaviourism focused on what could be measured experimentally. Emotion has been shied away from as a possible topic of serious scientific investigation because of their inevitable subjective nature. Panksepp (1998) has called for a serious reconsideration of this neglect because of the primary role affect plays in the organization of human behaviour. Current dominance of cognitive theory and its accompanying school of cognitive behaviour therapy mean there is scant prospect of redressing this bias in the near future. They support only a subsidiary role of affect in the organization of behaviour despite neuro-anatomical and phylogenetic evidence to the contrary (Panksepp, 1998). This neglect of the importance of affect is particularly detrimental in the study of acute responses to traumatic events where emotion is at the core of distress and its phenomenology.

The relationship between acute and chronic post-traumatic reactions

The perceived relationship between acute stress reactions and PTSD is complex and has shaped the way traumatic stress reactions are dealt with in clinical practice (Yehuda and McFarlane, 1995). The failure to understand the complexities of this relationship explains, in part, why formulations of PTSD pose such paradigmatic problems. During the First and Second World Wars immediate clinical concern was to treat acute stress disorders in men who had broken down in the course of combat (Glass, 1974). Many responded quickly to treatment and returned to combat. Others did not respond to acute interventions and required more intensive treatment away from the front where symptoms often became chronic (Kardiner, 1959). A variety of explanations are used to explain these outcomes.

For some acute reactions were seen as a failure of the 'stimulus barrier' to protect the ego from disintegration (Freud, 1955) and pre-morbid factors such as childhood conflict and an inadequate personality were seen as important aetiological factors (Bailey, 1918). Failure to resolve symptoms led to further hypotheses formulations that encompassed notions of secondary gain. Namely, that disorders allowed escape from battlefields. More accepted psychoanalytic notions of developmental psychopathology were thus evoked and Leri (1919, p. 118) argued a few cases 'deserved the rights and privileges of disease'. The vast majority of presentations were construed as failures of the will of patients. Failures of courage were claimed to be caused by some inherited trait making these men unable to survive the anvil of combat. When MacPather (1922, p. 28) appeared before a War Office Committee he argued that cowardice and shell shock were the same phenomena. 'Cowardice I take to mean action under the influence of fear, and the ordinary kind of shell shock to my mind was a chronic and persisting fear'.

The role of military medical officers was also thought to be critical in creating prolonged morbidity. Bailey, the head of neuropsychiatry in the US army emphasized the importance of suggestion that 'lays its crippling hand on conditions not primarily neurological'. He argued that 'classical symptoms of hysteria results from suggestion originating in medical examinations, or from misapplied medical or surgical treatment' (Bailey, 1918, p. 2150). The notion that empathy could dangerously reward patients was reflected in administrations of the disciplinary therapies that emerged from uses of galvanism to treat conversion disorders and neurosis in the late nineteenth century.

Yealland (1918) took the view that the therapist should persuade the patient to overcome his symptoms and '… resume his official soldierly and manly function'. To facilitate this outcome the consequences of symptom had to be arranged as to be painful to patients (Leed, 1979). Painful electrical currents were applied, whilst commands and admonitions were shouted at patients kept in an isolated environment. An alternative treatment developed by Bellin and Vernet for use in the French Army comprised taking soldiers to dugouts near the front where extremely painful subcutaneous injections of ether were administered (Leed, 1979).

These practices, rationales invoked to justify their use and the war setting were not conducive to reflective theorizing about the nature of emotions or psychopathology. Implied in these paradigms was the notion that upon cessation of war there would be no secondary gains and disorders would disappear. When patients remained ill secondary gain was again invoked as a desire for financial compensation. The observation that was never adequately addressed was that a significant majority of men who developed combat related disorders did not break down in battle, but presented their symptoms when attempting to re-enter civilian life. In 1945, the US psychiatrist Grinker noted 'To our astonishment the majority of the neuroses that are hospitalized today in the convalescent hospitals are people who have developed either the first signs of their neurosis on return to this country or have become worse after landing on these shores'. The then dominance of psychoanalytic theory prevented any serious attempt to deal with the fact there is no simple continuum between acute combat stress reactions and chronic traumatic pathology of combat. As Glass noted in 1974, 'The limited ability to cope with combat was deemed the result of faulty personality development and thus conformed to the psychoanalytic model of the psychoneuroses and was so generally diagnosed' (p. 802).

The enduring force of such attitudes to suffering as a result of war persisted into the Second World War. However, some important shifts in perspective occurred at this time. The extent to which 'peri-traumatic' reactions (e.g. dissociation, freezing-surrender, disorganization) predicted prolonged distress was more systematically examined in World War II (WWII). Grinker and Spiegel (1945, p. 82) proposed that some people develop excessive responses under stress and that such responses are often transformed into prolonged disorders. 'Fear and anger in small doses are stimulating and alert the ego, increasing efficacy. But, when stimulated by repeated psychological trauma the intensity of the emotion heightens until a point is reached at which the ego loses its effectiveness and may become altogether crippled'.

Grinker and Spiegel (1945, p. 84) also proposed a hierarchy of combat anxiety states including: '… mild anxiety states in which the subjective and motor signs of anxiety are present but function is not yet interfered with. In moderate anxiety states the same symptoms may have progressed to the point where the flier makes mistakes in flying and now has his own incapacity to fear as well. Finally severe anxiety states, with much regression of the ego, confusion in regard to the environment, mutism and stupor'.

In the post war period, the importance of extreme stress as a determinant of acute symptoms was accepted with the inclusion of 'gross stress reaction' in DSM-I (APA, 1952). The need for separate diagnoses to account for chronic disorders was not addressed. Interest in social psychiatry blossomed during this period, and led to the development of crisis theory and crisis interventions. This was not an era of phenomenological precision due to the pre-eminence of psychoanalytic ideas, where defence and conflict remained the organizing principles of observation. Also, there was a growing interest in the life events literature. Unfortunately, this failed to recognize aetiological differences between stresses involving horror and threat to life, and those comprising financial or relationship problems. This led to the recognition that acute disturbances in function can follow events other than combat.

In DSM-II (APA, 1968) a shift towards including less severe events was reflected in 'transient situational disturbance'. This diagnosis was used to describe acute symptomatic distress following a range of adverse events. More prolonged disorders were categorized as anxiety or depressive neuroses. Regardless of whether these conditions were attributable to developmental fixation or genetic predisposition the role of environmental stress was by implication considered a non-specific trigger that might serve to release, exacerbate or prolong a predictable diathesis to psychiatric symptoms.

The diagnosis of PTSD eventually filled the nosological gap by acknowledging that extremely traumatic events can produce chronic clinical disorders not necessarily tied to an acute disturbance. The prevailing notion that this disorder can arise in normal individuals represented a move away from the psychoanalytic notions of vulnerability and emphasized the importance of the event.

Inevitably, this formulation proved too simplistic a representation of the complex interplay between individuals and their environment (McFarlane, 1999).

Drivers of knowledge and theoretical interest

Against this background a series of pragmatic questions have motivated interest in acute reactions to traumatic events. The military has immediate concerns due to costs of combat stress reactions to fighting manpower, but history demonstrates how rapidly lessons learned in one war are forgotten. Amongst commanders great ambivalence has existed to the belief that combat stress is a major cause of loss of manpower. Commanders without experience of combat have an exaggerated faith in resilience created by training, and claim the issue is solely one of bravery and courage. However, field experience repeatedly demonstrates that even the most battle-hardened soldiers can break down after prolonged combat exposure.

Military perspectives about the nature of acute reactions to combat have by necessity been framed by questions about soldiers ability to continue fighting (Solomon *et al.*, 1996). This is a behavioural issue and not one of refined phenomenology. At the front line, the diagnosticians are not psychiatrists or psychologists, but platoon commanders and other service personnel. Observed behaviour disturbances take a variety of forms and tend to be highly fluid in their phenomenology. For instance:

1. Soldiers may become increasingly anxious so as to interfere with their ability to function or take commands. The demeanour and agitation of such individuals is characterized by high arousal, tremulousness and facial expressions of fear.
2. Individuals may become frozen in response to orders, commands and environmental demands for adaptive behaviour.
3. Soldier may adopt attitudes of inappropriate indifference to danger, and failure to integrate or process salient environmental information.
4. Distress and tearfulness may overcome soldiers so that they are unable to function.
5. Behaviour may become erratic thus creating a potential danger for other personnel.

These reactions are observed in the field and involve monitoring an individual's behavioural response to the demands being placed upon him. In essence, the individual's internal affects and distress come to override previously demonstrated capacities for efficient goal directed behaviour.

Horowitz' (1986) studies of traumatic bereavement have played a critical role in formulating both the dynamic theory about acute reactions and the nature of their phenomenology. In 'Stress Response Syndromes' he described the central role of intrusion and avoidance, and argued oscillations between these phenomena occur in the early stages of reaction to traumata. These ideas were very influential when initial criteria for PTSD were formulated and for improving understanding of immediate distress responses. This formulation represented an important conceptual shift because, for the first time, considerations of the internal modulation of distress took account of the importance of traumatic memories rather than affect alone. This led to an interest in various and fluctuating states of mind experienced during and after exposure to trauma.

Other states of mind

As a diagnosis, acute stress disorder is limited by the implication of it being an established mental state akin to other diagnostic categories. However, in the immediate aftermath of traumatic events fluid interactions occur between individuals and their environments that have many determinants. Important factors include continuation of threats, reactions of other people, the presence of physical injury and treatments provided plus whether or not survivors remain in a malevolent environment. During WWII, Marshall (1947) observed that the level of attachment between a soldier, and his immediate comrades can determine the difference between being able to fight or retreating into states of fear and inaction. Soldiers seldom fight effectively if not in the presence of other men they know and trust. It is interesting that in the nineteenth century, combat stress reactions were conceived of as nostalgia and distress was primarily attributed to separation from family and familiar attachments (Glass, 1974). In settings of extreme stress, individuals' states of mind are not fixed as in other psychiatric disorders. Rather they comprise a fluid pattern of orientation and self-organization involving critical struggles to master fear, organize reactions and behaviours to help secure survival. If the information available is overwhelming and cannot be stabilized by the presence of others, the mind mobilizes a set of adaptive coping mechanisms. Survival is promoted if all information salient to the individual can be sorted and organized. Panic occurs when the multitude of novel stimuli is overwhelming and cannot be prioritized. In this state anxieties evoked by the situation can freeze an individual's behaviour or can cause a progressive breakdown of the ability to integrate multiple stimuli and threats. The capacity to integrate these multiple layers of sensory stimuli is one of the key determinants of whether or not individuals dissociate in this setting. It may involve a process of disengaging the capacity of environmental influences to sustain emotional arousal and thereby evoking a state of numbing. In extreme forms, normal orientations to the self can be lost, both in terms of one's own body and the sense of being an agent in the world. In the latter instance, a state of 'de-realization' is experienced. These can be transitory states allowing rapid reintegration and performance of effective goal directed tasks once control of anxieties is regained.

Another critical frame of orientation can occur in the face of threat that determines the information fields that individuals react to. Chemtob (1999) refers to this state as 'survival mode'. This state of mind involves the suppression of affect and promotes a scanning of the environment for threat. Vigilance with its accompanying propensity to shift attention helps predict the most immediate threats to survival. At the same time constant re-orientations take place in assessments of person-to-person attachments centred on a powerful desire to remain within and protect an available group. The mode of cognition at these times is one of intense problem solving, rather than the more open style of associative thinking. This implies that individuals are entrapped in their immediate environment and outer reality at the expense of the more internal dialogues that typically allow subtle shifts between different affective states. Many aspects of the behaviour of individuals in situations of extreme stress are reflective of these mental states. For instance, the patterns of acute stress related symptoms observed in different individuals may reflect their ability to switch from one to the other. Those who remain in 'survival mode' after an environment of safety has been re-established will be at a considerable disadvantage and are prone to further affective intensifications of the sense of threat. To date, there has been no systematic study of these phenomena and the ways they impact on acute stress disorder symptoms. This is a critical issue since there is a great deal of difference between stressors like motor vehicle accidents, which may last for seconds and are typically followed by short periods of rescue, and combat during which very direct threats and demands for adaptive behaviour may last for days. In the latter context, the emergence of symptoms of psychological disorganization will have entirely different meanings to those experienced in the former. For these reasons, it is important that the acute stress disorder literature is not treated as homogeneous.

Trained professionals such as fire officers or soldiers who are regularly exposed to danger draw upon very different repertoires of behaviour, learning and memory when exposed to traumatic stressors than do individuals suddenly involved in car accidents. Development of symptoms in the aftermath of these situations is likely to have very different determinants that reflect the role of training, anticipation, motivation for re-exposure and group morale. For these reasons it is important not to generalize findings about acute stress reactions in one setting to those that may occur in other situations.

Acute stress disorder also should be separated from several other conditions. First, adjustment disorder as defined in *DSM IV* (APA, 1994), relates to events of a less severe nature than defined by the stressor criterion. There are many similarities about the fluctuating nature of the individual's distress and the mixed range of emotions. However, an adjustment disorder can also have a more prolonged duration than an acute stress disorder with the maximum duration being 6 months. Adjustment disorder carries the lineage of transient situational disturbance and describes the states of perturbation following situations of loss and conflict, for example, in relationships. Finally, there are some individuals where there will be an intense pattern of distress that has a phobic quality. In these individuals, a pattern of acute disorganization and anxiety follows the contemplation of having to again confront the situation that was highly traumatic. Once this possibility is removed, the distress and fear settles. This pattern of response again needs to be differentiated from an acute stress disorder.

The definition of acute stress disorder

The number of published observational studies that focus specifically on acute stress disorder has increased since its inclusion as a diagnosis in *DSM IV* (APA, 1994). Because wars and disasters are very difficult contexts for the conduct of research into early reactions to trauma there was a paucity of data to inform initial formulations of its diagnostic criteria. *DSM IV* criteria listed in Table 4.1 reveal their emphasis on the presence of acute dissociative reactions in combination with other PTSD symptoms. In part, the criteria selected reflect the role of acute dissociation as a critical component of long-term post-traumatic reactions.

In contrast, ICD-10 definitions are more reflective of descriptions accumulated from military psychiatry that are, perhaps, more specific to combat [ICD-10; World Health Organization (WHO), 1993]. This definition focuses on the polymorphic nature of symptoms and recognizes that anxiety, depression and lability are important features the phenomenology of which can fluctuate rapidly. This particular formulation of diagnostic criteria has, however, created a significant bias in observations made of symptoms that occur in the aftermath of trauma. The ICD criteria are more in keeping with the factor analysis conducted by Solomon *et al.* (1996) into the content and phenomenology of acute stress disorders evoked by combat. This included the development of severe psychosomatic reactions, such as diarrhoea or shaking, that are not part of the list of symptoms that comprise current diagnostic criteria. In essence, acute stress disorder is a form of PTSD that occurs within 2 days and 4 weeks after a traumatic experience. The critical conceptual difference between PTSD and acute stress disorder lies in the significance of dissociative symptoms at least three of which are required for a differential diagnosis.

Dissociation

Although of considerable historic importance the role of dissociation in the acute symptom profile has only since the introduction of *DSM IV* become an interest for clinicians and researchers. For instance early work by Charcot and Richter (1881), Freud (1933) and Janet (1889) described dissociation or double consciousness as a central psychopathological process in the onset of conversion symptoms and traumatic neuroses. It has many components including depersonalization, derealization, amnesia and time distortion. Classen *et al.* (1998) reviewed literature that investigated the relationship between acute reactions and PTSD. The difficulty in reviewing and describing the symptoms of acute stress disorder lies in the paucity of empirical work that preceded its

Table 1 *DSM IV* diagnostic criteria for acute stress disorder

A.	The person has been exposed to a traumatic event in which both of the following were present:
	(1) the person experienced, witnessed, or was confronted with an event or events that involved actual or threatened death or serious injury, or a threat to the physical integrity of self or others;
	(2) the person's response involved intense fear, helplessness, or horror
B.	Either while experiencing or after experiencing the distressing event, the individual has three (or more) of the following dissociative symptoms:
	(1) a subjective sense of numbing, detachment, or absence of emotional responsiveness
	(2) a reduction in awareness of his or her surroundings (e.g. 'being in a daze');
	(3) de-realization;
	(4) depersonalization;
	(5) dissociative amnesia (i.e. inability to recall an important aspect of the trauma)
C.	The traumatic event is persistently re-experienced in a least one of the following ways: recurrent images, thoughts, dreams, illusions, flashback episodes or a sense of reliving the experience; or distress on exposure to reminders of the traumatic event.
D.	Marked avoidance of stimuli that arouse recollections of the trauma (e.g. thoughts, feelings, conversations, activities, places, people).
E.	Marked symptoms of anxiety and increased arousal (e.g. difficulty sleeping, irritability, poor concentration, hypervigilance, exaggerated startle response, motor restlessness).
F.	The disturbance causes clinically significant distress or impairment in social, occupational, or other important areas of functioning or impairs the individual's ability to pursue some necessary task, such as obtaining necessary assistance or mobilizing personal resources by telling family members about the traumatic experience.
G.	The disturbance lasts for a minimum of two days and a maximum of 4 weeks and occurs within 4 weeks of the traumatic event.
H.	The disturbance is not due to the direct physiological effects of a substance (e.g. a drug of abuse, a medication) or a general medical condition, is not better accounted for by Brief Psychotic Disorder, and is not merely an exacerbation of a pre-existing Axis I or Avis II disorder.

Source: American Psychiatric Association, 1994.

inclusion in *DSM IV*, and subsequent studies have inevitably been biased by the particular formulations that describe this syndrome.

It has long been recognized that symptoms such as amnesia, psychological numbing and depersonalization occur in response to a range of traumatic stressors (Lindemann, 1944; Grinker and Spiegel, 1945; Kardiner and Spiegel, 1947). Embedded in the literature are a series of studies about the impact of dissociative reactions on short- and long-term functioning. An early realization was that these would be evoked by events of the type described in the *DSM IV* stressor criterion, especially if reactions included intense fear, horror or helplessness, re-experiencing, avoidance and hyper-arousal.

For ethical and pragmatic reasons it is extremely difficult to conduct research in the immediate aftermath of traumatic events, but reports of acute reactions are available for a nightclub fire (Lindemann, 1944), automobile accidents (Noyes *et al.*, 1977; Barton *et al.*, 1996), the Buffalo Creek dam disaster (Titchener and Kapp, 1976), riots in penitentiaries (Hillman, 1981), a collapsed hotel (Wilkinson, 1983), combat (Feinstein, 1989), tornadoes (Madakasira and O'Brien, 1987;

North *et al.*, 1989), bushfires (Berah *et al.*, 1984) and aircraft accidents (Sloan, 1988). Reported dissociative symptoms range from disorganization and sluggishness in thinking and decision-making, seen in the dam disaster (Titchener and Kapp, 1976), to the constricted affect in combat soldiers (Feinstein, 1989). Shock and bewilderment was reported after the Ash Wednesday bush-fire disaster (Berah *et al.*, 1984).

De-realization is the perception that the external environment is unreal or dreamlike. Thirty to 53% of witnesses to executions or earthquakes report some such change. In contrast, depersonal-ization is a state where individuals have a sense of observing themselves as if from the outside and being detached from their own bodies. This phenomenon is reported in victim populations affected by an earthquake (Cardena and Spiegel, 1993), witnesses to an execution (Freinkel *et al.*, 1994) and tornado survivors (Madakasira and O'Brien, 1987). Other dissociative symptoms observed in the acute trauma phase include a general constriction of awareness of the environ-ment and a sense of numbing. However, in an interview study of 200 subjects on the first day after involvement in motor vehicle accidents dissociative symptoms were not common in distressed individuals (Atchison and McFarlane, 1997). Dissociation was, however, associated with severe pain and the use of nitrous oxide.

From a theoretical perspective dissociation in such settings is considered a primary coping mechanism for managing traumatic experiences. Janet (1911) and, more recently, van der Kolk *et al.* (1996) have emphasized the critical role of dissociation as a mechanism that minimizes the disruptive effects of traumatic events by decreasing the individual's awareness of what is and has been confronted. This modification of awareness is associated with a series of perceptual shifts, including memory impairment, emotional detachment, de-realization and depersonalization. As such dissociative reactions may impede the linking of cognitive reappraisals that occur in the aftermath of trauma with fear structures that are embedded within memory representations of trauma. As a consequence, there is a fragmentation of memory, as well as an over-generalization of trauma related schemas resulting in disruption of normal processes involved in accessing other associative networks.

The clinical significance of dissociative symptoms in the immediate aftermath of a traumatic event is based upon their apparent predictive ability in relation to subsequent PTSD. Some researchers have suggested dissociative responses are common and serve potentially adaptive ends (Horowitz, 1986, Barton *et al.*, 1996). Other studies indicate some maladaptive conse-quences arise from dissociative responses. For instance Holen (1993) studied survivors of a North Sea oilrig disaster and found that survivors who had a dissociative reaction in the immediate set-ting of the event were more likely to report chronic symptoms. In a series of longitudinal studies of Israeli combat soldiers Solomon *et al.* (1989) established that 20% of the variance of subse-quent PTSD could be predicted by the presence of numbing during the acute phase of their trauma. A similar observation was made by Foa *et al.* (1995) in a study of assault victims. Numbing at the time of the assault predicted those who subsequently went on to develop PTSD at 3 months. In these studies, numbing covered a range of emotional reactions including the blunting of feelings, detachment from others, loss of interest and a sense of foreshortened future. Many of these observations were made retrospectively several months after the event. Clearly, this presents a significant potential for bias because the later development of more chronic symp-toms may dominate the individual's awareness.

Re-experiencing phenomena

Whilst re-experiencing symptoms have been seen as the core of PTSD, the diagnosis of acute stress disorder also requires their presence. These symptoms cover a number of dimensions that include recurring images of the terror experienced in a range of sensory domains, nightmares, dreams and flashbacks. All are associated with a sense of reliving some aspect of the traumatic experience. Psychological distress and physiological arousal triggered by these persistent intrusive re-experiencing phenomena typically arise on exposure to reminders of the trauma that may be either real or symbolic. Rachman and de Silva (1981) have highlighted that some individuals do not experience these thoughts as necessarily being unpleasant. These intrusive memories can settle in individuals who are able to exert some influence on their associations. In turn, this may lead to extinction of the fear networks associated with some traumatic memories. Thus, in survivors who do not go on to develop PTSD the frequency of intrusive re-experiencing symptoms may progressively decrease. In contrast individuals who do develop PTSD find that fears and distress associated with these memories persist or intensify over time. This suggests that in these survivors the activation of trauma related schemas progressively increases the sense of threat, and does not promote a sense of mastery or homeostasis.

Bryant and Harvey (1997) highlighted how PTSD as a diagnosis does not require that the recurrence of the unwanted memories of the traumatic experiences be involuntary. What appears to be critical is the struggle that the individual has with these memory structures and the feelings they evoke. As Rivers (1918) highlighted in his treatment of World War I soldiers, attempts to manage thoughts and reactions are critical to long-term outcomes. Hence, if an individual is severely distressed in the immediate aftermath of an event this process of gradually developing a sense of mastery may be significantly disrupted. In this regard, feelings associated with the traumatic experience may play a critical role in determining whether the individual does or does not develop an acute stress disorder.

Avoidance phenomena

A number of studies have highlighted the existence of avoidance phenomena in the immediate aftermath of traumatic events (Cardena and Spiegel, 1993; North et al., 1989; Bryant and Harvey, 1996). However, these reactions can be very difficult to demonstrate or articulate in the early aftermath of such events. For example, an individual who remains in hospital after a motor vehicle accident will not be exposed to behavioural cues, such as driving, that may evoke phobic avoidance. This type of avoidance reaction is often linked to the way individuals manage thoughts and feelings about traumatic events. Horowitz (1986) highlighted the phasic nature of post-traumatic phenomena, and suggests this is driven by attempts to modulate and lessen distress. Cognitive models (Foa and Kozak, 1986; Litz and Keane, 1989; Creamer et al., 1992) point out that avoidance phenomena allow temporary relief, but if excessive can impede emotional processing. According to these cognitive models avoidance is a primary predictor of the risk of later developing PTSD.

Diagnostic criteria for ASD reflect the instability of avoidance symptoms since the threshold for a differential diagnosis is not set at three specified symptoms as for PTSD. All an individual has to demonstrate is marked avoidance that may take the form of psychogenic amnesia, emotional numbing and interpersonal withdrawal. The latter can be difficult to judge in the setting of serious injury and where there has been major interpersonal losses. This further complicates inter-rater reliability in observations of these phenomena.

Arousal symptoms

These include insomnia, problems with concentration and memory, irritability and exaggerated startle responses. Comparison of diagnostic criteria demonstrates the non-specific nature of these symptoms, since they occur in a range of other psychiatric disorders. Weisaeth (1989), in a study of a factory explosion, found persistence of arousal symptoms to be a particularly important predictor of PTSD. To define what is, and what is not an abnormal arousal response in the immediate aftermath of traumatic events is difficult since these reactions mediate adaptive changes in vigilance and modulate expression of emotion. Most survivors experience irritability and disruption of sleep patterns following traumatic exposure. Given these difficulties in defining normative reactions and that an ASD diagnosis requires marked arousal there are, in this respect too, difficulties of inter-rater reliability.

Associated symptoms

Crisis theory emphasizes the importance of disturbed emotional modulation, disrupted decision-making capacity and impaired capability to relate to others. Feelings of grief, terror and disgust may also play a critical role in influencing an individual's mental state in settings where deaths or horror have occurred. Depression and a profound sense of loss can also be disruptive to an individual's immediate psychological orientation. Very little observation about these issues has been undertaken in relation to the ASD diagnosis. Observations of reactions that are manifest during the first few days after an event are significantly biased by symptoms included in the *DSM IV* diagnostic criteria. This is to the exclusion of more flexible and open-ended observational frameworks. Furthermore, the progressive sequence of emotions and phenomena requires systematic observation. For example, does hyper-arousal precede dissociation or vice versa? Or are these relatively independent phenomena? To what extent is it possible to have very high levels of intrusive memories in the relative absence of anxiety and distress? Until these matters are resolved it is important they be approached with an open mind. Once completed such research will probably lead to substantial revisions of ASD criteria.

Conclusions

The definition of diagnostic criteria for ASD has allowed the development of more reliable and valid instruments to explore early reactions to trauma. In the main research has involved careful exploration of the relationship between acute symptoms and later onset of PTSD following a limited range of traumatic exposures, e.g. motor vehicle accidents. However, *DSM IV* diagnostic criteria have limited the observational set applied to the investigation of these phenomena. They do not reflect the fluid and polymorphic nature of acute stress reactions defined in ICD-10 and described in the research of Solomon *et al.* (1996). From a pragmatic perspective the definition of ASD is a critical issue in settings where the behavioural disturbance of the individual carries a major disadvantage. This is particularly the case during combat, where it is not clinicians who make initial diagnoses, but the soldiers' comrades and officers. Often this occurs in the face of continued exposure to the primary triggering stressor where, typically, there are marked fluctuations in mental state. The meaning of and consequences arising from behavioural disturbance in this setting are obvious and will contrast with that of soldiers removed from the front line. Hence, there is a great need to further clarify the nature of people's behaviour and symptoms during immediate and ongoing exposure, and establish their relationship to both acute and chronic post-traumatic stress disorder.

References

American Psychiatric Association (1952) *Diagnostic and Statistical Manual of Mental Disorders.* Washington DC: APA.

American Psychiatric Association (1968) *Diagnostic and Statistical Manual of Mental Disorders*, 2nd edn. Washington DC: APA.

American Psychiatric Association (1994) *Diagnostic and Statistical Manual of Mental Disorders*, 4th edn. Washington DC: APA.

Atchison, M. and McFarlane, A. (1997) Clinical patterns of acute psychological response to trauma. In *The Aftermath of Road Accidents, Psychological, Social and Legal Consequences of an Everyday Trauma*. London: Routledge, pp. 49–57.

Bailey, P. (1918) War neuroses, shell shock and nervousness in soldiers. *J Am Med Ass* **71**, 2148–53.

Barton, K.A., Blanchard, E.B. and Hickling, E.T. (1996) Antecedents and consequences of acute stress disorder among motor vehicle accident victims. *Behav Res Ther* **34**, 805–13.

Berah, E.F., Jones, H.J. and Valent, P. (1984) The experience of mental health team involved in the early phase of a disaster. *Aust NZ J Psychiat* **18**, 354–8.

Bryant, R.A. and Harvey, A.G. (1996) Initial post-traumatic stress responses following motor vehicle accidents. *J Traumatic Stress* **9**, 223–34.

Bryant, R.A. and Harvey, A.G. (1997) Acute stress disorder: a critical review of diagnostic issues. *Clin Psychol Rev* **17**, 757–73.

Cardena, E. and Spiegel, D. (1993) Dissociative reactions to the Bay Area earthquake. *Am J Psychiat* **150**, 474–8.

Charcot, J.M. and Richter, P. (1881) *Les demoniaques dans l'art*. Paris: Macula.

Chemtob, C. (1999) *Survival mode theory*, paper presented at the ASTSS Annual Conference. Brisbane 15–16 September, 1999.

Classen, C., Koopman, C., Hales, R., and Spiegel, D. (1998) Acute stress disorder as a predictor of posttraumatic stress symptoms. *Am J Psychiat* **155**, 620–4.

Creamer, M., Burgess, P. and Pattison, P. (1992) Reaction to trauma: a cognitive processing model. *J Abnormal Psychol* **101**, 452–9.

Feinstein, A. (1989) Posttraumatic stress disorder: a descriptive study supporting DSM-III-R criteria. *Am J Psychiat* **146**, 665–6.

Foa, E.B. and Kozak, M.J. (1986) Emotional processing of fear: exposure to corrective information. *Psycholog Bull* **99**, 20–35.

Foa, E.B, Riggs, D.S. and Gershuny, B. (1995) Arousal, numbing, and intrusion: symptom structure of posttraumatic stress disorder following assault. *Am J Psychiat* **152**: 116–20.

Freinkel, A., Koopman, C. and Spiegel, D. (1994) Dissociative symptoms in media execution witnesses. *Am J Psychiat* **151**, 1335–9.

Freud, S. (1933) In Strachey, J. (ed. and transl., 1955) *The Standard Edition of the Complete Psychological Works of Sigmund Freud*, Vol 7. London: Hogarth Press.

Freud, S. (1955) Beyond the pleasure principle. In Strachey, J. (ed. and transl., 1955) *The Standard Edition of the Complete Psychological Works of Sigmund Freud*, Vol. 18 pp. 3–64. London: Hogarth Press.

Glass, A.J. (1974) Mental health programs in the armed forces. In Arieti, S. (ed.) *American Handbook of Psychiatry*, 2nd edn. pp. 800–809. New York: Basic Books.

Grinker, R. (1945) The medical, psychiatric and social problems of war neuroses. *Cincinnati J Med* **26**, 241–59.

Grinker, R.R. and Spiegel, J.P. (1945) *Men Under Stress*. Philadelphia: Blakistan.

Hillman, R.G. (1981) The psychopathology of being held hostage. *Am J Psychiat* **138**, 1193–7.

Holen, A. (1993) The North Sea oil rig disaster. In Wilson, J.P. and Raphael, B. (eds) *International Handbook of Traumatic Stress Syndromes*, pp. 471–8. New York: Plenum Press.

Horowitz, M.J. (1986) *Stress Response Syndromes*, 2nd edn. New York: Plenum Press.

Janet, P. (1889) *L'automatisme psychologique: essai de psychologie expérimentale sur les formes inférieures de l'activité humaine*. Paris: Félix Alcan

Janet, P. (1911) *L'état mental des hystériques*, 2nd edn. Paris: Alcan.

Kardiner, A. (1959) Traumatic neuroses of war. In Wilson, J.P. and Raphael, B. (eds) *American Handbook of Psychiatry*, Vol. 1, pp. 245–257. New York: Basic Books.

Kardiner, A. and Spiegel, H. (1947) *War Stress and Neurotic Illness*. New York: Hoeber.

Leed, E.J. (1979) *No Man's Land*. London: Cambridge University Press.

Leri, A. (1919) *Shell-shock, Commotional and Emotional Aspects*. London: University of London Press.

Lindemann, E. (1944) Symptomatology and management of acute grief. *Am J Psychiat* **101**, 141–8.

Litz, B.T. and Keane, T.M. (1989) Information processing in anxiety disorders: application to the understanding of posttraumatic stress disorder. *Clin Psychol Rev* **9**, 243–57.

MacPather, E. (1922) Report of the War Office Committee of Enquiry into 'Shell-shock'. In Leed, E.J. (ed.) *No Man's Land: combat and identity in World War I*. London: Cambridge University Press, pp. 163–92.

Madakasira, S. and O'Brien, K. (1987) Acute posttraumatic stress disorder in victims of a natural disaster. *J Nerv Ment Dis* **175**, 286–90.

Marshall, S.L.A. (1947) *Men Against Fire*. New York: William Morrow and Company.

McFarlane, A.C. (1999) Risk factors for the acute biological and psychological response to trauma. In Yehuda, R. (ed.) *Risk Factors for Posttraumatic Stress Disorder*. Washington DC: American Psychiatric Press, pp. 163–90.

North, C.S., Smith, E.M., McCool, R.E. and Lightcap, P.E. (1989) Acute post-disaster coping and adjustment. *J Traumatic Stress*, **2**, 353–60.

Noyes, R., Hoenk, P.R., Kuperman, S. and Slymen, D.J. (1977) Depersonalisation in accident victims and psychiatric patients. *J Nerv Ment Dis* **164**, 401–7.

Panksepp, J. (1998) *Affective Neuroscience: the foundations of human and animal emotions*. New York: Oxford University Press.

Rachman, S.J. and de Silva, P. (1981) Abnormal and normal obsessions. *Behav Res Ther* **16**, 101–10.

Rivers, W.H.R. (1918) The repression of war experience. *Lancet* Feb. 2.

Sloan, P. (1988) Post-traumatic stress in survivors of an airplane crash landing: a clinical and exploratory research intervention. *J Traumatic Stress*, **1**, 211–529.

Solomon, Z., Laror, N. and McFarlane, A.C. (1996) Acute posttraumatic reactions in soldiers and civilians. In van der Kolk, B.A., McFarlane, A.C. and Weisaeth, L. (eds) *Traumatic Stress: the overwhelming experience on mind, body, and society*. New York: Guilford Press, pp. 102–14.

Solomon, Z., Mikulincer, M. and Benbenistry, R. (1989) Combat stress reactions: clinical manifestations and correlates. *Military Psychol* **1**, 35–47.

Titchener, J.L. and Kapp, F.T. (1976) Family and character change at Buffalo Creek. *Am J Psychiat* **133**, 295–9.

van der Kolk, B.A., McFarlane, A.C. and Weisaeth, L. (1996) *Traumatic Stress: the overwhelming experience on mind, body, and society*. New York: Guilford Press.

Weisaeth, L. (1989) The stressors and the posttraumatic stress syndrome after an industrial accident. *Acta Psychiat Scand* **89** (Suppl. 355), 25–37.

Wilkinson, C.B. (1983) Aftermath of a disaster: the collapse of the Hyatt Regency Hotel skywalks. *Am J Psychiat* **140**, 1134–9.

World Health Organization (1993) *The ICD-10 Classification of Mental and Behavioural Disorders: diagnostic criteria for research*. Geneva: World Health Organization.

Yealland, L. (1918) Hysterical disorders of speech. In Yealland, L. (ed.) *Hysterical Disorders of Warfare*. pp. 1–30. London: Macmillan.

Yehuda, R. and McFarlane, A.C. (1995) Conflict about current knowledge about PTSD and its original conceptual basis. *Am J Psychiat* **152**, 1705–13.

5 Psychobiological perspectives on early reactions to traumatic events

Arieh Y. Shalev

Introduction

The neurobiology of human responses to extreme events involves mechanisms related to bodily survival, learned conditioning, autobiographical memory-formation and complex, socially modulated, adaptation to change. The breadth of the topic is revealed by examining the time frames of some of the typical responses. These extend from fragments of seconds (for defence reflexes, such as auditory startle), several seconds (for sympathetic activation), tens of minutes (for activation of the hypothalamic-pituitary-adrenal axis), hours (for early gene expression), days (for memory consolidation) and months (for permanent changes in the central nervous system; Post, 1992).

Furthermore, at each stage the biological responses to mental stressors are heavily modulated by appraisal (e.g. of perceived threat and available resources; Lazarus & Folkman, 1984), controllability, attribution of meaning, and by the relative success in coping with tasks related to survival and learning (see Shalev and Ursano, Chapter 11 of this book). Prior experiences, individual and group beliefs are also powerful modulators of the psychological and therefore the biological responses to adversities.

The inherent complexity of the resulting 'neurobiology' defies any systematic description. Yet, given the frequent occurrence of post-traumatic stress disorders in the aftermath of traumatic events it is important to outline what might go wrong. It is also important to challenge some simplistic views, according to which the neurobiology of mental trauma is mainly that of stress responses.

This chapter outlines several ways in which psychological reactions to traumatic are transduced into permanent alterations of the central nervous system (CNS). It posits a dual process in which the very early 'stress' responses trigger a cascade of potentially adaptive mechanisms, and secondary biological responses, mostly related to learning and strongly influenced by the environment determine the long-term outcome of the traumatic experience.

The many facets of human responses to traumatic events

Danger, threat, violent death and other major stressors have been the lot of the human species for millennia. Their salience, however, may never have been as pronounced as nowadays, when softer, more protected ways of living are shared by large human communities. The biological responses to extreme stress may, therefore, erroneously be perceived as 'exceptional' insofar as they engage mechanisms that are not evoked as regularly in our daily lives as they might have been in the more distant past. These responses, however, are fundamental attributes of every living organism, and therefore are 'hard-wired' in animal brains and bodies. Moreover, the smooth and efficient activation of the immediate responses to stress has truly assured the 'successful' survival of the human species. In this sense, it is very unlikely that the biology of the immediate response to stressful events would become the major cause of trouble.

Yet, in order to assure its long-term survival the human species developed another major adaptive mechanism namely that of learning from experience. Humans build mountains of newly-learned behaviour on top of rather limited repertoire of biogenetically predetermined templates. Our extensive capacity to learn from experience and the underlying amount of brain plasticity make us extremely sensitive to the environment and this can have major health related, including pathogenic effects. Most adverse mental health consequences of traumatic events might, therefore, result from our immense ability to learn, remember and re-shape our behaviour (and the underlying CNS functioning) on the base of new—including catastrophic experiences.

Additional biological dimensions related to disasters are our being social, familial and territorial beings. These core attributes of mankind make us reactive to harm done to others, vulnerable to the effect of loss and separation, affected by displacement and relocation. Such sources of vulnerability can amplify the direct effect of traumatic events, and add a distressful period of grief and re-adaptation to the horrors of the immediate exposure.

A current reductionism in psychiatry equates the term 'biological' with the body and the term 'survival' with the individual. Animal and human biology, however, encompasses higher mental functions such as communication language and appraisal. Survival (Segal and Macdonald, 1998) similarly exceeds the individual and extends to families, generations, tribes or other natural or psychologically defined groups (e.g. nations, military units, etc ...). Moreover, behaviour designed to assure the survival of the group (e.g. rescue, protection of one's children) may conflict with individual safety, leading to risk-taking behaviour, to denying aversive emotions and to overcoming avoidance. Such conflicting motivations can generate excessive distress and, thereby, also powerful bodily responses.

Human beings are also hungry for meaning, and require cognitive congruence in order to function smoothly and peacefully. Consequently, a cycle of bodily 'alarm' responses may be triggered and maintained by such abstract psychological factors as learning about a disaster, not having a clear plan of action, or being unable to convey coherent meaning to situations and experiences. This top-down effect, in which elaborate cognitive and linguistic functions activate the hard-wired mid-brain stress machinery, is a powerful modulator of bodily responses to stress. For example, the meaning conveyed to one's action (e.g. cowardice, heroism), as well as the meaningfulness of a group effort (e.g. unnecessary war) can either soothe and down-regulate fear responses, or maintain and reinforce them (Holloway and Ursano, 1984).

Finally, stressful events often include adverse physiological conditions, such as heat, hypothermia, pain, bleeding, starvation or dehydration. These add their direct bodily effects to the balance of psychological perturbations. Being wounded in combat, for example, adds to the likelihood of developing post-traumatic stress disorder (PTSD; Pitman et al., 1989).

The biology of the response to traumatic events, therefore, is very complex. It involves biological defences against excessive demands (the famous General Adaptation Response; Selye, 1956), mechanisms related to learning and adaptation, responses to social cues, reactions to loss and separation, and the effect of cognitive disarray and chaotic experiences.

For didactic purpose, we divide the biological responses into a relatively simple and safe response, related to actually surviving a threat, and a rather risky and prolonged one, related to 'post-processing' and learning from experience. The latter encompasses all the ways by which we elaborate, integrate and eventually turn off the powerful survival-related 'stress' machinery.

As will be shown below, failure to turn off that machinery, or to put it back into its proper temporal and spatial context, may lead to major mental and bodily disequilibrium. Specifically, it might lead to permanently responding to remote reminders of any threat by excessive alarm.

This chapter addresses the biological responses that might lead to mental disorders. Among those, the following are addressed:

- survival-related, immediate stress response;
- learning mechanisms engaged by stress responses;
- the neglected biology of loss, separation and grief;
- post-event habituation or sensitization.

The biology of stress responses

Extreme environmental demands immediately engage the body stress responses through activation of corticotropin releasing factor (CRF) at the hypothalamus and sympathetic 'alarm' activation involving the locus-ceruleus norepinephrine system (Chrousos and Gold, 1992). The former leads to secretion of adrenocorticotropin hormone (ACTH) from the pituitary gland and, subsequently, to secretion of cortisol from the adrenals into the blood stream. The latter leads to a surge of peripheral catecholamines and activation/deactivation of body organs, according to their relevance to defending the organism (e.g. digestion may be deactivated, whereas blood transport to the muscles is activated). Other responses include an activation of brain areas related to perceiving and responding to the environment. Other players in the immediate response include nuclei controlling facial expression, breathing rhythm, startle response and parasympathetic modulation of heart rate. This cluster of responses is controlled by the central nucleus of the amygdala—a powerful modulator of fear responses (Davis, 1994; LeDoux, 1995).

The hormonal stress response has a typical temporal course, and typical effects on behaviour, cognition and emotion. It follows the three phases described by Selye: alarm, resistance, and either return to equilibrium or exhaustion. The entire sequence, however, is rather short, such that in many traumatic events individuals quickly reach a state of depletion or exhaustion.

Behaviour under acute stress is likely to become sharp and goal directed. Yet, in the absence of clear goals (e.g. clear enemy to fight, obvious ways to escape from danger) behaviour may become ineffective or disorganized. *Cognition* equally becomes goal-directed and focused, yet distressed individuals also experience difficulties to shift goals, scan alternatives and change a plan of action. Persistence of ineffective action, loss of resourcefulness and increasing anxiety may create a mental situation of '*crisis*'. In such a situation, individuals are caught in a vicious cycle of ineffective coping, inability to disengage from so doing, failure to shift their attention, change a course of action and use other available resources, and increasing distress. *Crisis intervention*, at the early aftermath of traumatic events, can be construed as a systematic attempt to break the bio-psychological cycle of distressed cognition emotion and behaviour.

Excessive distress has the potential of disrupting cognition and action to the point of creating chaotic behaviour (and experiences). Importantly, under conditions of extreme stress attention may also be over-focused and incomplete. The 'gun barrel' memory, in which a victim clearly remembers the barrel of a gun pointed toward his or her, but does not recall the assailant's face, is an example of focused and incomplete attention. Dissociative experiences during stressful events (Shalev *et al.*, 1996; see also other chapters of the book) may also represent an extreme form of such altered cognition.

The two main stress hormones, cortisol and epinephrine have somewhat complementary roles in the acute response to stress. Adrenergic (or sympathetic) activation sustains the above-mentioned alarm response, while circulating cortisol, first, subserves this response by shutting off unnecessary bodily activities (e.g. immune response) and, secondarily, terminates the adrenergic response through negative feed back mechanism (Yehuda, 1998). Circulating cortisol, in fact, goes back to the hypothalamus and the pituitary and shuts off the secretion of its own modulators (CRH and ACTH), as well as that of the adrenergic response. Because of such property of cortisol, it has recently been theorized that a failure to mount appropriate levels of cortisol during traumatic events may lead to prolonged adrenergic activation and, thereby, increase the risk of developing post-traumatic stress disorders (Yehuda, 1998). Abnormally low cortisol levels following trauma were, in fact, reported in vulnerable rape victims and in road accident survivors who were at higher risk for developing PTSD (Resnick et al., 1995; McFarlane et al., 1997), but the causal link with PTSD has not been established. A combination of adrenergic activation and low levels of cortisol had been shown to significantly increase emotional learning in animals (Bohus, 1984; Munck et al., 1984). Importantly, the hormonal stress response seems to 'go wrong' in individuals whose prior life experience had been particularly stressful (Resnick et al., 1995)—yet this also requires further confirmation. The intensity of bio-psychological responses to traumatic events increases in circumstances that are uncontrollable and inescapable (Seligman and Meier, 1967; Anisman et al., 1981; Breier, 1989).

The biology of learning and adaptation

Immediate alarm responses are followed, in the brain, by a cascade of metabolic and genomic (i.e., expression of new genes) events (Post, 1992). Importantly, the cascade of neuronal changes includes areas of the brain that are not directly involved in stress response. Particularly interesting is the activation of protein synthesis in brain areas related to learning and memory, such as the hippocampus and the amygdala (Davis, 1994). Newly-synthesized proteins in these areas constitute the biological basis of long-term memories of stressful events.

The distribution of these biological changes, in the brain, suggests that there are two types of memory traces of stressful events: explicit memories (i.e. verbal and retrievable) and implicit memories (e.g. changes in habits, conditioned responses). This is very important, because non-verbal, implicit memories of traumatic events may shape future behaviour in the absence of conscious elaboration and verbal recall (e.g. by causing bodily alarm and emotional fear responses upon exposure to reminders of the traumatic event). Experimental work in animals (LeDoux et al., 1989) has shown that a subtype of emotional memories, based on 'quick and dirty' processing of sensory information, is acquired, and stored in the lateral and basal nuclei of the amygdala. LeDoux has also shown that such 'emotional' learning (indeed, fear conditioning) is relatively immune to change. Memory traces stored in the basal and lateral nuclei of the amygdala are subsequently used to interpret new sensory signals as to their aversive nature, such that when a stimulus is interpreted as immediately threatening, the central nucleus of the amygdala is activated (see above) and fear response is put in motion.

Despite the persistence of emotional learning, the behavioural expression of fear conditioning can be inhibited by the activity of cortical areas of the brain (Morgan et al., 1993). This is, in fact, what happens when aversive or conditioned responses subside: the information is not forgotten or erased, but rather put under inhibitory control. Brain areas involved in such inhibitory control include sensory association areas, areas in the frontal lobe and the hippocampus. Memories of traumatic events, therefore, are not suppressed, but rather controlled and neglected, such that they have no behavioural expression. Subsequent trauma may activate such memories, yet the strategy of controlling the effect of aversive learning may also be stronger in individuals who recover from traumatic events. Exposure to stressful events, therefore, may either 'sensitize' or 'immunize' survivors (Solomon et al., 1987).

Further experimental work has shown that aversive memories, at the level of the amygdala, can be reinforced by elevated plasma levels of the stress hormone epinephrine (McGaugh, 1985; Cahill and McGaugh, 1998). An initial hyper-secretion of the stress hormone epinephrine could be involved in an exaggeration and a consolidation of fear-related memories of the traumatic event (Cahill *et al.*, 1994; McGaugh *et al.*, 1990). Moreover, the intensity of the adrenergic 'stress' response can also foster emotional (and amygdala-mediated) learning at the expense of rational or declarative, hippocampus-mediated learning (Metcalfe and Jacobs, 1996). Supportive evidence for the link between an initial autonomic activation and subsequent post-traumatic stress disorder has been found in a recent study (Shalev *et al.*, 1998). In this study, heart rate levels upon admission to an emergency room following traumatic events were higher in subjects who subsequently developed PTSD.

What clinicians may wish to keep in mind from the above is the powerful and circular interaction between psychological and physiological components of the response to traumatic events. Perceived threat triggers intense bodily reactions that, in their turn, shape the subjective quality of mental traces of the aversive event (both implicit and explicit). The subjective quality of these memory traces will then be used to interpret subsequent adversity. This cycle of bio-psychological events can be self-limited and decay with time. Yet, additional adversity, such as often seen in the aftermath of major disaster, can create a chain of mutually reinforcing reactions, the memory of which may be etched forever in a person's brain. Efforts to reduce the stressfulness of events (e.g. by providing shelter, information, orientation, warmth and hope) have an essential role in mitigating this bio-psychological cascade. The social setting and human interaction of early intervention may also achieve such mitigation (for extended discussion, see Shalev and Ursano, Chapter 11 in this book).

The neglected biology of loss, separation and grief

Adversities often continue beyond the impact phase of disasters (e.g. a hurricane stops, but damage and destruction persist). Importantly, a phase of re-appraisal starts, at the aftermath of exposure, during which the physical and psychological consequences of the event are being re-evaluated in the light of the person's entire life experience and his or her future perspectives hopes and aspiration (Lazarus and Folkman, 1984). The optimal outcome of this phase is to achieve optimal integration of newly-learned information, as well as adaptation to loss and to having experienced a disastrous event. Such adaptation is seldom achieved without mental pain, best construed as a process of grief (Lindemann, 1944).

The biological features of grief and bereavement in adults are not well researched (Biondi and Picardi, 1996). In contrast, the effect of separation in infants has received extensive attention. Seminal animal studies (Levine *et al.*, 1997, for a review) show that early maternal separation is followed by life-long hormonal disturbances. Handling of recently born rodent pups by humans, for example, creates an alteration of the reactivity of the hypothalamic-pituitary-adrenal axis (HPA axis), which persists through adulthood (Meaney *et al.*, 1991). This effect is somewhat reversible, if mothers are allowed to give excessive bodily attention (licking) to the pups immediately following separation. Early parental loss in humans has similarly been shown to increase both the likelihood of adult depression (Agid *et al.*, 2000) and the intensity of depressive symptoms in healthy adolescents (Canetti *et al.*, 2000).

While one may argue that such long-lasting effects of separation may only occur during periods of excessive brain plasticity such as during infancy, recent work suggests that brain plasticity increases under stress in adults as well (Adamec, 1997; Kim *et al.*, 1996). Theoretically, therefore, separation during the catastrophic events may have a long-term neuroendocrine effect, analogous to that seen in earlier stages of brain development. This effect may be independent from that related to threat and aversive conditioning.

The behavioural response to unexpected and uncontrollable loss includes distressing longing for the lost object, and repeated attempts to retrieve its concrete or symbolic remnants. It also includes depressed mood and loss of interest in daily activities. Symptoms of traumatic loss in healthy adults (Lindemann, 1944) are very similar to those observed in PTSD. This also suggests that loss might be essential for PTSD to develop. Furthermore, the phenomenon of painful ruminations, which is common to PTSD, depression and normal grief mentally re-exposes survivors to aversive experiences. To the extent that such repeated mental exposure are intense or uncontrollable (Shalev *et al.*, 1993; Ehlers *et al.*, 1998), they may become a secondary source of trauma and reinforce the initial effect of the traumatic event. Depressive symptoms, in recent trauma survivors, increase the likelihood of subsequent PTSD (Freedman *et al.*, 1999). Interestingly, the effects of uncontrollable stress and concurrent depression on the HPA axis are additive (Breier, 1989). The biological model proposed here posits, therefore, that the threat of a traumatic event triggers a normal 'survival' response, which, when augmented by subsequent depression, disarray or loss becomes interminable and self-sustaining, and ends by permanently modifying the CNS. In line with this model a recent meta-analysis of risk factors for PTSD has shown that adversity during the trauma and adversity after the traumatic event are the major determinants of subsequent PTSD (Brewin *et al.*, 2000).

The role of habituation and sensitization following exposure

The above discussion of the complementary roles of initial stress responses and subsequent depression and loss suggests that some of the pathogenic effects of traumatic events occur during the phase of recovery and adaptation. Accordingly, the likelihood of developing prolonged stress disorders is significantly affected by factors that follow the initial exposure. Two types of factors can be isolated:

- the occurrence of concrete 'secondary' stressors (e.g., = physical pain, physiological deprivation, relocation, etc. ....);
- departure of the bio-psychological reparative processes from their normal and essentially protective course.

Instead of 'progressive reparation', PTSD may be the consequence of 'progressive temporal sensitization' (Antelman, 1988; Yehuda and Antelman, 1993).

A recent study of physiological responses to startle exemplifies such progressive sensitization (Shalev *et al.*, 2000). The abnormal startle response, which is typically observed in patients with chronic PTSD is not found in recent trauma survivors but becomes manifest only after some four months following exposure to a traumatic event. At an earlier stage (i.e. 1 week and 1 month following exposure) individuals who later develop PTSD have a normal responses to startling tones and do not differ from survivors who will not develop PTSD. Once the disorder has developed, the abnormal startle response of PTSD persists and constitutes part of the clinical picture of PTSD—as well as one the disorders biological markers. This finding points to the great importance of the quality of recovery environment during the stages that follow the impact phase of traumatic events in re-shaping the neurobiology of traumatized survivors.

Synthesis

This review points to a dual pathogenic mechanism in trauma survivors. First, the immediate response to a traumatic event acts as a necessary, but not sufficient trigger for a cascade of psycho-biological changes. In and of itself, this 'triggering' effect cannot cause prolonged bio-psychological disorders. At a second stage, learning and adaptation responses can lead to either resolution and positive learning, or prolonged and redundant expressions of distress. The latter may, within few weeks, sensitize the CNS, and change its basic routines of stimulus discrimination and responses, to the point of creating irreversible changes.

The social mediators of the recovery from traumatic exposure are extremely important. The human group conveys meaning to the event and to subsequent grief. Human presence is necessary to soothe trauma survivors and such soothing may have profound biological effects. The early aftermath of traumatic events, therefore, is a critical period both in the medical and the biological sense. It is a period of enhanced neuronal plasticity, during which psychological factors are inseparable from bodily 'physiological' ones, and the two concur to either 'kindle' chronic stress disorders or foster a sense of meaningfulness, adaptation and resilience. Herein lies the true challenge of early interventions after trauma.

Acknowledgements

This work was supported by a PHS research grant NH-50379.

References

Adamec, R. (1997) Transmitter systems involved in neural plasticity underlying increased anxiety and defense-implications for understanding anxiety following traumatic stress. *Neurosci Behav Rev* **21**, 755–65.

Agid, O., Shapira, B., Zislin, J., Ritzner, M., Hnin, B., Murad, H., Troudart, T., Bloch, M., Heresco-Lecy, U., Lerer, B. (2000) Environment and vulnerability to major psychiatric illness: a case control study of early parental loss and schizophrenia. *Mol Psychiat* **4**, 163–72.

Anisman, H., Ritch, M. and Sklar, L.S. (1981) Noradrenergic and dopaminergic interactions in escape behaviour: analysis of uncontrollable stress effects. *Psychopharmacol* **74**, 263–8.

Antelman, S.M. (1988) Time-dependent sensitization as the cornerstone for a new approach to pharmacotherapy: drugs as foreign/stressful stimuli. *Drug Devel Res* **14**, 1–30.

Biondi, M. and Picardi, A. (1996) Clinical and biological aspects of bereavement and loss-induced depression: a reappraisal. *Psychother Psychosomat* **65**, 229–45.

Bohus, B. (1984) Humoral modulation of learning and memory processes: physiological significance of brain and peripheral mechanisms. In Delacour, A. (ed.) *The Memory System of the Brain*. Singapore: World Scientific, pp. 337–64.

Breier, A. (1989) Experimental approaches to human stress research: assessment of neurobiological mechanisms of stress in volunteers and psychiatric patients. *Biolog Psychiat* **26**, 438–62.

Brewin, C.R., Andrews, B. and Valentine, J.D. (2000) Meta analysis of risk factors for posttraumatic stress disorder. *J Consult Clin Psychol* **68**, 748–66.

Cahill, L. and McGaugh, J.L. (1998) Mechanisms of emotional arousal and lasting declarative memory. *Trends Neurosci* **21**, 294–9.

Cahill, L., Prins, B., Weber, M. and McGaugh, J.L. (1994) Beta adrenergic activaion and memory for emotional events. *Nature* **371**, 702–4.

Canetti, L., Bachar, E., Bonne, O., Agid, O., Lerer, B., Kaplan, De-Nour, A. and Shalev, A.Y. (2000) The impact of parental death versus separation from parents in the mental health of Israeli adolescents. *Comprehensive Psychiatry* **41**, 360–68.

Chrousos, G.P. and Gold, P.W. (1992) The concepts of stress and stress system disorders: overview of physical and behavioural homeostasis. *J Am Med Ass* **267**, 1244–52.

Davis, M. (1994) The role of the amygdala in emotional learning. *Int Rev Neurobiol* **36**, 225–66.

Ehlers, A., Mayou, R.A., Bryant, R.F. (1998) Psychological predictors of chronic posttraumatic stress disorder after motor vehicle accidents. *J Abnorm Psychol* **107**, 508–19.

Freedman, S.A., Peri, T., Brandes, D. and Shalev, A.Y. (1999) Predictors of chronic PTSD—a prospective study. *Br J Psychiat* **174**, 353–9.

Holloway, H.C. and Ursano, R.J. (1984) The Vietnam veteran: memory, social context and metaphor. *Psychiatry* **47**, 103–8.

Kim, J.J., Foy, M.R. and Thompson, R.F. (1996) Behavioural stress modifies hippocampal plasticity through N-methyl-D-aspartate receptor activation. *Proc Nat Acad Sci* **93**, 4750–3.

Lazarus, R.S. and Folkman, S. (1984) *Stress, Appraisal and Coping. Chapter 2: cognitive appraisal processes.* New York: Springer.

LeDoux, J.E. (1995) Setting stress into motion: brain mechanisms of stimulus evaluation. In Friedman, J.M., Charney, D.S. and Deutch, A.Y. (eds) *Neurobiological and Clinical Consequences of Stress.* Philadelphia: Lippincott-Raven, pp. 125–134.

LeDoux, J.E., Romanski, L. and Xagoraris, A. (1989) Indelibility of subcortical emotional networks. *J Cognit Neurosci* **1**, 238–43.

Levine, S., Lyons, D.M. and Schatzberg, A.F. (1997) Psychobiological consequences of social relationships. *Annl NY Acad Sci* **807**, 210–18.

Lindemann, E. (1944) Symptomatology and management of acute grief. *Am J Psychiat* **101**, 141–8.

McFarlane, A.C., Atchison, M. and Yehuda, R. (1997) The acute stress response following motor vehicle accidents and its relations to PTSD. *Annl NY Acad Sci* **821**, 437–41.

McGaugh, J.L. (1985) Peripheral and central adrenergic influences on brain systems involved in the modulation of memory storage. *Annl NY Acad Sci* **444**, 150–61.

McGaugh, J.L., Introini-Collison, I.B., Nagahara, A.H., Cahil, L., Brioni, J.D. and Cartellano, C. (1990) Involvement of the amygdaloid complex in neuromodulatory influences on memory storage. *Neurosci Biobehav Rev* **14**, 425–31.

Meaney, M.J., Mitchell, J.B., Aitken, D.H., Bhatnagar, S., Boduoll, S.R., Iny, J.L. and Sarrieah, A. (1991) The effects of neonatal handling on the development of the adrenocortical response to stress: implications for neuropathology and cognitive deficits in later life. *Psychoneuroendocrinol* **16**, 85–103.

Metcalfe, J. and Jacobs, W.J. (1996) A 'hot-system/cool-system' view of memory under stress. *PTSD Res Q* **7**, 1–3.

Morgan, M.A., Romanski, L.M. and LeDoux, J.E. (1993) Extinction of emotional learning: contribution of medial prefrontal cortex. *Neurosci Lett* **163**, 109–13.

Munck, A., Guyere, P.M. and Holbrock, M.J. (1984) Physiological functions of glucocorticoids in stress and their relations to pharmacological actions. *Endocrinol Rev* **93**, 9783–99.

Pitman, R.K., Altman, B. and Macklin, M.L. (1989) Prevalence of posttraumatic stress disorder in wounded Vietnam veterans. *Am J Psychiat* **146**, 667–9.

Post, R.M. (1992) Transduction of psychosocial stress into the neurobiology of recurrent affective disorder. *Am J Psychiat* **149**, 999–1010.

Resnick, H.S., Yehuda, R., Pitman, R.K. and Foy, D.W. (1995) Effect of previous trauma on acute plasma cortisol level following rape. *Am J Psychiat* **152**, 1675–7.

Segal, N.L. and MacDonald, K.B. (1998) Behavioural genetics and evolutionary psychology: unified perspective on personality research. *Hum Biol* **2**, 159–84.

Seligman, M.E.P. and Meier, S.F. (1967) Failure to escape traumatic shock. *J Exp Psychol* **74**, 1–9.

Selye, H. (1956) *The Stress of Life.* New York. McGraw-Hill.

Shalev, A.Y., Peri, T., Canneti, L. and Schreiber, S. (1996) Predictors of PTSD in recent trauma survivors: a prospective study. *Am J Psychiat* **153**, 219–25.

Shalev, A.Y., Peri, T., Brandes, D., Freeman, S., Orr, S.P. and Pitman, R.K. (2000) Auditory startle in trauma survivors with PTSD: a prospective study. *Am J Psychiat.*

Shalev, A.Y., Sahar, T., Freedman, S., Peri, T., Glick, N., Brandes, D., Orr, S.P. and Pitman, R.K. (1998) A prospective study of heart rate responses following trauma and the subsequent development of posttraumatic stress disorder. *Arch Gen Psychiat* **55**, 553–9.

Shalev, A.Y., Schreiber, S. and Galai, T. (1993) Early psychiatric responses to traumatic injury. *J Traumatic Stress* **6**, 441–50.

Solomon, Z., Garb, R., Bleich, A. and Grupper, D. (1987) Reactivation of combat related posttraumatic stress disorder. *Am J Psychiat* **144**, 51–5.

Yehuda, R. and Antelman, S.M. (1993) Criteria for rationally evaluating animal models of posttraumatic stress disorder. *Biolog Psychiat* **33**, 479–86.

Yehuda, R., McFarlane, A.C. and Shalev, A.Y. (1998) Predicting the development of post-traumatic stress disorder from the acute response to a traumatic event. *Biolog Psychiat* **44**, 1305–13.

6 Learning theory perspectives on early reactions to traumatic events

Sean Perrin

Introduction

The term 'learning theory' as used in this chapter refers to classical and operant conditioning theories. Both approaches view reinforcement as the central process by which the environment acts upon the organism to produce complex behaviour patterns (Donahoe, 1998). The differences between the two theories are evident in the procedures used to demonstrate learning. In the classical conditioning procedure (Pavlov, 1927) a reflex-eliciting stimulus (e.g. food) is presented to the animal following an environmental event (e.g. a tone). In the operant procedure (Thorndike, 1911), the eliciting stimulus is presented following a particular behaviour (e.g. pressing a lever). In both cases, the eliciting stimulus acts as a reinforcer because it changes the way the environment guides behaviour. For instance, in the presence of the tone the animal salivates (a reflex), in the presence of the lever the rat presses it (an instrumental response; Donahoe, 1998). Modern learning theorists recognize that the natural environment often provides both types of contingencies simultaneously (Donahoe, 1998). This is certainly the case with traumatic events that involve presentations of aversive stimuli.

Over the last 100 years the effects of aversive stimuli on animals have been studied using both classical and operant procedures. In the classical approach, animals are delivered an electric shock following some environmental stimulus (e.g. a tone). Subsequent presentation of the stimulus produces arousal, analgesia to pain, orientation or startle responses, and the so-called 'fight-or-flight' response. In the operant approach shock is delivered dependent upon a particular behaviour of the organism. If the behaviour terminates or delays the shock it increases in frequency over time (i.e. active avoidance). If the behaviour is followed by the shock it decreases in frequency (i.e. conditioned suppression).

The remainder of this chapter concentrates on classical conditioning theories of fear and Post-traumatic Stress Disorder (PTSD). Operant principles are discussed, but no purely operant view of traumatization has been put forward so far. The learning theory principles discussed hear apply equally well to Acute Stress Disorder (ASD). ASD differs from PTSD largely in terms of the duration of symptoms. Finally, the implications for early treatment that derive from learning theory are discussed.

Mowrer's two-factor theory of fear

The early learning theorists had little use for emotion in their models. Pavlov thought they were overly 'mentalistic', while Skinner (1938) considered feelings imprecise and 'fictional' as causes of behaviour. By contrast, O. H. Mowrer was a conditioning theorist who found such views, and the strict adherence of the early theorists to one learning paradigm or the other to be overly restrictive. In his view, learning involved both classical and operant principles, i.e. a two-factor theory (Mowrer, 1947, 1960). Moreover, he believed that "it is by means of emotions that we internalize or 'treasure up' … a knowledge of the external world …" (Mowrer, 1960).

In the first factor of his theory, Mowrer (1960) argued that classical conditioning trials bring about two categories of conditioned reflexes or responses (CRs): those involving the smooth muscles and glands (e.g. salivation) and emotions (e.g. fear). To illustrate, a rat is placed in a white compartment (the context), where it hears a tone (the neutral stimulus) and is then shocked (the unconditioned stimulus—US). After several trials the rat learns to fear the tone (now the conditioned stimulus—CS) and the white compartment. In Mowrer's view fear helps the rat anticipate and respond to the potential US (the shock), which was signalled by the CS (the tone) and the compartment (the context).

In the second factor of his theory, Mowrer argued that escape behaviours, and generally all behaviours involving the musculo-skeletal system, are far too complex to be reflexes. Like Thorndike, he saw escape behaviour as instrumental. During repeated trials with the both the CS (the tone) and US (the shock) together in the compartment, the tone produces and emotional response (fear) that guides the animal's behaviour (escape). Behaviour that led to a reduction in fear and escape from the shock were negatively reinforced. In subsequent trials, the CS was presented alone, but the rat continued to engage in escape behaviour. This is due to the fact that the escape behaviour prevented the rat from learning that the CS (tone) did not always lead to the US (shock; Mowrer, 1960).

The importance of Mowrer's two-factor theory to our understanding of emotion learning, phobias and PTSD cannot be understated. He introduced into learning theory the concept of fear as an organizing principle for animal and human behaviour. This approach was to have a tremendous impact on later accounts of Pavlovian fear conditioning and avoidance learning (Rescorla and Solomon, 1967; Levis and Hare, 1977). Nevertheless, two-factor and classical conditioning theories of fear have been the subject of much criticism (Ayres, 1998). However, many of the criticisms made are no longer applicable given modern perspectives on processes involved in Pavlovian conditioning (Rescorla, 1988) or the increased complexity of conditioning paradigms now used (McAllister and McAllister, 1995; Ayres, 1998; Kehoe and Macrae, 1998). Indeed, there is considerable evidence in the animal literature that fear can be independently measured, reliably elicited, and shown to both motivate and reinforce avoidance behaviour (Ayres, 1998). Fear and anxiety are central to our understanding of Acute Stress Disorder (ASD) and PTSD.

Learning theory perspectives on early reactions to traumatic events

As defined under the DSM-IV criteria for PTSD and ASD [American Psychiatric Association (APA), 1994] a traumatic event is one where: 'The person … [was] … confronted with an event or events, that involve actual or threatened death or serious injury, or a threat to the physical integrity of oneself or others … [and] involved intense fear, helplessness, or horror'. Both conditions are characterized by persistent re-experiencing of the event, avoidance of stimuli associated with the trauma and numbing of general responsiveness, and persistent symptoms of arousal (APA, 1994). This stated it must be recognized ASD and PTSD are not the only outcomes of traumatic events, but PTSD-like symptoms are common among a high proportion of survivors. All the same, the diagnoses provide a useful framework for viewing early reactions to traumatic events. In the following sections each of the three symptom clusters listed above will be discussed from a conditioning perspective.

Persistent symptoms of increased arousal

Keane *et al.* (1985) invoke the conditioning principles described by Pavlov and Mowrer to explain persistent symptoms of increased arousal following trauma. Stimuli present during the trauma become conditioned to elicit startle, arousal and fear. Fear, in this case, is an emotional construct that might also be denoted as vigilance. It is important to note that in the animal literature the appearance of 'freezing' following an aversive US (e.g. a shock) is seen to be a defence against predatory attack and a state of 'vigilance' (Fanselow and Lester, 1988). In addition to the direct conditioning of previously neutral stimuli during the traumatic incident, other neutral stimuli, which closely resemble the trauma-related CSs, may come to elicit fear, arousal and startle in the aftermath of the event (via stimulus generalization; Keane *et al.*, 1985). Likewise, neutral stimuli that have been paired with trauma-related CSs *after* the event can also become conditioned to elicit anxiety (via higher-order conditioning; Keane *et al.*, 1985).

Intrusive recollections of the traumatic event are additional sources of distress because they include many of the CSs present during the trauma. While not explicitly stated by learning theorists it is reasonable to assume that intrusive recollections may higher-order condition anxiety to the situations or places in which they occur (e.g. being in bed). Thus, through direct and higher-order conditioning plus stimulus generalization it is possible for a traumatized individual to be confronted with a wide array of cues that elicit fear and distress (Keane *et al.*, 1985).

To this account can be added two further principles. First, it has been repeatedly demonstrated that the presence of one CS can potentiate responding to another CS so that the overall intensity of the resultant fears, arousal and startle responses are greater than to any one CS alone (Bouton *et al.*, 2001). Given the wide array of eliciting stimuli that emerge from the processes described by Keane *et al.* (1985) it is easy to explain the very high degrees of fear and arousal found in ASD and PTSD. Secondly, studies indicate that uncontrollable or unpredictable aversive events (like most traumas) can produce stronger and more easily generalizable CRs than controllable and predictable events (Foa *et al.*, 1992). Thus, the literature suggests that traumatic events that occur in places or situations that were previously associated with safety and security have the potential to produce particularly intense and widespread symptoms of fear and arousal (Foa *et al.*, 1992). However, precise predictions about the early impact of traumatic events that derive from these two aspects of learning theory are beyond the scope of this chapter.

Having identified potential sources of fear, vigilance, arousal and startle, it is possible to give account of the remaining symptoms within this cluster of trauma symptoms. For instance, it seems reasonable to assume that sleep and concentration difficulties arise as a function of recent trauma survivors being in a heightened state of conditioned arousal and vigilance, both of which are maintained in part by the occurrence of intrusive recollections. Keane *et al.* (1985) suggest that anger and irritability found in combat veterans with chronic PTSD can be attributed to the fact that these responses are likely to be incompatible with anxiety and, as such, are negatively reinforced so as to make their recurrence more likely.

Avoidance of traumatic cues and general numbing of responsiveness

Following Mowrer, Keane *et al.* (1985) argued that the avoidance symptoms found in PTSD occur because they reduce or terminate conditioned fear. The persistence of avoidance responses in humans (when compared to animals exposed to electric shock) is explained by two factors. First, traumatic events rarely involve a single CS-US pairing. Rather they involve the presentation of several neutral stimuli just prior to the US that may be any number of aversive stimuli associated with the trauma (Keane *et al.*, 1985). Studies have shown that a serial presentation of stimuli (i.e. at intervals less than one second apart, with the last occurring close to the US) produce avoidance responses in animals comparable to those found in humans (Levis and Hare, 1977; Kehoe and Macrae, 1998). Secondly, avoidance symptoms are frequent because of the wide array of eliciting stimuli in the affected individuals' environments and the occurrence of intrusive recollections (Keane *et al.*, 1985). Avoidance or escape from the CSs and the traumatic recollections, along with a failure to recall all of the CSs present during the trauma, prevent extinction of the conditioned fear response (Keane *et al.*, 1985). Likewise, the social community of PTSD sufferers may discourage discussion of the traumatic event and actively prevent contact with eliciting stimuli (Keane *et al.*, 1985). A further consideration is that the failure of extinction might be due not only to avoidance or incomplete recall of the trauma-related cues in memory (Keane *et al.*, 1985), but also the important role of context. Briefly stated, studies have shown extinction of conditioned responses to be more likely if eliciting stimuli are presented in a context that closely resembles the original conditioning experience (Bouton and Nelson, 1998).

The term 'general numbing of responsiveness' refers to decreased interest in activities, detachment from others and a restricted range of affect. While these may reflect active and passive avoidance, Foa *et al.* (1992) have suggested that the analgesia found in animals following exposure to uncontrollable or unpredictable shock might explain numbing symptoms in PTSD survivors. Indeed, analgesia to pain is found in individuals with PTSD under certain conditions of stress (van der Kolk *et al.*, 1989). However, general numbing of responsiveness may be most relevant to the restriction of affect (Foa *et al.*, 1992). Decreased interest in activities and detachment from others may reflect the influence of other emotional states resulting from the traumatic event (i.e. guilt, shame and depression), as well as skills deficits (Keane *et al.*, 1985). To this explanation one might reasonably add that detachment from others may reflect a true state of affairs, i.e. the traumatized person is frequently avoided because their PTSD symptoms are aversive to others. Additional research into the precise mechanisms that underlie the numbing of general responsiveness is needed (Litz, 1993).

Persistent re-experiencing of traumatic events

Conditioning theories do not predict the occurrence of intrusive recollections, but attempts have been made to fit them within this framework. One widely held view is that during conditioning trials (e.g. the traumatic event) a CS-US/UR representation is made in memory (e.g. a tone that has become associated with shock and pain). Subsequent presentation of the CS alone (a tone or other stimuli that have been paired to the CS), activates the original CS-US/UR memory representation (Bouton and Nelson, 1998; Falls, 1998; Wagner, 1979, 1981). In the aftermath of trauma recollections occur when the individual encounters trauma-related CSs. In addition, encounters with stimuli that have become associated with the trauma-related CS through stimulus generalization and higher-order conditioning also elicit the traumatic memory. In either case recollections are often experienced as *unintentional* because the individual is not consciously aware of the stimuli that elicit them. Such a view is consistent with research demonstrating that people often do quite poorly when asked to identify the CSs to which they have been exposed in conditioning trials (Morgan and Riccio, 1998; Bouton *et al.*, 2001). Finally, the recollections are experienced as *intrusive* because they include CSs, which elicit unpleasant emotional states and physiological reactions (Keane *et al.*, 1985).

Using the perspective of a conditioning framework it is therefore possible to seek an answer to the question of why PTSD suffers have intrusive recollections. Perhaps they are just epiphenomena. Alternatively, Keane *et al.* (1985) argue that recall of the event is functional in so far that they may help consolidate memory and initiate adaptive responding. For instance, it can be assumed that reviewing the contingencies that brought about an intensely fearful state might help a traumatized person deal more adaptively with a present fear state. Others have invoked information-processing theory to explain recollections (Foa and Kozak, 1986; Brewin, 2001). For the present, much support appends to Foa *et al.*'s (1992) position that intrusive recollections, flashbacks and nightmares are analogous to a conditioned fear response, and may share similar underlying mechanisms of acquisition.

Clearly, traumatic recollections are less well understood from a conditioning perspective than other symptoms of PTSD. Nevertheless, accounting for event related reactions and symptoms evoked by a trauma, whether these conform to diagnostic criteria for ASD or PTSD is not outside the grasp of learning theorists. As Foa *et al.* (1992) have pointed out, a diagnosis of PTSD does not actually require the presence of either intrusive recollections or nightmares. The presence of distress upon exposure to stimuli resembling the event is sufficient to fulfil the re-experiencing criteria under Category B in DSM-IV (APA, 1994). Indeed, it is the arousal, distress and avoidance that occur in response to traumatic recollections and reminders that are so central to our understanding of PTSD, and its effective treatment (Foa *et al.*, 1992). As has been explained in the above review symptoms of avoidance and arousal that make up the bulk of criteria for a differential diagnosis of PTSD can, indeed, be adequately accounted for using the paradigms of learning theory.

Implications for treatment and early responses to traumatic events

The argument put forward in this chapter is that conditioning is the mechanism by which most PTSD symptoms arise in the aftermath of trauma. From this it follows a reasonable intervention is to effect extinction of conditioned responses via controlled re-exposure to trauma-related cues (including memories). Extinction rests on the premise that repeated exposure to a CS in the absence of the aversive US will lead to a gradual fading away of the conditioned fear, arousal and startle responses. However, it is essential that the subject be exposed to all of the stimuli conditioned during the traumatic event and its aftermath. In other words, the therapist should try to maximize the patient's recall of all stimuli present during the trauma (e.g. thoughts, physical sensations, visual, auditory and olfactory cues). It is also important to try and maximize the similarity between the context of therapeutic exposure, and the context in which the traumatic event occurred (Bouton and Nelson, 1998). Specifically, the patient should be encouraged to engage in therapeutic exposure outside of the therapist's office and, if possible, near the sight of the trauma, at similar times, and either alone or with others who were present. Failure to maximize the similarity between the context in which therapeutic exposure occurs and the original trauma may prevent generalization of treatment gains beyond the therapist's office. For this reason, it is essential that a detailed history or narrative of the event be gathered from the client in order to ascertain all potential traumatic and contextual cues (e.g. the place, time of day, the activities they were engaged in, any thoughts they had just prior to the traumatic event and what they were intending to do). Such information obtained by interview can be supplemented with direct observations of patient responses in session and self-monitoring by the patient.

There are several techniques in common use for bringing someone into contact with trauma-related CSs. They include direct exposure to the CSs (i.e. *in vivo*), imaginary exposure to the CSs, as well as writing and talking about the traumatic events. Conditioning theory predicts that these methods will not necessarily and inevitably achieve the desired therapeutic effects, but are likely to be characterized along a continuum of effectiveness (i.e. from more to less effective). Therapeutic exposures may take the form of flooding (Levis and Hare, 1977) or be graduated as in systematic desensitization (Wolpe, 1958). Alternatively, therapists may help clients deal more effectively with their traumatic reactions by teaching relaxation, deep breathing, positive self-talk, distraction and social skills (Suinn, 1974). Such training involves the strengthening of conditioned responses that are incompatible with anxiety, but does not address the mechanisms that support anxiety. However, in their review of the PTSD treatment literature, Foa and Meadows (1997) found that therapies involving prolonged exposure to traumatic cues and treatments aimed at anxiety management are reported to be effective in reducing PTSD symptoms. It should be noted cognitive theory-based early interventions described elsewhere in this volume incorporate some forms of exposure.

Questions about the ideal or optimum timing of interventions for traumatized survivors is the subject of much controversy and has a particular bearing upon the provision of early interventions. Conditioning theory is neutral on this issue. In experiments with animals, extinction trials often begin within a day or two of conditioning trials. However, no systematic research has been directed at the effect of bringing forward or delaying extinction trials. We do know that while a high percentage of individuals initially suffer PTSD-like symptoms in the early aftermath of traumatic events this proportion typically drops fairly precipitously within the following days or weeks. It seems likely that extinction of responses initially evoked by trauma occurs naturally for the individuals concerned. In this respect, it is possible that the quality of their recovery environments is such as to provide opportunities to discuss the trauma and reinforcers that facilitate recovery (e.g. social support). It could prove most informative to carry out systematic investigations, using learning theory perspectives, on trauma survivors to identify the naturally occurring contingencies that support recovery or mitigate against it. Factors to be considered in such studies would be those that arise in connection with providing early intervention services.

References

American Psychiatric Association (1994) *Diagnostic and Statistical Manual of Mental Disorders*, 3rd edn. Washington DC: APA.

Ayres, J.J.B. (1998) Fear conditioning and avoidance. In O'Donohue, W. (ed.) *Learning and Behaviour Therapy*. Massachusetts: Allyn and Bacon, pp. 122–45.

Bouton, M.E. and Nelson, J.B. (1998) The role of context in classical conditioning: some implications for cognitive behaviour therapy. In O'Donohue, W. (ed.) *Learning and Behaviour Therapy*. Massachusetts: Allyn and Bacon, pp. 59–84.

Bouton, M.E., Mineka, S. and Barlow, D.H. (2001) A modern learning theory perspective on the etiology of panic disorder. *Psycholog Rev* **1**, 4–32.

Brewin, C.R. (2001) A cognitive neuroscience account of posttraumatic stress disorder and its treatment. *Behav Res Ther* **39**, 373–93.

Donahoe, J.W. (1998) Positive reinforcement: the selection of behaviour. In O'Donohue, W. (ed.) *Learning and Behaviour Therapy*. Massachusetts: Allyn and Bacon, pp. 169–187.

Falls, W.A. (1998) Extinction: a review of theory and the evidence suggesting that memories are not erased with nonreinforcement. In O'Donohue, W. (ed.) *Learning and Behaviour Therapy*. Massachusetts: Allyn and Bacon, pp. 205–29.

Fanselow, M.S. and Lester, L.S. (1988) A functional behaviouristic approach to aversively motivated behaviour: predatory imminence as a determinant of the topography of defensive behaviour. In Bolles, R.C. and Beecher, M.D. (eds) *Evolution and Learning*. Hillsdale: Erlbaum, pp. 185–212.

Foa, E.B. and Kozak, M.J. (1986) Emotional processing of fear: exposure to corrective information. *Psycholog Bull* **99**, 220–35.

Foa, E.B. and Meadows, E.A. (1997) Psychosocial treatments for posttraumatic stress disorder: a critical review. *Ann Rev Psychol* **48**, 449–80.

Foa, E.B., Zinbarg, R. and Olasov-Rothbaum, B. (1992) Uncontrollability and unpredictability in post-traumatic stress disorder: an animal model. *Psycholog Bull* **112**, 218–232.

Keane, T.M., Zimmering, R.T. and Caddell, J.M. (1985) A behavioural formulation of PTSD in Vietnam veterans. *Behav Therap* **8**, 9–12.

Kehoe, E.J. and Macrae, M. (1998) Classical conditioning. In O'Donohue, W. (ed.) *Learning and Behaviour Therapy*. Massachusetts: Allyn and Bacon, pp. 36–58.

Levis D.J. and Hare, N. (1977) A review of the theoretical rationale and empirical support for the extinction approach of explosive (flooding) therapy. In Hersen, M., Eisler, R.M. and Miller, P.M. (eds) *Progress in Behaviour Modification*, Vol 4. New York: Academic Press, pp. 299–376.

Litz, B.T. (1993) Emotional numbing in combat-related post-traumatic stress disorder: a critical review and reformulation. *Clin Psychol Rev* **12**, 417–32.

McAllister, W.R. and McAllister, D.E. (1995) Two-factor theory: Implications for understanding anxiety based clinical phenomena. In W. O'Donohue, L. Krasner (eds) *Theories of Behaviour Change: exploring behaviour change*. Washington DC: American Psychological Association, pp. 145–71.

Morgan, R.E. and Riccio, D.C. (1998) Memory retrieval processes. In W. O'Donohue, L. Krasner (eds) *Theories of Behaviour Change: exploring behaviour change*. Washington DC: American Psychological Association, pp. 464–82.

Mowrer, O.H. (1947) On the dual nature of learning: a reinterpretation of 'conditioning' and 'problem-solving'. *Harvard Educat Rev* **17**, 102–48.

Mowrer, O.H. (1960) *Learning Theory and Behaviour*. New York: John Wiley and Sons.

Pavlov, I.P. (1927) *Conditioned Reflexes*. London: Oxford University Press.

Rescorla, R.A. (1988) Pavlovian conditioning: it's not what you think it is. *American Psychologist*, **43**, 151–160.

Rescorla, R.A. and Solomon, R.L. (1967) Two-process learning theory: relationships between Pavlovian conditioning and instrumental learning. *Psycholog Rev* **74**, 151–82.

Skinner, B.F. (1938) *The Behaviour of Organisms*. New York: Appleton-Century-Crofts.

Suinn, R. (1974) Anxiety management training for general anxiety. In Suinn, R. and Weigel, R. (eds) *The Innovative Therapy: critical and creative contributions*. New York: Harper & Row, pp. 66–70.

Thorndike, E.L. (1911) *Animal intelligence*. New York: MacMillan Co.

Van der Kolk, B.A., Greenberg, M.S., Orr, S.P. and Pitman, R.K. (1989) Endogenous opioids, stress induced analgesia, and posttraumatic stress disorders. *Psychopharmacol Bull* **25**, 417–21.

Wagner, A.R. (1979) Habituation and memory. In Dickinson, A. and Boakes, R.A. (eds) *Mechanisms of Learning and Motivation*. New Jersey: Erlbaum, pp. 5–47.

Wagner, A.R. (1981) SOP: a model of automatic memory processing in animal behaviour. In Spear, N. and Miller, R. (eds) *Information Processing in Animals: memory mechanisms*. San Francisco: Academic Press, pp. 301–36.

Wolpe, J. (1958) *Psychotherapy by Reciprocal Inhibition*. Stanford: Stanford University Press.

7 Cognitive perspectives on early reactions to traumatic events

Hazel Pilgrim

Introduction

Cognitive theory has inspired and informed a number of distinct forms of psychological interventions generically referred to as cognitive therapy. In recent years they have been subjected to systematic evaluation with encouraging results for clinically significant expressions of anxiety, phobias, depression and obsessive-compulsive disorders. It has also been demonstrated as a valid therapy for PTSD (Marks *et al.*, 1998; Tarrier *et al.*, 1999). Development of cognitive theories has often followed clinical observations in such a way that the theory, in turn, engenders suggestions as to which types of interventions may be useful in therapeutic practice. This being the case, cognitive therapies and theories are in a process of continuous evolution.

This chapter will describe current cognitive models for PTSD and briefly summarize research supporting their use in the implementation of early intervention programs for survivors of recent trauma. Particular emphasis will be placed on understanding the general cognitive principles that apply during the various stages of post-trauma response. These are derived from research that has examined the role of survivors' cognitions after such events, and related these to the subsequent course and development of traumatic stress reactions.

Cognitive models of PTSD

Cognitive models of PTSD are concerned with the conscious personal significance of traumatic events for each survivor. Different models offer specific accounts of how information processing takes place, but a common theme is that each survivor is confronted with a challenge to integrate trauma-related impressions into existing cognitive structures.

Cognitive structures comprise the working beliefs and assumptions that we all hold about ourselves and the world in which we live. It is via these cognitive structures that we are able to make sense of our lives and daily make adaptive decisions that promote survival (Mahoney, 1991; Beck and Emery, 1985; Hollon and Garber, 1988). Situations do occur, however, when information or impressions formed by an individual is seemingly incongruous or irreconcilable with existing cognitive structures. When this happens the tendency is to attempt to distort information in order to protect established cognitive structures and obviate a need for change. However, if the new information is indisputable, individuals have to change and adapt their cognitive structures so as to facilitate its assimilation.

In the early aftermath of trauma it is conceivable that neither of these processes can occur. Assimilation may not occur readily if impressions are so incongruous as to be outside the realm of the individual's previous experiences. Alternatively, experiences may have been so personally threatening that no pre-existing cognitive structures exist for making sense of what has happened (Janoff-Bulman, 1985; Horowitz, 1986). Epstein (1990) and Horowitz (1990) have suggested that as long as trauma-related information remains unassimilated, it will be maintained in an active state that can create information overload resulting in intrusive thoughts, flashbacks and nightmares. Related cognitive constructs are used to account for post-trauma avoidance of stimuli associated with the event, hyper-vigilance and high levels of arousal.

The model also proposes that when attempts are made to avoid processing trauma-related information cognitive structures will, nevertheless, have been disrupted. Janoff-Bulman (1985) and Epstein (1990) have also proposed that traumatic events can disrupt basic cognitive structures. In either case, the result may be distorted beliefs. Resick and Schnicke's (1993) Cognitive Processing Model suggests distortion of trauma-related information can lead to disassociation and a sense of unreality.

Emotional processing

Emotional processing models originate from Lang's theories of emotion (1985). He posited a semantic network of related and interconnected information from which subjective meanings are derived that influence responses evoked by particular events. In keeping with this Foa *et al.* (1989) suggested that in order for processing to occur a fear network must be activated. However, trauma may engender over-generalization of event-related cues associated with danger. This may create a fear network with a capacity to trigger fear reactions to relatively innocuous cues.

Rachman (1980) has suggested emotional processing may be influenced by four factors. They are stimulus-related factors, factors relating to the individual's state at the time of the trauma, survivors activity at the time and factors of their personality. Their inter-relationship also influences subsequent reactions.

Dual representation

A recent model proposed by Brewin *et al.* (1996) suggests traumatic memories take two forms: one that is verbally accessible and one where the individual is consciously aware. The other is an automatic response to stimuli (e.g. flashbacks). They base their theory on the notion that sensory information is subject to conscious and unconscious processing (Epstein, 1994) and also that information is stored and represented differently in various parts of the brain. As a consequence of this, emotional processing may be explicit or implicit (Broadbent *et al.*, 1986).

Psychosocial models

Joseph *et al.* (1995) have proposed that intrusive re-experiencing phenomena evoke strong emotions, such as fear and anger, and that these emotions are subject to appraisals related to a survivor's personality. The resulting distress is likely to lead to avoidance coping in the form of worry and ruminations as described by Wells and Matthews (1994). They go on to suggest that a certain amount of avoidance may be of benefit initially, in so far as it defers processing to a more appropriate phase of post-trauma reactions. In excess, however, avoidance may lead to emotional numbing and dissociation.

Trauma-related cognitions

Thoughts, appraisals, beliefs, assumptions and attributions

Recent studies have investigated assumptions, beliefs and cognitions associated with the development and maintenance of traumatic stress reactions (Perloff, 1983; Janoff-Bulman, 1985; McCann *et al.*, 1988; Dutton *et al.*, 1994). Cognitive-behavioural theorists have suggested that thoughts, beliefs, attitudes, expectations, appraisals, assumptions and attributions exert fundamental influences on human behaviour generally (Beck and Emery, 1985; Hollon and Garber, 1988; Mahoney, 1991). These factors should therefore also feature in our considerations of early reactions to trauma. In this context, it is interesting to note that changes in emotional states can exert a decisive influence on cognitive reactions to unfolding events (Hollon and Kendall, 1980; Giles *et al.*, 1989). For instance, research by Ehlers and Clark (2000) demonstrates how catastrophic thinking and negative appraisals in the wake of the emergence of symptoms can lead to avoidance and safety-seeking behaviour akin to those found for panic disorders. They also found strong associations between initial interpretations of PTSD symptoms, and subsequent persistence and severity of PTSD.

The relationship of trauma-related cognitions to the subsequent course of post-trauma reactions has so far been studied from three main perspectives. Namely, cognitive reactions to traumatic events and stimuli associated with those trauma. Examples would be intrusive or avoidant responses that are often recognized as signs of a developing disorder (Horowitz, 1986; Cassidy *et al.*, 1992; Creamer *et al.*, 1992). Secondly, a number of researchers have considered the cognitive processes that come into play following trauma (Horowitz, 1986; Brewin *et al.*, 1996; Joseph *et al.*, 1995; Foa *et al.*, 1989, 1991). This includes research on cognitive processes involved in suppression of trauma-related thoughts and intrusions. For example, Ehlers and Steil (1995) suggest the extent of evoked distress and the control strategies each trauma survivor may use can be predicted by establishing idiosyncratic meanings attributed to intrusions. Linked to the same, attentional bias may be the result of seemingly voluntary attempts to monitor threat-related stimuli evolving into over-control and general reduction in awareness. Thirdly, research that demonstrates how cognitions contribute to the development and maintenance of reactions to traumatic events. This line of investigation encompasses 'cognitive appraisal variables', such as survivors' attributions, memories, subjective appraisals and perceptions (Joseph *et al.*, 1991, 1995; Resnick and Newton, 1992; McNally, 1993; Dunmore *et al.*, 1997, 1998), as well as their cognitions about the events. Research indicates trauma can change, or even shatter some cognitive assumptions and core beliefs held by survivors (Herman, 1992a,b; Janoff-Bulman, 1992; McCann and Pearlman, 1990a,b).

Cognitions, coping styles and vulnerability

Joseph *et al.* (1991) discuss the role of attributions to the emergence of particular post-trauma coping styles and the findings that those views of the world emphasize an external locus of control tend to have poorer outcomes for PTSD. Similarly, negative cognitions about the self or emergent reactions evoked by trauma may result in more frequent attempts to avoid addressing the personal repercussions of what has happened that, in turn, inhibit cognitive assimilation of impressions (Dunmore *et al.*, 1997, 1998). Poorer outcomes are said to be associated with situations in which trauma provoke a changed sense of self (Ehlers *et al.*, 1998), especially if this is in a negative direction (Dunmore *et al.*, 1997).

The importance of these research findings for early intervention is that cognitive structures have often been disrupted by traumatic events and that this can result in distorted beliefs, even if survivors try to avoid processing recently formed impressions. An example of such a distorted belief would be a statement to the effect of 'I will never be safe anywhere again'.

Theoretical speculation has also centred on the possibility that certain beliefs and assumptions render some individual particularly vulnerable to the effects of trauma, whilst others are more resilient to their effects. For the former a common subject of speculation is that their beliefs are more likely to be shattered by a traumatic event and the tolerance levels for such change is particularly low. Janoff-Bulman (1985) identified three themes that may make beliefs vulnerable to trauma. They are presumptions of personal invulnerability, that the world is meaningful and comprehensible, and that the self is perceived in a positive way. Epstein (1990) also tried to identify beliefs associated with vulnerability to developing enduring post-trauma reaction. He labelled these as believing the world is benevolent and a source of joy, that it is meaningful and comprehensible, and that the self can be perceived as worthy. Janoff-Bulman and Epstein assume that these beliefs are most likely to be challenged to the point of disintegration if a traumatic experience provides compelling evidence not reconcilable with these fundamental beliefs. In an elaboration of these speculations Williams (1999) has suggested that over-generalized beliefs held with rigid conviction may be most readily shattered by traumatic experiences. Dalgleish (1999) purports that people with more flexible beliefs may encounter fewer difficulties when trying to assimilate new trauma-related impressions and adjust more successfully to what has happened.

McNally (1993) suggests that, although it may appear that shattered cognitions about the world are difficult to process, the most important adjustments each individual survivor has to make, tends to centre on how they redefine their view of self.

Safety, trust, power, esteem and intimacy as cognitive themes

It has been suggested by McCann *et al.* (1988), that disrupted beliefs associated with victimization can be categorized into five main themes: safety, trust, power, esteem and intimacy. In turn, these categories are linked to basic human needs expressed during progressive life stage developmental phases (Piaget, 1971; Eysenck, 1976).

The importance of beliefs held at the time of trauma and during its aftermath is demonstrated in a study by Pilgrim (1999). The study used the Personal Beliefs and Reactions Scale (PBRS) (Resick *et al.*, 1991), which incorporated themes suggested by McCann *et al.* (1988). The questionnaire was administered to a mixed population of 570 adults with and without a current diagnosis of PTSD. Of this total, 119 subjects had been recruited as part of a study carried out by Tarrier *et al.* (1999). In total 322 respondents reported involvement in some traumatic event. Of these, 159 had symptoms consistent with a diagnosis of PTSD. Pilgrim found a strong relationship between symptoms evoked by trauma and survivors' cognitions rooted in themes of safety, trust, control, esteem, intimacy and self-blame. Factor analysis grouped cognitions into six categories. Four of these contained negative cognitions about self as being 'vulnerable and flawed', 'holding unrealistic ideas', 'feeling out of control' and 'wanting to change what had happened'. The remaining two categories comprised of 'positive regard for others' and 'positive regard for self'. A perception of self as 'vulnerable and flawed' seems to place an individual at particular risk, since this category accounted for the largest proportion of variance in relation to subsequent PTSD symptoms and also a lack of response to therapeutic intervention. Cognitions about 'being out of control' also contributed significantly. Positive cognitions about self and others were shown to have an inverse relationship with both symptom level and change after therapy. Pilgrim (1999) went on to retrospectively analyse 33 PTSD patients' notes to further identify relevant cognitions. She then developed a semi-structured interview administered to 12 patients referred with a diagnosis of PTSD who described the meaning of the traumatic event, their symptoms and changes in self provoked by what happened. A consistent pattern emerged showing that patients felt their previously held assumptions had been violated by the trauma. These findings reinforce the importance of cognitive processing during the aftermath of trauma. Patient returns also indicated that individuals tend to be avoiding memories of these events because to do otherwise evoked intense emotions that disrupted adjustment. For some, fear produced classic panic type cognitions with beliefs that the individual may go mad, lose control or have a heart attack. For others, fear was interpreted to indicate cowardice and weakness. Anger was perceived as dangerous, might lead to a loss of control and becoming violent. Distress, grief and sadness were perceived as unacceptable because they involved losing control indicated weakness and made the individuals feel vulnerable. Pilgrim has continued to find this pattern with PTSD patients throughout clinical practise. In her opinion, identifying the avoided emotions and associated cognitions is generally the key to successful therapy.

Hyper-vigilance and exaggerated startle response in the aftermath of trauma were seen as normal reactions to perceived danger, and were often felt most keenly by individuals with distorted beliefs about safety and trust.

Cognitions and avoidance

Most of the strategies for coping reported by subjects in Pilgrim's (1999) study involved some form of avoidance. This included using distraction and suppressing feelings, as well as avoidance of reminders. For some this involved taking numbing agents such as alcohol. Those who continued to re-experience their trauma interpreted this as evidence there was something deeply wrong with them for having lost control and they were going mad. Often this led to feelings of guilt and shame, and this was particularly relevant where some time had lapsed since the trauma.

Loss of interest in activities regularly enjoyed before the trauma was construed as a way of avoiding others. Detachment from colleagues, friends and family occurred for the same reason and a belief was held that others would not understand or would pass unfavourable judgement. Similarly, sleep difficulties were often the result of deliberate avoidance of nightmares. Many subjects reported not wanting to sleep, since they were likely to have nightmares, which would evoke intense emotions and unsettling cognitions. Loss of concentration and irritability were typically rationalized as resulting from lack of sleep.

These findings are particularly important for reconstructing early intervention after trauma. At a theoretical level at least, there is reason to believe that if steps are taken to mitigate the development of beliefs about being 'vulnerable and flawed' or 'out of control' a positive influence may be exerted on trauma-related reactions. Service providers should also note the observation that positive beliefs about self or others can negate the effect of negative cognitions about emotional responses.

Pilgrim's model of development and maintenance of PTSD

A new way of construing factors that influence the course and development of trauma evoked reactions can be proposed by integrating findings from Pilgrim's study with an earlier model formulated by Joseph *et al.* (1995; Fig. 7.1).

The model is premised by the accepted ideas, promoted by cognitive theory, that basic assumptions or schema exert important influences on expectations, beliefs and ideas about the self, others and the world. They are constantly used to interpret new information and some will relate to survival.

Information that threatens the integrity of these cognitions is typically disregarded or distorted as suggested by cognitive dissonance models. However, if impressions are formed that are perceived as threatening, a fear reaction will be evoked. Similarly, if information is also perceived as

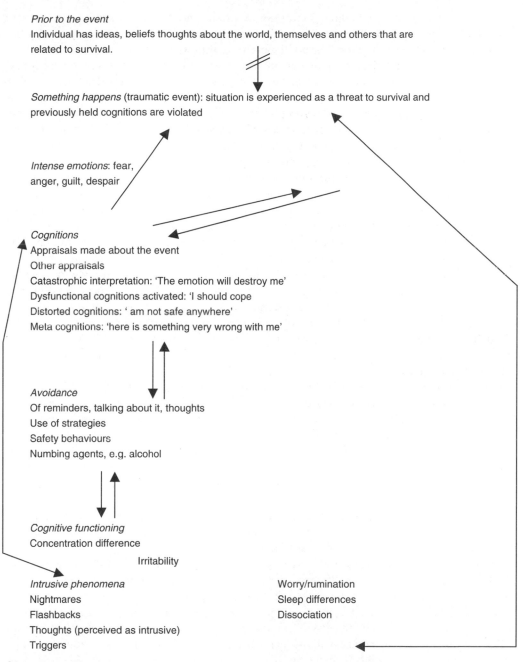

Prior to the event
Individual has ideas, beliefs thoughts about the world, themselves and others that are related to survival.

Something happens (traumatic event): situation is experienced as a threat to survival and previously held cognitions are violated

Intense emotions: fear, anger, guilt, despair

Cognitions
Appraisals made about the event
Other appraisals
Catastrophic interpretation: 'The emotion will destroy me'
Dysfunctional cognitions activated: 'I should cope
Distorted cognitions: ' am not safe anywhere'
Meta cognitions: 'here is something very wrong with me'

Avoidance
Of reminders, talking about it, thoughts
Use of strategies
Safety behaviours
Numbing agents, e.g. alcohol

Cognitive functioning
Concentration difference
                                    Irritability

Intrusive phenomena   Worry/rumination
Nightmares   Sleep differences
Flashbacks   Dissociation
Thoughts (perceived as intrusive)
Triggers

Figure 7.1 Pilgrim's model of development and maintenance of PTSD.

not fitting with assumptions relating to survival or other important assumptions, cognitive confusion will arise. This may also engender emotional reactions. The appraisals individual survivors make during the early aftermath of trauma may be crucial to subsequent development, particularly if the event may activates dysfunctional cognitions.

According to this model, it is the emotional reactions evoked by a trauma that define the experience as traumatic. To some extent, this explains why different individuals may or may not perceive the same event as a trauma. So, if prior experience has led recent survivors to expect a particular type of event, it will not be difficult for them to integrate the new information into existing cognitive structures. The experience will merely confirm what they already know.

On the other hand, individuals whose cognitive structures do not anticipate a particular type of experience may perceive the event as a threat to all they have previously learned about themselves and the world. An individual sustained by ideas of personal invulnerability, and being able to control themselves and their world will be deeply affected if implicated in events over which they had no control and felt vulnerable. Individuals who expect the unpredictable and are not concerned about always being in control might be less likely to interpret an event as traumatic.

It is likely if the amount of conflicting threatening information exceeds that which can be integrated into existing cognitive structures the individuals in question may experience numbing, derealization, a sense of unreality or dissociation as described for Acute Stress Disorder. Over a period of time, it is possible for the cognitive structures to gradually accept the new information and the survivor will begin to feel the true emotions evoked by the event.

The next aspect of the model seeks to describe the processes that account for some survivors developing PTSD, whilst others do not. According to Horowitz's (1986) model and to the learning theory formulations, intense emotions experienced during a trauma elicit a natural aversion that causes individuals to attempt to avoid emotions. Avoiding similar and associated events may be part of the evolutionary and biological functions of emotions. For some it will be seemingly reflexive, but survivors can also make active choices as to whether or not to avoid emotions. This will depend on the interpretations that each individual makes. Patients with PTSD seem to interpret their emotions as being dangerous with a perceived capacity to engulf them, drive them mad, destroy them or be dangerous.

A decision to avoid emotions may be re-enforced by others who say 'try not to think about it' or 'distract yourself'. Survivors may therefore seek to avoid all reminders of the event in an attempt to avoid emotional responses, but this is countered by an apparently inherent need to process and integrate new information, particularly if impressions are personally relevant or threatening, and the information is stored by sensory structures in the brain in an active form prior to being integrated into existing cognitive structures. Individuals who continue to avoid emotions and reminders may block this process, but events will become manifest as intrusive re-experiences.

Emotional triggers tend to generalize so that information that is only vaguely associated with an event can engender emotional responses leading to their avoidance. For example, someone involved in a car accident may begin avoiding walking on busy streets. When survivors are reminded of a trauma they consciously experience fear that is interpreted as danger being present. However, with so many new triggers fear may be experienced in many different situations and survivors may reason that nowhere is safe. This same process may operate in relation to other beliefs, such as trust, control, esteem and intimacy, resulting in survivors becoming hyper-alert, constantly on the look out and hyper-vigilant with a propensity to exaggerated startle responses.

Being aware of their experiences individual make meta-cognitive appraisals about their experiences within the framework of believing it is in their best interests to avoid their emotions. So the tendency is to regard the self as odd, different or strange. Many survivors report that they are not the same persons they used to be, and this difference is generally regarded negatively. Often the interpretation will be 'there is something wrong with me' or 'I am going mad'. This may result in loss of self-esteem and increase the inclination to protect oneself from negative evaluations made by others.

The consequences of these processes are likely to be detrimental to survivors' relationships, their work and status in life. Knowing this to be the case they interpret unfolding events as further evidence there is something very wrong. As the individual struggles to make sense of what is happening to them they perceive their difficulties as being related to the traumatic event, which then gains in importance and the associated emotions become more intense.

So over time the system continues to maintain and feed the disorder. This explains why symptoms tend to get worse over time and people reach a state of despair before seeking help.

Further study is obviously needed to test various aspects of this model. If the suggestion is correct that those individuals who are best able to tolerate strong emotions are more likely to recover from trauma then reconstructed early intervention may seek to help survivors contain or control their initial emotional reactions. Underlying cognitive processes may be addressed at a later stage.

Implications for reconstructing early intervention after trauma

Previous processing models for trauma have emphasized a perceived need to help survivors confront what has happened and address emotions evoked by it so as to make personal sense of the event. In part, this gave rise of Critical Incident Stress De-briefing (Mitchell, 1983). However, recent research shows this approach is not consistently successful. There are strong theoretical and practical reasons why one-off discussions are insufficient for adequate cognitive processing of impressions mediated by trauma (Joseph et al., 1995; Pilgrim, 1999).

Pilgrim adds another explanation for the limitations of past prescriptive approaches to early intervention. Namely, individuals with deep fears of the consequences of experiencing emotions are likely to wish to avoid experiencing them in the context of a group meeting.

From a theoretical point of view processing models suggest early intervention might usefully set out to support survivors with their initial emotional reactions so that these do not become overwhelming or engender unhelpful beliefs. Only if adjustment difficulties are reported at a later stage is it appropriate to offer more structured forms of cognitive behaviour therapy.

However, some level of continuous monitoring of survivors is indicated because as time goes on distorted beliefs become more entrenched and as further adjustment difficulties are encountered they may become more resistant to offers of help and support.

Cognitive assessment should ideally be carried out once symptoms are identified. Its focus may be the extent to which the individual regards emotional responses evoked by trauma as unacceptable. Once identified, cognitions associated with these emotions can be challenged using cognitive and behavioural techniques conducive to effective processing of the event.

A most important first step for enabling survivors to undertake this work is to build up therapeutic trust. Someone who strongly believes in the harmful effect of emotions is not likely to welcome or accept challenges to their cognitive beliefs, assumptions, etc. It is therefore good practice to allow individual survivors to decide when they wish to engage in the therapeutic process. In the early aftermath of trauma, survivors may not recognize that avoidance is not likely to help bring an end to intrusive reminders and their associated emotions. If levels of dissociation are particularly high, early interventions should be provided so as to allow survivors to proceed at a slow pace.

References

Beck, A.T. and Emery, G. (1985) Anxiety Disorders and Phobias. New York: Basic Books.

Brewin, C.R., Dalgleish, T. and Joseph, S. (1996) A dual representation theory of post-traumatic stress disorder. Psycholog Rev 103, 670–86.

Broadbent, D.E., Fitzgerald, P. and Broadbent, M.H.P. (1986) Implicit and explicit knowledge in the control of complex systems. Br J Psychol 77, 33–50.

Cassidy, K.L., McNally, R.J. and Zeitlin, S.B. (1992) Cognitive processing of trauma cues in rape victims with post-traumatic stress disorder. Cognit Ther Res 16, 283–95.

Creamer, M., Burgess, P. and Pattison, P. (1992) Reactions to trauma: a cognitive processing model. *J Abnorm Psychol* **101**, 452–9.

Dalgleish, T. (1999) Cognitive theories of post-traumatic stress disorder. In Yule, W. (ed.) *Post-Traumatic Stress Disorders: concepts and therapy*. Chichester: Wiley, pp. 193–220.

Dunmore, E., Clark, D.M. and Ehlers, A. (1997) Cognitive factors in persistent versus recovered post-traumatic stress disorder after physical or sexual assault: a pilot study. *Behaviour Cognitive Psychother* **25**, 147–59.

Dunmore, E., Clark, D.M. and Ehlers, A. (1998) *The Role of Cognitive Factors in Posttraumatic Stress Disorder Following Physical or Sexual Assault: findings from retrospective and prospective investigations*, Paper presented at British Association of Behavioural and Cognitive Therapies Meeting, Durham, July 9–11.

Dutton, M.A., Burghardt, K.J., Perkin, S.G., Chrestman, K.R. and Halle, P.M. (1994) Battered women's cognitive schema. *J Traum Stress*, **7**, 237–55.

Ehlers, A. and Clark, D.M. (2000) A cognitive model of posttraumatic stress disorder. *Behav Res Ther* **38**, 319–45.

Ehlers, A. and Steil, R. (1995) Maintenance of intrusive memories in post-traumatic stress disorder: a cognitive approach. *Behaviour Cognitive Psychother* **23**, 217–49.

Ehlers, A., Mayou, R. and Bryant, B. (1998) Psychological predictors of chronic post-traumatic stress disorder after motor vehicle accidents. *J Abnorm Psychol* **107**, 508–19.

Epstein, S. (1990) Beliefs and symptoms in maladaptive resolutions of the traumatic neurosis. In Ozer, D., Healy, J.M. and Stewart, A.J. (eds) *Perspectives on Personality*, Vol. 3. London: Jessica Kingsley Publications.

Epstein, S. (1994) Integration of the cognitive and the psychodynamic unconscious. *American Psychologist*, **49**, 709–724.

Eysenck, H.J. (1976) The learning theory model of neurosis—a new approach. *Behav Res Ther* **14**, 251–67.

Foa, E.B., Steketee, G. and Rothbaum, B.O. (1989) Behavioural-cognitive conceptualizations of post-traumatic stress disorder. *Behav Ther* **20**, 155–76.

Foa, E.B., Feske, U., Murdock, T.B., Kozak, M.J. and McCarthy, P.R. (1991) Processing of threat related information in rape victims. *J Abnorm Psychol* **100**, 156–62.

Giles, D.E., Etzel, B.A. and Biggs, M.M. (1989) Long term effects of unipolar depression on cognitions. *Comprehens Psychiat* **30**, 225–30.

Herman, J.L. (1992a) Complex PTSD: a syndrome in survivors of prolonged and repeated trauma. *J Traum Stress*, **5**, 377–91.

Herman, J.L. (1992b) *Trauma and Recovery*. New York: Basic Books.

Hollon, S.D. and Garber, J. (1988) Cognitive therapy. In Abramson, L.Y. (ed.) *Social Cognition and Clinical Psychology: a synthesis*. New York: Guilford Press, pp. 204–253.

Hollon, S.D. and Kendall, P.C. (1980) Cognitive self-statements in depression: development of an automatic thought's questionnaire. *Cognit Ther Res* **4**, 383–95.

Horowitz, M.J. (1986) *Stress Response Syndromes*, 2nd edn. New York: Jason Aronson.

Horowitz, M.J. (1990) A model of mourning: changes in schema's of self and others. *J Am Psychoanalyt Ass* **38**, 297–324.

Janoff-Bulman, R. (1985) The aftermath of victimization: rebuilding shattered assumptions. In Figley, C.R. (ed.) *Trauma and its Wake: the study and treatment of post-traumatic stress disorder*. New York: Brunner/Mazel, pp. 15–34.

Janoff-Bulman, R. (1992) *Shattered Assumptions: towards a new psychology of trauma*. New York: Free Press.

Joseph, S.A., Brewin, C.R., Yule. W. and Williams, R.M. (1991) Causal attributions and psychiatric symptoms in survivors of the herald of free enterprise disaster. *Br J Psychiat* **159**, 542–6.

Joseph, S., Williams, R. and Yule, W. (1995) Psychosocial perspectives on post-traumatic stress. *Clin Psychol Rev* **15**, 515–44.

Lang, P.J. (1985) The cognitive psychophysiology of emotion: fear and anxiety. In Tuma, A.H. and Maser, J.D. (eds) *Anxiety and the Anxiety Disorders*. Hillsdale: Erlbaum, pp. 131–70.

Mahoney, M.J. (1991) *Human Change Processes: the scientific foundations of psychotherapy*. New York: Basic Books.

Marks, I., Lovell, K., Noshirvani, H., Livanou, M. and Thrasher, S. (1998) Treatment of posttraumatic stress disorder by exposure and/or cognitive restructuring: a controlled study. *Arch Gen Psychiat* **55**, 317–25.

McCann, I.L. and Pearlman, L.A. (1990a) *Psychological Trauma and the Adult Survivor: theory, therapy and transformation*. New York: Brunner/Mazel.

McCann, I.L. and Pearlman, L.A. (1990b) Constructivist self development theory as a framework for assessing and treating victims of family violence. In Stith, S., Williams, M.B. and Rosen, K. (eds) *Violence Hits Home: treating victims of family violence*. New York: Springer, pp. 305–329.

McCann, I.L., Sakheim, D.K. and Abrahamson, D.J. (1988) Trauma and victimization: a model of psychological adaptation. *Counselling Psychol* **16**, 531–94.

McNally, R.J. (1993) Self-representation in post-traumatic stress disorder. A cognitive perspective. In Segal, V.Z. and Blatt S.J. (eds) *The Self in Emotional Distress: cognitive and psychodynamic perspectives*. New York: Guilford Press, pp. 71–79.

Mitchell, J. (1983) When disaster strikes: the critical incident stress debriefing process. *J Emerg Med Serv* **8**, 36–9.

Perloff, L.S. (1983) Perceptions to vulnerability to victimization. *J Soc Iss* **39**, 41–61.

Piaget, J. (1971) *Psychology and Epistemology: towards a theory of knowledge*. New York: Viking.

Pilgrim, H. (1999) *Cognitive Aspects of PTSD*. PhD Thesis, University of Manchester.

Rachman, S. (1980) Emotional processing. *Behav Res Ther* **18**, 51–60.

Resick, P.A., Schnicke, M.K. and Markway, B.A. (1991) *The Relationship Between Cognitive Content and Post-traumatic Stress Disorder*, Paper presented at the Annual Meeting of the Association for Advancement of behaviour Therapy, New York.

Resick, P.A. and Schnicke, M.K. (1993) *Cognitive Processing Therapy for Rape Victims*. London: Sage.

Resnick, H.S. and Newton, T. (1992) Assessment and treatment of post-traumatic stress disorder in adult survivors of sexual assault. In Foy, D.W. (ed.) *Treating PTSD: cognitive-behavioural strategies*. New York: Guilford Press, pp. 96–126.

Tarrier, N., Pilgrim, H., Sommerfield, C., Faragher, B., Reynolds, M., Graham, E. and Barrowclough, C. (1999) A randomized trial of cognitive therapy and imaginal exposure in the treatment of chronic posttraumatic stress disorder. *J Consult Clin Psychol* **67**, 13–18.

Wells, A. and Matthews, G. (1994) *Attention and Emotion: a clinical perspective*. Hillsdale: Lawrence Erlbaum.

Williams, R. (1999) Personality and post-traumatic stress disorder. In Yule, W. (ed.) *Post-traumatic Stress Disorders: concepts and therapy*. Chichester: Wiley, pp. 95–115.

8 Systemic approaches to early interventions in a community affected by organized violence

Dean Ajduković and Marina Ajduković

Reviews of the literature on the effectiveness of early interventions with individuals and groups show the importance of the social context in which healing should progress. When describing the initial stage of psychological first aid Freeman *et al.* (2000) list activities that involve active, organized and supporting environments. This includes forms of practical help, provisions of food and shelter, protection from further threat, immediate care for physical needs, etc. Herman (1992) maintains that restoring connections with the environment, which emphasizes the importance of the social network of a victim, is among the critical points of trauma recovery. This is even more important in the event of massive organized violence that brings about large numbers of trauma victims, massive losses and disruption of the social fabric. All the same, the crucial role of the social context in the aftermath of traumatic event has frequently been overlooked (Kleber, 2000).

Wars are an extreme form of organized mass violence that have a profound impact on communities, families and individuals. They include all possible elements of trauma. The consequences are multiple, including large numbers of traumatized individuals and groups, high levels of deprivation, anger and aggression, mixed with fear, despair, hopelessness and loss of control. In cases of ethnic conflict all this is additionally aggravated by feelings of betrayal by neighbours and even by relatives. The affected people typically suffer a whole range of losses, whole villages or city communities are destroyed, social networks and other support mechanisms are shattered. As Blackwell (1989) points out, networks, just like families, may be largely wiped out. Where members of networks have survived, their relationships may become burdened by suspicion and mistrust, so they can no longer function as before. Man-made disasters, especially those that are characterized by high levels of long-lasting stress, are socially disruptive (Allen, 1995) and weaken inherent capacities for providing support. This contrasts with single though major events like natural disasters when communities are typically brought closer together.

This is particularly true if war is waged in a multi-ethnic and multi-religious context where the trauma has a specific symbolic meaning that questions, perhaps more dramatically than other traumatic events, the very fundamental view of the world as a predictable, just and meaningful place to live. This is amplified by the fact that organized violence is intentional, it has a political agenda, and is meant to destroy, hurt and create terror. Such instances are typically heavily loaded with human rights violations in the form of persecutions of people because of their political, ethnic, religious or other affiliations. These events that are intentionally perpetrated are often specifically chosen to affront important symbolic meanings of the populations being violated: rape, destruction of places of worship, graveyards, cultural heritage, ethnic cleansing, burning of homes, ritual slaughter and mutilation of the most vulnerable. The consequences both for individuals and the community are long lasting and survivors feel that gross injustice has been done to them. This easily leads to revenge and increases the likelihood of trans-generational transmission of violence within communities (Punamaki, 1987; Awwad, 1999; Gutlove, 1999). As within families, the re-establishment of meaningful patterns of interactions in the community after trauma is the vehicle through which it may be possible to begin to reconstruct a sense of meaning and purpose. To do this is, however, extremely difficult.

Three sets of factors have been recognized as key determinants of social and psychological consequences of traumatic events. Namely, characteristics of the events and context in which they take place, characteristics of individuals affected and their personal histories, plus characteristics of the prevailing social situation, e.g. the extent to which people get support from others (Brom and Kleber, 1989). Just as massive trauma exposure occurs within a given community social context so it is the very same, but altered context that is essential for the healing process to occur. For instance, making some sense of what has happened, why and how, and searching for meaning may be much more difficult after organized violence than after traffic accidents or random violence.

Community as a healing context

The essence of 'community' is the feeling of togetherness, participation in activities, sharing a culture and history. Heller (1990) points out that the term *community* is used in at least two ways. As a locality where the meaning refers to an identifiable territory. The second meaning is relational, and emphasizes networks of individuals who interact with formal organizations and institutions, as well as members of informal groups. The latter meaning is essential not only for understanding the damaging effects of massive violence, but also for appreciating that the recovery of individuals within such communities cannot proceed without addressing the broader needs of the community. To do so, calls for the provision of comprehensive interventions.

Early interventions in such contexts need to promote change, rather than simply providing support to clients. One of the main healing functions of a community is to contain and support both family systems and individual members (Ayalon, 1998). In community-based interventions, we seek to identify resources that are still remaining more or less intact and then work to strengthen the healing influence they can exert. It is worth keeping in mind that psychosocial interventions have both immediate and delayed effects on the empowerment of the affected people and communities. Community-based early intervention approaches focus on effects of trauma and on treatment resources that are available for individuals, but also for the community as a whole (Wessells, 1999). The distinctiveness of this strategy derives from taking a systemic approach rooted in an assumption that communal wounds, inflicted by circumstances such as armed conflict, require communal healing. Such a strategy emphasizes local participation, community mobilization and empowerment, and the use of local, culturally appropriate resources (Peddle *et al.*, 1999). These may include extended family and neighbour support, informal networks, parent groups, informal councils comprising community elders or *ad hoc* task groups, as well as ceremonies and rituals. Both early interventions and longer-term follow-up help, and support need to take this into account.

Early interventions in a traumatized community

Most of those who have suffered from trauma perpetrated as a part of organized violence, such as war, are likely to hold sets of beliefs that reflect a mixture of unsatisfied needs, high levels of uncertainty, insecurity and lack of hope. We have seen this in refugees and veterans, children, adolescents, adults and the elderly. During the stage of acute danger the priority for all is basic safety and survival. Once this is relatively secured, other needs emerge that are both existential and psychological. Once manifest, these needs are typically left frustrated and unfulfilled for a prolonged period of time. All too often, therefore, the people in question are re-exposed to further traumatic events.

This raises several crucial questions for the notion of early interventions. For instance, when does a traumatic event actually start and does it have a clear time line with a clear ending? When should early interventions be implemented? What is really an 'early intervention' under circumstances of repeated traumatization? It has to be acknowledged that healing cannot start if trauma victims are forced to functioning in 'survival mode' for prolonged periods because of prevailing adversities (Chemtob, 1996).

The core assumption that underpins provision of early interventions after trauma is that it should be provided in the immediate aftermath of an event. In a situation such as war it is very difficult to satisfy this criterion. Thus, early interventions during armed conflict and other massive destabilization of communities imply putting in place a sequence of activities, rather than a single intervention. These frequently have to be repeated or readjusted according to changing and often reoccurring circumstances that lead to repeated traumas. Terr (1990, 1991), who worked with traumatized children, distinguishes 'single blow' traumas from repeated traumas. Whilst the former type have limited effect on children, repeated traumas may lead to serious and long-term consequences (i.e. denial, numbing, anger, despair, fatalism about their lives) that, in turn, can result in major personality changes. According to Terr, children who are exposed to repeated trauma begin to prepare mentally for the next assault. They expect future trauma and develop psychological defences to protect themselves. The same is true for many adults in times of war (Allen, 1995).

Under such circumstances 'early interventions' in communities may qualify as such, irrespective of the length of time that has passed since a first trauma was endured. For other beneficiaries early intervention will be 'repeated' as part of ongoing provision and sometimes may actually be a 'late' intervention. In fact, within the same community context, some such interventions may be provided immediately and early in a chronological sense, whilst others follow at a later stage when they are, in fact, early relative to new traumatic events. Furthermore, in a community exposed to massive violence, we typically deal with people who have been exposed to different traumatic events at different points in time. For example, in one refugee centre we were able to start providing interventions within a week after the group of some 600 people had fled from their home communities. In another, much larger centre, this became possible only 18 months after fleeing, because the population displacement extended over a 6-month period. All the same, the range of interventions was similar in both cases: building social structures and networks, providing individual and group treatment, structuring leisure time for children, recruiting providers from within the refugee community and so on (Ajdukovic and Joshi, 1999). These examples illustrate some of the practical implications of seeking to offer help and support to destabilized communities. They reinforce recognition that under such circumstances early intervention is not a one-off event, but should be ongoing and often repeated. This requires advanced planning, not only so as to mobilize resources for a protracted period of time, but also to ensure a whole range of interventions can be offered. This notion is illustrated by the sequence in Fig. 8.1.

It is not uncommon for a refugee career cycle to feature this circular relationship between repetitive trauma exposure and repeated early interventions. This cycle begins with the pre-flight period, extends over the flight and refugee periods, whatever their duration, and ends with the resettlement process (Ben-Porath, 1991). During the first two phases, refugees are commonly exposed to multiple traumatic experiences. These events tend to occur in a quick succession, but

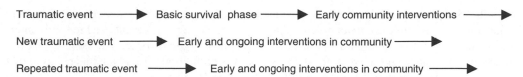

Traumatic event ———▶ Basic survival phase ———▶ Early community interventions ———▶

New traumatic event ———▶ Early and ongoing interventions in community ———▶

Repeated traumatic event ———▶ Early and ongoing interventions in community ———▶

Figure 8.1 Sequence of events and interventions in a community destabilized by organized violence.

at other times they reoccur after periods of relative safety. Return to and resettlement in the original communities is typically idealized as a solution to almost all the problems with which refugees are faced. However, an actual return can prove a highly re-traumatizing experience, when survivors are confronted with the realities of the destruction perpetrated on the fabric of their community. This reaction can be aggravated by contrasts between actual realities and long held idealizations that may have supported a displaced community during war (Ajdukovic, 1993).

At times therefore, the provision of early intervention under changing and complex circumstances can mean that those involved in delivering services may have to start all over again once the social context changes. A dramatic example of such a scenario arose when the 'Gaza' refugee centre in Croatia was shelled during the autumn of 1993. The attack went on for days until the refugees had to be evacuated to another location, where they remained for several months. The psychosocial support team that had been working with this refugee community since its original displacement found that, after this evacuation, both adult and child clients had regressed to a low level of functioning characteristic of their state when first admitted to the original refugee centre. Efforts to re-establish community structures and recreate a sense of community, whilst also continuing work with re-traumatized clients were dwarfed by a re-emergence of instability, insecurity and exposure to further life-threatening events. In fact, this proved true both for the refugees and care staff.

Preconditions for early interventions in a disrupted community

The degree of safety offered by a situation in which people live, as well as prevailing social and political circumstances, set contexts that allow trauma recovery to take place, but these considerations also set limits for what can be achieved by early intervention. Only when violence is no longer being perpetrated can trauma-healing processes begin. This consideration has substantial conceptual and practical implications for early interventions.

Since trauma recovery after armed conflict takes place in a specific social context, it is essential that the defining characteristics of the prevailing situation be acknowledged, and taken into account by those wishing to offer early help and support to affected populations. Under such circumstances healing should be seen as an interactive process that seeks to develop a range of relationships with affected communities. Their aims extend beyond those explicitly focusing on fostering mastery over post-traumatic symptoms. Therefore, healing of trauma is unlikely to be accomplished by any individual acting alone. Early intervention should seek to take account of all of life's relevant dimensions manifested within families, peer groups, communities and whole societies (Reichenberg and Friedman, 1996; Ayalon, 1998). How to start re-establishing supportive environments under circumstances where the very notion of belonging to a community has been disrupted is the critical challenge addressed by both early intervention and follow-up care.

For instance, under circumstances of organized violence we had to consider several such factors all at once or in close succession. In a western part of Croatia large numbers of people were affected and their needs were as great as they were diverse. The communities in question had been destabilized, uprooted and had become dysfunctional. Natural support resources were severely limited and trust within the communities had been broken. There was urgent need for early intervention, especially to promote trauma healing for the most highly exposed individuals, families and groups that had been forced to flee their homes. A precondition for making this possible was to promote normalization of functioning of the whole communities in exile.

Under such extreme conditions communities typically need outside help. This is because inner resources are insufficient to meet increased needs in the aftermath of organized violence. Help from the outside may include material resources (e.g. basic life provisions like food, clothing, heating, sanitation and building materials) and expertise to direct trauma-related work (e.g. identification and screening of trauma victims, psycho-education, counselling, trauma treatment, medication). However, the aim of this help should be to encourage local capacity building that leads to empowerment of the community. This is not an easy outcome to achieve, and we have encountered several situations where local care-providers have been insufficiently skilled to cope with new and immediate needs and demands for psychological first aid, trauma treatment, life skills building and reducing the increased prevalence of family violence.

Considering a strategy for early interventions

In communities destabilized by armed conflict, the symptoms exhibited by local people should not be viewed only through the lens of a particular trauma experienced by an individual leading to PTSD. An alternative and complementary conceptualization takes account of the social context of trauma, and the community construction of trauma and its sequelae. Wessells (1999) has argued that to pursue the former option is likely to lead to an inclination to advocate setting up mental health clinics and other specialist venues for delivering psychological and psychiatric services for trauma reactions. Although beneficial and necessary, specialized trauma care provision, with its narrow clinical focus, encounters serious limitations. For instance, such approaches tend to individualize problems and construe trauma as a phenomenon pertaining only to the individual. In turn, this distracts attention from wider social factors affecting the situation. Exclusively clinical conceptualization of trauma tends to overlook the hindering influences exerted by ongoing political oppression and discrimination.

A further consequence of such biases is that it can lead to over-simplified problem formulations resulting in under-estimation of resources required to promote community recovery. At worst, it may even result in resource misappropriation. Caution is appropriate so as not to impose ill-advised medicalized concepts that may lead to impositions of ready-made early intervention protocols developed in altogether different cultural contexts. The imperative for those seeking to offer early intervention after traumatization of whole communities is to be aware of systemic changes evoked by early interventions in the initial phase of an emergency and how these can facilitate empowerment of destabilized communities. Help that promotes community resources may be the intervention of choice.

Planning early community interventions

When planning both for early and follow-up interventions it is necessary to take into account that needs of individual members of a community may vary greatly. Some interventions will therefore not require high-level therapeutic skills. These interventions recommend themselves for typically serving many clients in a short time. Examples include providing information about missing ones, helping access other services, raising awareness about survivors' legal status, working towards early family reunification, providing basic emotional and social support, collecting narratives about traumatic experiences, guidance in structuring free time for children, adolescents and adults, etc. In these instances, providers can come from within the affected communities subject to their being given simple training and support. Other interventions requiring more sophisticated expertise are, generally speaking, indicated for the more limited number of community members who have reacted with extreme distress. This is important to bear in mind when planning the allocation of limited resources in the early aftermath of major social disruptions. Our experience (Ajdukovic, 1997) and advice offered by others (Koss and Harvey, 1991; MacQueen *et al.*, 1996; Awwad, 1999) suggest the following early intervention strategies can yield good results:

1. Provide direct services as soon as is feasible after the event. To do so may involve using mainly experienced service providers. Their complementary function is to serve as a resource to facilitate first-line capacity building that will in time become the platform for further help and support. Since destabilized communities lack inner resources, help may have to be temporarily brought in from the outside. However, it is of the greatest importance that needs assessment, planning and service delivery be done in full co-ordination with and explicit knowledge of local providers. Otherwise, importing resources into resource-scarce environments can increase competition and suspicion between the local authorities and providers. By giving early support to local providers and institutions attention is given to immediate needs. The strategy also provides opportunities for local resources to be rebuilt and strengthened. Outside help should at no time be imposed and calls for cultural understanding so as to effect respectful interfacing with indigenous resources, however limited these may be. In our opinion the challenge of coping with and adjusting constructively to the systemic destabilization of an affected community ultimately rests with the individuals and groups that comprise this very same community.

2. Empower local care-providers to assume ever-greater responsibilities for delivering services in their community. This can be achieved by providing in-field training from the beginning of an intervention. This increases professional self-esteem and helps local resources grow fast.

3. Work with key community figures and leaders, local media and governmental institutions, so that these are made aware of the benefits to be derived from early community-based interventions. This is crucial for increasing the likelihood of support for long-term follow-up and the sustainability of intervention programmes. Such approaches also recommend themselves for taking account of the importance of local value systems, resources that may be at the disposal of key figures and/or exist within their larger communities, and sets out to build upon these to once again restore more normal functioning.

When planning allocation of resources for community-based programmes that seek to target a range of needs, we have found the framework of public health policies to be very useful. Based on accumulated experience we have proposed a model named 'The pyramid of community psychosocial interventions'. It has evolved from earlier proposals by Richman (1996) and Ajdukovic (1998) and is described in Fig. 8.2.

Our model illustrates that most people in a community affected by organized violence are likely, in the first instance, to need basic psychosocial support. Typically, this can be successfully provided by 'natural helpers' and by putting in place systems for non-professionalized care provided by members of the community. The 'natural helpers' are individuals to whom other community members sometimes turn for advice and support when distressed. They are usually trusted members of the community who typically have good social skills and a capacity for empathy. They are well placed to communicate common wisdom that may be usefully thought of as 'reframing interventions' that help survivors see their situation from a more constructive perspective.

It is important for designated helpers to have access to basic information relevant to their assigned tasks. This can be arranged through short and inexpensive training courses and workshops. They should also have at their disposal leaflets and brochures to disseminate to a number of clients as a part of their designated work. It is also essential that they have access to consultation with mental health professionals when help and support is needed. In the case of early interventions, such provision typically needs to be provided by care-providers brought in from outside to help communities overcome the most acute phases of crises. Moving towards the top

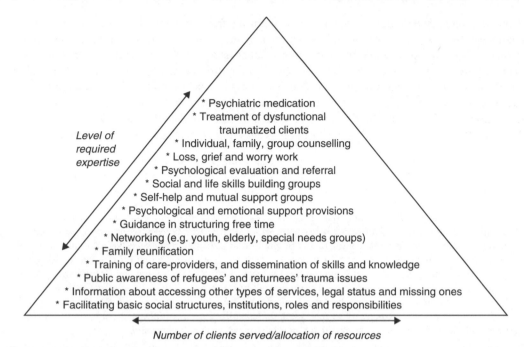

Level of required expertise

* Psychiatric medication
* Treatment of dysfunctional traumatized clients
* Individual, family, group counselling
* Loss, grief and worry work
* Psychological evaluation and referral
* Social and life skills building groups
* Self-help and mutual support groups
* Psychological and emotional support provisions
* Guidance in structuring free time
* Networking (e.g. youth, elderly, special needs groups)
* Family reunification
* Training of care-providers, and dissemination of skills and knowledge
* Public awareness of refugees' and returnees' trauma issues
* Information about accessing other types of services, legal status and missing ones
* Facilitating basic social structures, institutions, roles and responsibilities

Number of clients served/allocation of resources

Figure 8.2 Pyramid of community psychosocial interventions.

of 'The pyramid of community psychosocial interventions' further services targeted at a smaller number of community members should be supported by higher levels of expertise.

It is important to acknowledge that care-providers from within a community may themselves be traumatized. This is a serious limiting factor for the planning and delivery of help since key personnel can more easily become overwhelmed with their assigned work (Ajdukovic and Ajdukovic, 1998, 2000). However, because of the scale of community disruptions and the extent of actual need, there is no feasible alternative to involving community members in the provision of early intervention services, and ensuring that thorough professional support and supervision are available to attend to their mental health needs.

Early community interventions and prevention

Early community interventions should be comprehensive and not piecemeal. A community is a social structure and it is this that is the target of interventions. At the same time, this structure can be the facilitator for early interventions that address the needs of its individual members and con-stituent groups. There are many similarities between community-based programmes in general (e.g. prevention of youth delinquency, health prevention) and community interventions after massive violence. However, the major differences are that at times of peace community interventions seek to facilitate desirable social changes under conditions where active community agents are in place to help bring about transformations. When a community is traumatized through systematic violence, early interventions should be designed to facilitate constructive responses to the social changes that have been imposed. These are the first steps that help normalize community life through strengthening existing networks and structures, restoring old networks and establishing new ones (Segerstrom, 1995).

In unstable regions it is helpful to acknowledge the risks of future community disruptions and, from an early stage, set in place preventive approaches that anticipate disruptions that are likely to follow. In this respect, experiences gained within Israel (Lahad and Cohen, 1998) show that disruptions can be reduced by preparing civilian populations to cope with crises and disasters. For instance, by training local authorities to cope with critical situations and handle these effectively before, during and after they occur, as well as training professionals in emergency intervention techniques.

Early interventions as a means of social reconstruction after violence

The systemic community-based concept of early interventions presented here is embedded in the framework of empowerment of individual clients, families and whole communities. The core principle for this approach to early intervention after trauma is that it presumes a measure of resilience and coping in service users and their networks (Ayalon, 1998). It also looks for salutogenic effects that arise from such interventions. These may be conducive to longer-term post-traumatic growth of individuals and communities. This can occur not only at the level of symptoms engendered by trauma exposure (Antonovsky and Bernstein, 1986; Joseph *et al.*, 1993; Krizmanic and Kolesaric, 1996), but also at the level of re-establishing basic social structures and strengthening community coherence. The means for doing so may include providing immediate educational opportunities, providing non-formalized skills training for adolescents and adults, seeking to effect early family re-unification and re-establishing mutually supportive relationships (i.e. youth, women, elderly, single parents). Early supportive interventions are most useful when they restore or enhance normal role functioning, and especially so when they reinforce, rather than bypass, existing social structures (Heller, 1990).

To establish meaningful activities for adults, together with opportunities for developing new livelihoods and creating work opportunities are further provisions that have strong recovery effects in the early phase of assisting destabilized communities. In this regard, it is salutary to note that some early intervention initiatives that started with a medical orientation towards trauma treatment have recently recognized this. In Bosnia, the trauma project implemented by the Harvard Program in Refugee Trauma is now implementing a micro-enterprise component in its provision (Mollica, 2000).

The following list describes interventions that can usefully be implemented as part of the early phase of community-based psychosocial interventions:

- provide support that re-establishes basic social structures, roles and responsibilities;
- disseminate information (e.g. about legal status, missing family members, plans of community institutions);
- psycho-education for specific groups of beneficiaries (e.g. adolescents, children, elderly, parents, teachers, volunteer helpers, veterans);
- the provision of social and emotional support to families through a network of trained non-professional providers;
- the establishment of mutual support groups with similar interests, backgrounds or experiences;
- screening, identification and triage of the most highly affected individuals, families and groups;
- provisions for referral in highly specific cases (e.g. chronic psychiatric patients, dysfunctional torture victims);
- provide support and consultation to staff in community institutions (e.g. schools, community health clinics, churches, youth clubs) to re-establish their normal routines and re-empower staff to become able to provide specific support to community members;

- informal, recreational and creative activities;
- in-service training and follow-up support to local care-providers;
- meetings with community authorities and advising them on the status of mental health in the community and on planning priorities;
- network with all relevant community institutions, agencies and non-governmental organizations (e.g. community health clinics, centres for social work, schools, libraries, women's groups, scouts, relief organizations, etc.);
- briefings for the media and actively seek their participation in dissemination of basic knowledge that is helpful to affected populations (e.g. regular radio contact shows, writing articles for the local newspapers, printing and disseminating leaflets, etc.).

Community recovery and perception of justice

Another important condition that can facilitate or hinder community recovery after war relates to perceptions of justice and accountability. Most particularly, that individuals who are guilty of acts of violence, war crimes or atrocities should be brought to justice. It is with this consideration in mind that the International Crime Tribunal for Former Yugoslavia (ICTY) and the International Crime Tribunal for Rwanda (ICTR) were created by the UN Security Council to investigate and prosecute war criminals. These judicial initiatives presume that survivors of atrocities can begin to heal if truths about the recent past are acknowledged in public.

This introduces another challenge to care-providers involved in early interventions. Namely, that they must be prepared for and trained to deal with personal accounts of what has happened. Victims' narratives can help make sense of traumatic events, as in individual trauma therapy, and also meet the need of deeply hurt people to be heard. Traumatized victims of organized violence typically need to know the truth about 'missing important others' and also to find their own 'truths' about what has occurred. Unlike other types of traumatization, where facts and truths are usually much more self-evident and clear (i.e. traffic accidents, random sniper shooting), this is typically not as straightforward in instances of mass violence. The need to know facts and ascertain truths are connected to the social belief that accounting for past crimes, and bringing about justice is important for the process of achieving some measure of stabilization and safety for communities and their members. Truth and Reconciliation Commissions have been established in over 20 countries (Hayner, 1996) to collect testimonies from victims of organized violence with a view to facilitating some level of healing. In time, it is also hoped that this process might lesson tensions and hostilities between former adversaries. Therefore, early interventions might encompass making provision for trauma narratives both on the part of individual and community groups.

Assistance brought to a traumatized community from the outside should always aspire to be time limited. Therefore, it is essential that such help that is to be provided interfaces with and strengthen services that are available locally and help increase local competence. When planning delivery of outside assistance that responds to acute needs, the longer-term goal of community development should be kept in mind right from the very beginning. To do otherwise is to violate the key concept of empowerment as a core value for early intervention after trauma. In communities disrupted by organized violence, the ultimate goal is to re-establish and maintain peace. It is our belief that a crucial aspect of promoting this aim is to focus on social reconstruction of relational dimensions of communities. Its achievement depends on characteristics of the broader socio-political context, and it is through the reconstruction, strengthening and mobilization of these that systemic approaches to early intervention seek to exert its positive influences on communities traumatized by organized violence.

References

Ajdukovic, D. (1993) Model of psychological assistance to displaced people [Model pruzanja psiholoske pomoci prognanicima]. In Ajdukovic, D. (ed.) *Psychological Dimensions of Displacement* [*Psiholoske dimenzije progonstva*]. Zagreb: Alinea, pp. 25–42.

Ajdukovic, D. (1997) Challenges of training for trauma recovery. In Ajdukovic, D. (ed.) *Trauma Recovery Training: lessons learned*. Zagreb: Society for Psychological Assistance, pp. 27–37.

Ajdukovic, D. (1998) *Levels of Psychosocial Assistance to Returnees*, paper presented at the international conference 'Psychosocial support in post-war communities', Graz, April 17–20.

Ajdukovic, D. and Ajdukovic, M. (ed.) (2000) *Mental Health Care for Helpers*. Zagreb: Society for Psychological Assistance.

Ajdukovic, D. and Joshi, P.T. (ed.) (1999) *Empowering Children: psychosocial assistance under difficult circumstance*. Zagreb: Society for Psychological Assistance.

Ajdukovic, M. and Ajdukovic, D. (1998) Mental health care for helpers: experiences from a training program. In Arcel, L.T. (ed.) *War Violence, Trauma and the Coping Process*. Copenhagen: International Rehabilitation Council for Torture Victims, pp. 314–18.

Allen, J.G. (1995) *Coping with Trauma*. Washington DC: American Psychiatric Press.

Antonovsky, A. and Bernstein, J. (1986) Pathogenesis and salutogenesis in war and other crisis: who studies the successful coper? In Milgram, A.N. (ed.) *Stress and Coping in Time of War*. Philadelphia: Brunner/Mazel.

Awwad, E. (1999) Between trauma and recovery: some perspectives on Palestinian vulnerability and adaptation. In Nader, K., Dubrow, N. and Stamm, B.H. (eds) *Honoring Differences: issues in the treatment of trauma and loss*. Philadelphia: Brunner/Mazel, pp. 234–66.

Ayalon, O. (1998) Community healing for children traumatized by war. *Int Rev Psychiat* **10**, 224–33.

Ben-Porath, Y.S. (1991) The psycho-social adjustment. In Westermeyer, J., Williams, C.L. and Nguyen, A.N. (eds) *Mental Health Services for Refugees*. Washington DC: US Government Printing Office, pp.1–23.

Blackwell, R.D. (1989) *The Disruption, and Reconstitution of Family, Network and Community Systems Following Torture, Organized Violence and Exile*. London: Medical Foundation.

Brom, D. and Kleber, R.J. (1989) Prevention of post-traumatic stress disorders. *J Traumat Stress*, **2**, 335–51.

Chemtob, C. (1996) *Dynamic Processing in Trauma*. Unpublished lecture, Society for Psychological Assistance, Zagreb.

Freeman, C., Graham, P. and Bowyer, D. (2000) *Psychological First Aid Replacement for Psychological Debriefing*. Edinburgh: Rivers Centre.

Gutlove, P. (1999) *Conflict, Conflict Management and Trauma Recovery*. Cambridge: Institute for Resource and Security Studies.

Hayner, P. (1996) Commissioning the truth: further research questions. *Third World Q* **17**, 19–29.

Heller, K. (1990) Social and community intervention. *Ann Rev Psychol* **41**, 141–68.

Herman, J. (1992) *Trauma and Recovery*. New York: Basic Books.

Joseph, S., Williams, R. and Yule, W. (1993) Changes in outlook following disaster: the preliminary development of a measure to assess positive and negative responses. *J Traumat Stress*, **6**, 271–9.

Kleber, R.J. (2000) *Psychosocial Acute Care: current state of research on coping with trauma and acute stress interventions*. Paper presented at Psycho-social Acute Care in the Event of a Crisis Workshop, Vienna, 14–22 May 2000.

Koss, M.P. and Harvey, M.R. (1991) *The Rape Victim: clinical and community interventions*. San Francisco: Sage.

Krizmanic, M. and Kolesaric, V. (1996) Salutogenic model of psychosocial help. *Rev Psychol* **3**, 69–75.

Lahad, M. and Cohen, A. (1998) 18 years of community stress prevention. In Ayalon, O., Lahad, M. and Cohen, A. (eds) *Community Stress Prevention*, Vol. 3. Kiryat Shmona: Community Stress Prevention Centre.

MacQueen, G., Neufeld, V., Peters, M.A. and Barbara, J.S (1996) *A Health-To-peace Handbook*. Hamilton: War and Health Program of McMaster University.

Mollica, R. (2000) Invisible wounds. *Scient Am* **282**, 54–7.

Peddle, N., Monteirlo, C., Guluma, V. and Macauley, T.E.A. (1999) Trauma, loss and resilience in Africa: a psychosocial community based approach to culturally sensitive healing. In Nader, K., Dubrow, N. and Stamm, B.H. (eds) *Honoring Differences: issues in the treatment of trauma and loss*. Philadelphia: Brunner/Mazel, pp. 121–49.

Punamaki, R.L. (1987) *Children in the Shadow of War: a psychological study on attitudes and emotional life of Israeli and Palestinian children*, Research Report 23. Tempere: Tempere Peace Research Institute.

Reichenberg, D. and Friedman, S. (1996) Traumatized children. In Danieli, Y., Rodely, N. and Weisaeth, L. (eds) *International Response to Traumatic Stress*. New York, Baywood, pp. 307–26.

Richman, N. (1996) *Principles of Help for Children Involved in Organized Violence*. London: Save the Children.

Segerstrom, E. (1995) *Focus on Refugee Children*. Stockholm: Radda Barnen.

Terr, L. (1990) *Too Scare to Cry*. New York: Harper Collins.

Terr, L. (1991) Childhood traumas: an outline and overview. *Am J Psychiat* **148**, 10–20.

Wessells, M.G. (1999) Culture, power, and community: Intercultural approaches to psychosocial assistance and healing. In Nader, K., Dubrow, N. and Stamm, B.H. (ed.) *Honoring Differences: issues in the treatment of trauma and loss*. Philadelphia: Brunner/Mazel, pp. 267–82.

Section 3 The new evidence base for reconstructing early intervention after trauma

Early intervention after trauma will not be reconstructed by only broadening its theoretical base. Equally important for developing informed practice is an emergent evidence base from modern psychotraumatology. Some of this derives from studies focusing specifically on aspects of early intervention. Also to be incorporated is other recent evidence that has helped improve understanding of trauma and reactions evoked in their aftermath. Section 3 reviews this body of new evidence and considers its relevance for service improvement.

Early intervention has a track record of enthusiastic promotion, but a core weakness inherent in such advocacy is that scant regard has been given to adjustments achieved by survivors who do not receive formal help and support. In the absence of this elementary baseline information it is not possible to foster informed debate about the potential of early intervention to change the course of trauma reactions and improve prognosis. Evidence engendered by non-intervention studies generates benchmarks against which a case for reconstructed early intervention can be made.

The value of such studies is demonstrated in the chapter authored by Professor Ulrich Schnyder and Dr Hanspeter Moergeli of University Hospital, Zurich, Switzerland. Their results do not support a case for routine early intervention for all accident victims since an overwhelming majority made satisfactory adjustments to unfolding events. However, some subjects reported accident-related difficulties characterized by marked fluctuations during the follow-up period. For these individuals a case can be made for reconstructed early intervention. But the veracity of this argument hinges on screening instruments being developed to correctly identify individuals at greatest risk and conducting randomized controlled trials to establish which early interventions are effective and efficacious. By implication, evidence-based practice is no simple aspiration for reconstructed early intervention. The complexities and uncertainties with which it wrestles are legion.

Given the magnitude of difficulties engendered by these complexities anyone might be forgiven for feeling despondent or hopeless about the prospects of ever reconstructing early intervention. For Professors Arik Shalev and Robert Ursano, respectively, at Hadassah University Hospital in Jerusalem, Israel and the Uniformed Services University of the Health Sciences in Bethesda, Maryland, USA, a lack of initial clarity has inspired a resolve to structure and make sense of the evidence at hand. In this regard they have been commendably successful. By elucidating the phased, but not necessarily sequential, nature of acute traumatic stress reactions they help redefine early intervention as a broad repertory of flexibly administered services.

Conceptually, they shift these forms of help and support towards the notion of psychological first aid, defer considerations of symptom elimination and psychological therapy to a later stage. A distinct advantage of this perspective is that decisions about what to do in the early aftermath of trauma can be informed, to a considerable extent, by the predominant needs expressed by survivors during each progressive phase of post-trauma adjustment. These authors transform an apparently confusing body of evidence into a sensible set of rationales for what to do and when.

By implication, assessment of need becomes central to reconstructed early intervention. This can take many forms, but as mentioned above, screening for risk of longer-term problems is a particularly important challenge. Professor Chris Brewin of University College, London, Suzanna Rose who founded the West Berkshire Traumatic Stress Service and Bernice Andrews at Royal Holloway, Surrey, England detail the principles for doing so and describes techniques serving this end. Data secured from assault victims soon after the crime and at follow-up suggests that three or more intrusive re-experiencing symptoms predict longer-term adjustment difficulties. This is a line of investigation that holds great promise for reconstructed early intervention in so far that resources can be mobilized to help and support those in greatest need.

This new, systematic and evidence-based approach to assessment recognizes all trauma carry their own distinct risks and also that each incident creates a survivor population whose characteristics are far from uniform. Emergent needs may usefully be construed as belonging to a spectrum ranging from extreme dependence on help and support to autonomous coping conducive to positive adjustment. The latter group warrants more detailed study because reconstructed early intervention should aspire to foster adaptive coping strategies in all survivor groups. This recognition led Roderick Ørner, who established a staff support service for emergency services personnel in Lincolnshire, England, to conduct a survey of coping and adjustment strategies habitually used by experienced officers to mitigate reactions evoked by work-related trauma. Findings reported in his chapter amount to a new evidence base for early intervention. It engenders radically different recommendations about how best to help and support emergency responders. Further investigations will establish if the coping and adjustment strategies used to good effect amongst these survivors can engender similar benefits for other individuals or groups recently exposed to trauma.

9 A psychodynamically orientated intervention strategy for early reactions to trauma

Lionel Bailly

Introduction

The type of therapeutic intervention used by an institution at any particular time depends upon the state of the science and theory that inform its leading clinicians. Also important are their status within the wider scientific establishment, and also the traditions and history of its founding institutions.

Psychiatric early intervention for individuals exposed to potentially traumatic situations was initiated in periods of war by military medical services. It was the Russian army that first started front-line psychiatry during the Russo-Japanese war in 1904–5. Towards the end of the World War I, the British and US armies also took up this practice. France was a latecomer on the scene, instituting early intervention services for its troops only after the World War II. By then, the clinicians heading the French military mental health teams were psychiatrists, mostly with a psychodynamic training (Crocq, 1999). Consequently, the theoretical approaches that have most influenced early intervention practice in France have been psychoanalysis and phenomenological psychiatry (Crocq 1999).

Mitchell's formal prescriptions for Critical Incident Stress Debriefing (CISD) in 1983 (Mitchell, 1983) were noted with interest in France and provided an incentive to develop early intervention services in non-military settings. However, because local practitioners were committed to a different theoretical position from that which underpinned CISD, the type of early intervention that has evolved in France differs from that of many other countries. Furthermore, the development in the 1980s of Non-Governmental Organizations (NGOs) like Médecins Sans Frontières, Médecins du Monde, Handicap International, etc., provided arenas for delivering and evolving this particular form of practise (Moro and Lebovici, 1995). In 1996, after several terrorist bombing campaigns in France (especially Paris), the French President ordered the creation of a national network of teams that could be mobilized to provide early interventions after major critical events (Crocq, 1998). The functional units of this network are called *Cellules d'Urgence Médico Psychologiques* and their operational brief is to work in close co-operation with the emergency services. Their creation confronted practitioners and planners with such key issues as which methods of early intervention to use, what kinds of professionals should lead the services, how to train newcomers and how to assess the outcomes of these interventions.

Theory and rationales for psychoanalytic early intervention (PEI)

Some of the concepts traditionally used in psychoanalytic psychotherapy are used unchanged in PEI, others have been adapted in recognition of the particularities of early intervention in trauma cases.

Stress, trauma and traumatic stress

Psychoanalytic theory makes a clear distinction between stress and trauma. Stress is construed as a psychophysiological reaction to an external threat (Barrois, 1989; Briole *et al.*, 1996; Lebigot *et al.*, 2001). An individual in this state can identify the stressor and talk about it. Traumatic events are said to be those external situations that confront the psyches of individual survivors with their own death (Briole *et al.*, 1996). Psychoanalytic theory also distinguishes between the traumatic event and trauma. The latter is the subjective experience of the external event. Immediately after the event the traumatized subject will experience fear and anxiety, but not stress as defined above. Post-trauma psychopathology is therefore not considered to be a stress disorder (Barrois, 1989; Briole *et al.*, 1996; Crocq, 1999; Lebigot *et al.*, 2001). This hypothesis is supported by recent research into the psychobiology of PTSD, which demonstrates that evoked changes in cortisol levels after traumatic events are the opposite of those found for stress reactions (Yehuda, 1999).

The place of language in trauma and the role of speech in PEI

It is not uncommon for trauma victims to say that no words can describe what they have been through. For practitioners of PEI this is the crux of the matter. For instance, Lacan has attributed to the psyche of the fields of the Real, the Imaginary and the Symbolic. Language is the architecture and medium of the Symbolic, while the Real refers to the raw sensorial input that may have no place in the Imaginary and may not ever be symbolizable. In this model of the psyche, the traumatic response represents an eruption of the Real and therefore unsymbolizable (or unspeakable) into consciousness (Lacan, 1966). The individual who experiences trauma is overwhelmed with terror and cannot describe the subjective experience in words. Typically, too, the traumatized individual has experienced a failure of psychological defence mechanisms and is left with the raw sensorial memory of the event. This will be re-experienced until such time that it can be encoded into a symbolic form, i.e. expressed in language and, subsequently, be stored as a memory. In Lacanian theory, this difference between re-experiencing and remembering is the difference between a psychological event existing in the Real or the Symbolic fields. The task of therapists is to facilitate the transition from the former to the latter. The process of healing or working through is usually achieved through the construction of a discourse (a position as revealed through language), which gives expression to the subjective experience evoked by the traumatic incident.

It is because trauma 'is beyond' discourse that PEI makes a special point of offering victims an opportunity to create discourse during the initial phase for processing traumatic experiences (Daligand, 1997). PEI encourages victims to create a narrative of subjective experiences of the event as a bridge to becoming aware of the incomprehensible emotions triggered by it. Once this has been achieved victims are considered to have taken a major step towards realizing the possible subjective meanings of what has happened.

Transference and counter-transference

Transference is a concept proposed by Freud (1895) to describe some central features of the relationship that unfolds between patient and therapist. In particular, attention is drawn to the affective component of that link, the establishment of which is automatic and largely unconscious. Transference creates a 'new edition' of relationships rooted in the individual's past. So, in patients imagination therapists comes to represent different aspects of characters that have played important roles in shaping the course and development of their own lives. Transference can be positive or negative. In the former case, patients may experience warm and friendly feelings towards their therapists. Positive transference will support the patient's efforts to work through critical and formative life events, and will facilitate disclosure of intimate thoughts. When transference is negative patients may experience anger and suspicion towards therapists, and this can interfere with the therapeutic process.

In PEI transference demands particularly careful management for two important reasons: first, clinical practice with trauma cases suggests that the transference unfolds in a particularly marked manner. Therapists are often idealized as 'saviours' and the only persons 'who understand' what has happened. Negative transference may be equally strong, with the patient thinking that the therapist is motivated by curiosity, does not really care and is part of some conspiracy to hurt.

Secondly, according to psychoanalytic theory transference becomes more complex in group therapy situations (Briole *et al.*, 1996). In PEI, where these two factors are reunited, particular attention must be paid to the process.

Counter-transference describes feelings of therapist toward their patients and may in some cases interfere with therapeutic interventions. For instance, if a therapist is too pleased to be perceived as a saviour or is hurt by a patient's suspicion or rejection. In the context of group early intervention, uncontrolled counter-transference may compromise the whole intervention (Bailly, 1996).

Trauma and grief

Although loss is often associated with trauma it is not an objective of PEI to facilitate the mourning process. This form of intervention is therefore not prescribed for bereaved people who have not been exposed to a traumatic event. Confusion may arise from the fact that in common parlance, bereavement is often described as 'traumatic' in itself. However, unless the bereaved have witnessed the death of loved ones in traumatic circumstances it does not fulfil the criterion of 'confronting the psyche with its own death'. So, for instance in the aftermath of a plane crash PEI should be offered to survivors of the incident, but not to the people who were waiting at the airport for the plane to arrive. The bereaved have particular needs that may be addressed through support offered in groups, but their suffering is qualitatively different to *trauma* in the terms described above. Their plight is not the result of exposure to a concrete scene of destruction and death, but is the consequence of a loss experienced within the norms of human society.

PEI: a talking cure—but will any form of discourse do?

According to the theory that informs Psychoanalytic Early Intervention the mere act of talking about traumatic events does not in itself have a therapeutic effect (Crocq, 1999). A 'journalistic' discourse may concentrate on factual aspects of the experience at the expense or in total denial of emotions evoked by the incident. The point of PEI is to help subjects give expression to their subjective experience of the trauma and arrive at a symbolic representation of it. A narrative that does not contain subjects' reactions and emotions contributes nothing towards this aim.

In some cases, a focus on factually informative, but non-emotional discourse may be a symptom of the trauma itself in so far that subjects avoid painful feelings associated with the event.

Another type of narrative which PEI regards as pathological is when individuals fall into an increasingly dissociative state, while telling their experiences in a highly dramatic way.

Trance like discourse does not facilitate the symbolization of the traumatic experience because the individual is not fully conscious of what is being said. There is also a danger that those who listen to such accounts, particularly if they are not properly trained may become enthralled or so impressed by what they hear they become unable to perform their therapeutic role. Untrained non-mental health professionals, such as NGO workers, deployed in war zones have reported this phenomenon. Their accounts may be excessively empathic and expressed as hugging primary victims or crying with them. Near the other extreme of reactions is a strongly felt urge to reject victims.

So, in PEI therapists encourage subjects to make a conscious effort to find the best available words (signifiers) to describe a unique set of subjective experiences. A PEI group session involves a therapist asking survivors to tell what they have experienced and will steer them, through questions and comments, away from purely factual descriptions of the event towards descriptions of feelings and thoughts. On occasions when the emotional content of narratives run particularly high therapists will try to reduce the inclination subjects to use dissociation as a defence mechanism. They do this by intervening when discourse switches from enunciation of the trauma to a re-experiencing of it.

Do survivors have to ask to be debriefed?

In psychoanalytical therapy, it is considered crucial that patients make explicit their wish to undertake treatment. However, in trauma cases, it is often difficult to apply this rule because survivors often believe that nothing can be done and nobody can really help (Barrois, 1989). Therefore, a third party who is mindful of survivors' best interests frequently makes the initial request for professional help. That third party may be an institution or an organization (e.g. an airline or the military), and if they order all implicated personnel to attend for mandatory early intervention, the 'compulsory' character of the service procured may interfere with the survivors' motivation to participate. Survivors may also feel that the organizational response is partly an attempt to stop recriminations or absolve itself of responsibility for what has happened.

As practised, while PEI does not require that all individuals demonstrate an eagerness to take part in the group treatment. The issue of whether participation is voluntary or enforced is therefore routinely addressed at the beginning sessions. From the start therapists must make clear both their independence, and that the primary aim of the intervention is to serve the interests of all individuals present and not the commissioning organization.

Aim of intervention

The aim of PEI is to prevent post-traumatic psychopathology. It provides a setting in which the early symbolization of traumatic experiences can begin. Victims are offered opportunities to find words that go some way towards describing their subjective experiences of the traumatic event. The group dynamic should facilitate the creation of individual narratives in which each subject discovers that other group members may also have experienced similar emotions. This insight can help resolve feelings of isolation harboured by participants.

The many perspectives provided by group members for the same event aid each individual's search for a personal interpretation of what has happened. Whether it is the differences of the others' accounts or their similarity, the various points of view, and responses that are articulated may help each participant realize the completely personal and unique nature of their reactions, and also that in large measure, traumatic events are random and senseless. For example, survivors may find themselves struggling to discover personal meanings linked to their involvement in a train crash. A PEI meeting will therefore seek to help them separate out those elements of their personal histories that relate to their presence on that train and their reactions during the incident itself, as well as the external elements of chance that led to the crash.

Who is qualified to facilitate Psychoanalytical Early Intervention?

Given its distinct theoretical framework PEI is a highly specialized and sophisticated treatment. It addresses the aftermath of psychological trauma, which should be regarded as one of the most complex areas in mental health, and can involve exposure of therapists to disturbing stories of violence or destruction. In France, PEI therapists are mental health professionals (psychotherapists, psychiatrists, psychologists and family therapists) who have had training in psychotherapy and are experienced in the management of strong emotional reactions expressed in a group context. Questions of responsibility, blame, ethics and justice are commonly at the forefront of the minds of survivors who often challenge therapists on these issues so that PEI may require particularly delicate and experienced handling.

Technical considerations for the provision of psychoanalytic early intervention (PEI)

Preconstituted groups versus groups of victims

PEI is usually easier to administer to groups constituted before their exposure to potentially traumatic events (e.g. emergency service staff, military personnel) than to groups of survivors with no common background. The guiding principle of military psychiatrists in France is that 'Only briefed individuals can be debriefed' (Lebigot et al., 2001). This aphorism derives from the fact that PEI was initially designed for established groups of people deployed for a common purpose strengthened by a common history, shared standards of professional practice, agreed ideals etc. It is assumed such groups will have a strong group identity that is strengthened by facing danger together so as to provide reassurance and support. When group members have known one another before the traumatic event it is possible for each individual's psychological condition at the time of or immediately prior to a PEI to be compared with pre-incident adjustments and functioning (Lebigot 2001).

When PEI is offered to individuals not pre-constituted as established groups the principal link between members will be the shared traumatic incident. Apart from this event members may have nothing in common and, consequently, therapists may have to address strong group conflicts. For instance, with no formalized common aim at the time of an incident (no briefing) and no rank-related guidance (no leadership) during the event survivors may have behaved and responded in completely different ways. Some may have tried to help fellow victims, whilst others were preoccupied with ensuring their own survival. There may also have been conflicts between victims during the incident that had serious material consequences. This was illustrated during the inquest into the sinking of the Herald of Free Enterprise in Zeebrugge harbour. It interviewed some passengers who had survived by denying fellow travellers access to safe platforms, as well as survivors who were relatives of those who perished for this very reason.

In either type of group, PEI therapists sometimes find survivors identify so strongly with one another that low tolerance is shown towards emergent differences in accounts given by group members. A powerful pressure is exerted towards identifying a single definitive and common narrative that describes everybody's experience as one. This lofty ideal is an impossibility, which runs the danger of denying the individuality of each group member.

Group PEI versus individual PEI

It is possible to adapt the group PEI technique for single subject sessions. In certain circumstances individual PEIs may be strongly indicated. Therapists do not provide a 'classical' psychodynamic therapy session that generally lasts around 50 minutes and involve non-directive styles of interviewing. Instead, the session follows the same framework as used for group PEI (see sub-section on practical organization of PEI group sessions and contraindications below), and explores the objective and subjective perceptions of the traumatic event without necessarily emphasizing the person's critical life events pre-trauma.

Compared with group PEI a one-to-one relationship tends to promote deeper reflections about what has happened. It can also facilitate more personal disclosures about pre-existing conflicts experienced at a subjective or institutional level. Survivors also talk to therapists about matters relating to the future of their jobs or their private lives that should not be addressed in group sessions.

The one-to-one session is typically much longer than a psychotherapy session (approximately 90 minutes) and therapists take a less neutral stance in the proceedings. Complete neutrality could be experienced by survivors as lack of empathy or even to condone perpetrators. Therapists intervene more, ask more questions, make comments and formulate hypotheses relevant to the situation. In one-to-one PEI, a dialogue is created through which therapists come to symbolically represent a prototypical listener for the survivor.

The confidentiality and closeness associated with the one-to-one relationship is particularly useful when shame and guilt are experienced, or when important issues of responsibility and ethics are involved. An example would be a war veteran who shot a wounded friend during their escape from an ambush because he could not run to a departing rescue helicopter. The traumatized veteran said he was complying with an order not to leave any prisoners, but the experience was making him reassess the entire ethical basis of his involvement in the war. It is doubtful that group PEI, particularly that offered to his pre-constituted group, would have helped this man address these issues.

When and where?

It is not necessary to provide PEI immediately after traumatic events when survivors' primary needs are security, comfort and rest. Interventions should ideally take place between 2 and 5 days post-incident, but each instance should be considered on its own merits and characteristics. There may be occasions when an 'early intervention-like' session might be appropriate a long time after traumatic incidents. For instance, if the individuals concerned have been subjected to long-term traumatization or have been unable to access PEIs sooner (e.g. with victims of torture released from prison or people who have been trapped for some time in a war zone; Bailly, 1996). Such sessions are often a means to initiate longer-term treatment or to formally acknowledge that, on available evidence, survivors have managed to resolve their traumatic experiences without professional help.

PEI with pre-constituted groups should take place at venues that gives the organization to which they belong some form of symbolic or actual representation. This helps emphasize group identity shared by individuals participating in PEIs and demonstrates that the institution considers early intervention to be good professional practice. The institution must be cognisant of felt worries within the groups about confidentiality. A practical example is that venues allocated for PEI meetings should ensure participants will not meet their colleagues or managers.

Survivors with no pre-trauma group identity are usually offered venues for PEI sessions that anticipate the therapeutic process. So, it is not recommended that survivors of a public transport disaster meet in premises belonging to the company that runs the service in question. To do so might focus anger felt by participants to such an extent as to compromise the full process of PEI sessions.

Ideally, organizations most directly implicated in traumatic events should meet costs of holding PEI meetings and provide suitable premises for this purpose. Participants should be told who is paying for PEI services before sessions begin, and that this is consistent with sensible organizational practices intended to show concern for survivors and that this is a first step towards reparation.

In practical terms, premises must be comfortable, soundproofed and allow enough privacy for proceedings to be carried out without interruption. Care should be taken to exclude physical reminders of the ordeal (pictures on the wall, the sound of planes or trains, etc.) and it should be possible for participants to temporarily leave the main session room without meeting outsiders.

For who is PEI indicated?

All those who have experienced a potentially traumatic event should be offered PEIs and survivors should ideally be seen together. In practice, this means that those who belong to an organization connected with a traumatic incident, but not directly present and subject to it should not be invited to take part. Outsiders other than therapists should be excluded and media representatives should never attend. Given the military origins of PEI much experience has been gained about how hierarchical issues affect its practice. Line managers and superiors should only be included in group sessions if they were present at the traumatic event. While relationships of rank may inhibit self-expression within groups, trained therapists can use their presence to facilitate discussion. Exclusion of trauma survivors may lead to distorted or biased narratives that engender myths and fantasies about the event. This may inhibit recovery.

The same considerations apply to pre-constituted groups of juveniles (school groups, playgroups, scouts, etc.). It is not recommended that anyone not present during critical events be present at PEIs. This includes parents and other carers who typically have their own, but different needs. To address these, independent group meetings may be convened to run concurrently with PEIs. In preparation, the process is explained to parents and consent is required before children are asked if they wish to participate. Similarly, pupils absent during traumatic events endured by classmates should not be offered PEI. Instead, group or one-to-one counselling can be offered, as would be the case for other pupils at the same school. Exclusion of those not directly exposed to critical events is intended to create a clear space to express themselves and recognize they have been through something exceptional. The presence of others might obfuscate rationales informing PEIs and raise questions in the minds of survivors about why they are there (control? voyeurism?).

It is in the spirit of PEI to try to arrange for all survivors to be seen together when large numbers of people have been exposed to traumatic events. The rationale is that each participant had a unique role in unfolding incidents and a complete narrative can be formed only if all are present. This guidance prevents situations arising in which questions raised by survivors in one group can only be answered by someone participating in another. A further consideration is that the process of splitting large groups is rarely random and may therefore unintentionally contribute to the formation of subgroups. Each may form a 'biased' view of an event and the reactions that it has provoked. However, this guidance has to be balanced against the consideration that PEI with groups comprising more than thirty members presents considerable technical difficulties.

Practical organization of PEI group sessions

Pre-session arrangements

A minimum of two therapists is required to conduct PEI group interventions. One will lead groups through the therapeutic process in accordance with technical imperatives that will have been discussed and agreed beforehand by the therapists. Paramount amongst these technical considerations are agreements about who will lead sessions, what time limitations may apply, the suitability of assigned rooms and their general location. Attention should also be given to other users of the building to ensure privacy for group participants is respected throughout meetings and that interruption will not be tolerated.

The preliminary phase

Sessions start when therapists ask all present to switch off mobile phones and pagers so as to avoid unwelcome intrusions and disruptions. Next they introduce themselves before briefly stating why it is felt that PEI is indicated. Participants are told no time limit has been set for treatment sessions (unless otherwise agreed), but that PEI rarely lasts less than an hour-and-a-half and only occasionally exceeds 3 hours. Reassurance is offered that normal rules of confidentiality apply. To reinforce this point therapists explain the nature of their relationship with managers of the employing institution or organization, and policies agreed for the storage of notes taken during sessions, who can access these and for how long they will be kept, etc.

The clinical phase

Group members are then encouraged to describe, in their own words and drawing on their own experiences, what has happened. No pre-set order is followed for survivors to volunteer their contributions. If necessary, therapists will gently encourage reluctant members to offer their accounts, whilst subtly restraining the more talkative ones. Group members who start talking about emotions at this early stage will *not* be stopped. No common or group narrative is looked for at this stage. Each person's story is a subjective account rich in emotional nuance drawing on different aspects of what has happened. These different perspectives combine to engender a progressively more precise picture of the event for each participant, in both its objective and subjective dimensions.

Therapists intervene if participants dissociate during sessions and take steps to prevent other than verbally articulated re-experiencing of events during group meetings. Such re-experiencing by one group member might disturb other participants and has limited therapeutic effects. Thus, PEI is not a cathartic method in the usual psychoanalytical sense. It is 'cathartic' only in accordance with ancient historical meanings given to the word. In Greek tragedy the moment of Catharsis occurs towards the end of a play at the point at which the chorus moves from one side of the stage to the other and presents the audience with the hidden message of that play (Crocq, 1999). PEI engenders this process to help survivors negotiate a transition from the chaos of incomprehension to an elaborated discourse and narrative about personal experience.

To engender this process therapists seek to minimize deviations into non-trauma related matters or pre-existing conflicts that may have existed within the groups. Participants are also strongly dissuaded from disclosing plans and projects they may have regarding their future jobs or private lives.

Therapists offer no early interpretations based on survivors' narratives. When therapists realize some critical aspect events are systematically avoided by participants, they will guide their groups towards addressing these issues by fielding questions alluding to them.

At no point should therapists seek to de-dramatize description that bear witness of the real drama endured by survivors. If this guidance is transgressed participants may suspect the realities of individual experience are being denied, possibly in the service of therapists' own needs to protect themselves (Damiani, 2001).

The closure phase

Towards the end of PEI sessions therapists may intervene in different ways. Still avoiding personal interpretations therapists introduce their own hypotheses of each traumatic event and encourage group members to formulate their own formulations. For example, if after a 2-hour group meeting participants have difficulties coming to terms with the meaning of a particular event, a therapist may suggest that the event may not, in itself, have a meaning.

Since groups usually work without imposed time limits sessions will come to an end when participants have had a reasonable opportunity to express themselves and, in so doing, have created a complex and emotionally truthful story. This can take several hours, and should neither be hastened nor allowed to continue for too long. If therapists or survivors feel sessions are ending prematurely, this indicates they may be trying to avoid difficult aspects of critical events. On the other hand, extended sessions may signal a failure on the part of therapists to stop the participants' discourse becoming re-experiencing or have failed to provide guidance necessary for groups to arrive at useful understandings of events.

If, at the end of a session, some participants want to talk more, it is usual practice to offer one-to-one sessions within a few days. Group PEI should be limited to one session only since further meetings cannot capture the specificity of the original sessions. One-to-one consultations initially involve an exploration of the reasons why a person has asked for more professional help. In practice, the survivors in question will often have been reluctant to publicly address the more disturbing aspects of their own experiences or disclose relevant aspects of their own past life histories. If they ask for more than two additional sessions discussions should focus on the possibility of embarking on a course of psychotherapy.

It is not unusual for managerial hierarchies of organizations to seek information about what happened during PEIs. However, the guarantee of confidentiality given to the group is a crucial condition for the success of this form of early intervention. The rule should therefore not be compromised. To allays concerns expressed in some PEIs that managers may use information shared during meetings to promote or dismiss staff implicated, it is common practice for sessions to be facilitated external professionals at venues away from the organizations central offices or headquarters. This is now a formally sanctioned policy of the French non-governmental organization Médecins Du Monde.

Contra-indications of Psychoanalytical Early Intervention

PEI is contra-indicated for any group containing a member who is partly responsible or is perceived by the others to be responsible for or in some way contributed adversely to its unfolding and outcome. If a therapist realizes during the course of a session that such circumstances are at play the session should be stopped immediately. There are also practical difficulties inherent in conducting PEIs if serious conflict existed within the group before the trauma and therapists must make sure that early intervention should not be used as an opportunity to settle scores.

PEI is also contraindicated for groups where a strong ideology has fostered a view of some members as infallible heroes. This may occur in some extreme political or religious groups for whom discourse cannot be as free as is required for PEI. Group denial may produce a fake narrative of what happened that is akin to propaganda. Members of such a group may perceive feelings of fear or helplessness as unforgivable weaknesses or even as a betrayal of the core values and purposes of the organization.

Families should not be offered PEI because the discourse of each participant does, generally speaking, not carry equal weight within the group. The setting itself might also expose children to their parents' fears and sense of helplessness so as to render this a further trauma. Parents may also experience great difficulties when faced with the intensity of their childrens' distress.

Clinicians trained in PEI can use of some of its techniques during sessions with traumatized families. For instance, by recommending that details of traumatic events be addressed early rather than later and by emphasizing the importance of each individual's subjective account of what happened. There may also be a need to explore emotions and thoughts, rather than facts alone, but families should not be offered single extended early interventions with several PEI therapists present. A better alternative is a more classic form of therapeutic family intervention provided within the usual prescribed contexts by appropriately trained and experienced professionals.

Convening a one-to-one PEI session

With single survivor meetings one therapist facilitates long sessions that will typically be shorter than group sessions. The phases are the same as in group PEI (see section C-5), but therapists have to be more active because there are no other survivors with whom to discuss the event. A challenge for therapist in this situation is not to treat a session as if it were the first of a long series.

Future perspectives

CISD from a psychodynamic perspective

A comparison between CISD and PEI reveals several significant differences. First, CISD is a protocol-driven technique, rather than a highly specialized form of psychotherapy. Therefore, CISD meetings have been advocated as appropriate for a large variety of survivor populations and can be facilitated by individuals with very little experience of mental health care. A possible reason for poor outcomes in some CISD evaluations (Rose and Bisson, 1998; Conlon *et al.*, 1999; Rose *et al.*, 1999) could be attributed to using non-mental health professionals as debriefers.

The strictly defined phases of CISD meetings may frustrate survivors who feel a desire to talk freely about what they have been through at a time of their own choosing. In CISD disclosures of reactions and impressions are more likely to occur at times deemed appropriate by group facilitators. Attempts made in CISD to offer reassurance may be experienced by survivors as promises unlikely to be fulfilled. An implied de-dramatization of what has happened can also be perceived as a denial of suffering. In comparison, PEI allows survivors to tell their stories at their own pace and in the way that suits them best. One of the guiding principles of PEI is to anticipate survivors' emotional turmoil and help them overcome fear that may be experienced about exploring feelings. PEI also recognizes that particular reactions such as guilt and shame are not necessarily misplaced, and sets out to explore their meaning and function, rather than treating them as erroneous cognitions. PEI uses the relationship that builds up between groups of survivors and therapists (transference) as a driving force for sessions. It also recognizes the risk that therapists' own feelings towards the group (counter-transference) can interfere with therapeutic processes.

Is PEI an evidence-based practice?

To date, outcomes achieved by PEI have not been systematically assessed and evaluated. However, two randomized controlled trials are currently being carried out in Brussels and Paris.

In the latter, activities of Cellules d'Urgences Medico Psychologiques are assessed as part of a longitudinal study using the Impact of Events Scale (Horowitz *et al*. 1979) and a newly validated French instrument.

Conclusion

Applications of psychoanalytical theory to therapeutic practice do not necessarily translate into four sessions a week on an analyst's couch. The theory also provides a model for understanding the human psyche that in some ways is closer to Chaos Theory than to Newtonian physics (Gleick, 1987). If the theory behind psychoanalytic practice is useful it should be applicable to a wide variety of situations including those that involve trauma. The relatively recent development of PEI presents a special opportunity to systematically test the underlying theory and evaluate its clinical effects.

References

Bailly, L. (1996) *Les catastrophes et leur conséquences psychothérapeutiques chez l'enfant*. Paris: ESF Pb.

Barrois, C. (1989) *Les Névroses Traumatiques*. Paris: Dunod Pb.

Bisson J.I., Jenkins P., Alexander J. and Bannister C. (1997) Randomised controlled trial of psychological debriefing for victims of acute burn trauma. *Br J Psychiat* **171**, 78–81.

Briole, C., Lebigot, F., Briole, G., Lebigot, F., Lafont, B., Faure, J.D. and Vallet, D. (1996) *Le Traumatisme Psychique: rencontre et devenir*. Paris: Masson Pb.

Conlon. L., Fahy, T.J. and Conroy, R. (1999) PTSD in ambulant RTA victims: a randomized controlled trial of debriefing. *J Psychosom Res* **46**, 37–44.

Crocq, L. (1998) La Cellule d'Urgence Médicopsychologique. Sa création, son organisation, ses interventions. *Ann. Medico Psychol* **156**, 48–54.

Crocq, L. (1999) *Les Traumatismes Psychiques de Guerre*. Paris: Odile Jacob Pb.

Daligand, L. (1997) Analyse critique du debriefing. *Rev Franc Psychiat Psychol Med* **10**, 46–7.

Damiani, C. (2001) Le debriefing Psychologique: Modalités et Déroulement. In M. De Clercq (ed.), *Les Debriefing Psychologiques en question*, Actes du colloque de Bruxelles 11–12 February, 2000. Paris: Masson Pb.

Freud, S. (1895) *Studien Über Hysterie*. Leipzig & Vienna: Deuticke.

Gleick, J. (1987) *Chaos: making a new science*. London: Viking Penguin.

Horowitz, M.J., Wilner, N. and Alvarez, W. (1979) Impact of Event Scale: a measure of subjective stress. *Psychosomatic Medicine* **41**, 209–18.

Lacan, J. (1966) *Ecrits*. Paris: Seuil.

Lebigot, F., Damiani, C. and Mathieu, B. (2001) Le debriefing psychologique des victimes. In M. De Clercq (ed.), *Le Traumatisme Psychique*. Paris: Masson Pb.

Mitchell, J.T. (1983) When disaster strikes. The critical incident debriefing process. *J Emerg Med Serv* **8**, 36–9.

Moro, M.R. and Lebovici, S. (1995) *Psychiatrie Humanitaire en ex-Yougoslavie et en Armenie*. Paris: PUF Pb.

Rose, S. and Bisson, J. (1998) Brief early psychological interventions following trauma: a systematic review of the literature. *J Traum Stress*, **11**, 697–710.

Rose, S., Brewin, C., Andrews, B. and Kirk, M. (1999) A randomized controlled trial of psychological debriefing for victims of violent crime. *Psychol Med* **29**, 793–9.

Yehuda, R. (1999) Risk Factors for Post-traumatic Stress Disorder. Washington DC: APA Press.

10 The course and development of early reactions to traumatic events: baseline evidence from a non-intervention follow-up study

Ulrich Schnyder and Hanspeter Moergeli

Introduction

In the immediate aftermath following exposure to a traumatic event, the majority of people affected have at least short periods in which they feel distressed or show some sort of psychological disturbance. For instance, in accident survivors, dysphoric-depressed emotions, anxiety and dissociative symptoms, such as de-realization occur quite frequently during the first few days post-accident (Malt and Olafsen, 1992; Shalev *et al.*, 1996; Schnyder and Malt, 1998). High levels of dissociation were also found in recent victims of sexual and non-sexual assault (Dancu *et al.*, 1996), and in victims of natural disasters (Koopman *et al.*, 1994). With regard to the symptom clusters of post-traumatic stress disorder (PTSD), re-experiencing symptoms have been reported by up to 71% of survivors of disasters and violent assaults (Sloan, 1988; Feinstein, 1989; Cardena and Spiegel, 1993). Avoidance has been found in 30% of earthquake survivors (Cardena and Spiegel, 1993) and 50% of motor vehicle accident victims (Bryant and Harvey, 1996). Similarly, high levels of arousal have been reported in subjects who had been exposed to different types of traumatic events (Sloan, 1988; Feinstein, 1989; Cardena and Spiegel, 1993). Taken together, the current literature provides clear evidence for the significant levels of distress that may occur across a range of different traumas within the first days and weeks of the traumatic event.

Before the diagnosis of acute stress disorder (ASD) was introduced in the DSM-IV (APA, 1994), a number of studies investigated the occurrence of PTSD symptoms in the first month post-trauma. Incidences of PTSD (without the duration criterion) ranged from 8% in motor vehicle accident victims (Green *et al.*, 1993) to 94% in rape victims (Rothbaum *et al.*, 1992) and 100% in ambushed soldiers (Feinstein, 1989). A number of more recent studies reported incidences of ASD, ranging from 7% in typhoon survivors (Staab *et al.*, 1996), to 19% in a sample of victims of violent crime (Brewin *et al.*, 1999), to 33% in bystanders of a mass shooting (Classen *et al.*, 1998). Three studies used the only currently available structured interview schedule with known psychometric properties that provides diagnostic information relating to the presence of ASD, the Acute Stress Disorder Interview (Bryant *et al.*, 1998). These three studies yielded similar rates of ASD in different trauma populations: 13% in a sample of motor vehicle accident (MVA) victims (Harvey and Bryant, 1998b); 14% in a study on MVA victims with mild traumatic brain injury

(Harvey and Bryant, 1998a); and 13% in a mixed sample of survivors of violent assault, burns and industrial accidents (Harvey and Bryant, 1999).

According to a recently published meta-analysis of risk factors for post-traumatic stress disorder in trauma-exposed adults (Brewin et al., 2000), risk factors such as gender, age at trauma and race predict PTSD in some populations, but not in others. Education, previous trauma and general childhood adversity predict PTSD more consistently, but to a varying extent according to the populations studied and the methods used. More uniform predictive effects were found for variables such as psychiatric history, reported childhood abuse and family psychiatric history. Individually, the effect size of risk factors appears to be modest, but risk factors operating during and/or after the trauma, such as trauma severity, lack of social support and additional life stress, have somewhat stronger effects than pre-trauma factors (Brewin and Lennard, 1999). In other words, in spite of recent qualifications of the original concept of PTSD as a healthy person's normal response to an abnormal traumatic event (Yehuda and McFarlane, 1995), peri-traumatic variables, i.e. factors directly related to the traumatic event and its immediate aftermath continue to play an important role in the development of PTSD (Yehuda, 1999). Moreover, there is growing evidence suggesting that the development of PTSD may be facilitated by an atypical biological response in the immediate aftermath of a traumatic event, which in turn leads to a maladaptive psychological state (Yehuda et al., 1998).

In summary, there is now a solid body of knowledge regarding the medium- to long-term consequences of traumatic experiences in terms of incidence of post-traumatic stress disorder and other trauma-related disorders. There are also a growing number of studies reporting on the incidence of acute stress disorder and other psychological disturbances in the acute stage after a traumatic event. However, the development of early reactions to traumatic events over time, and their relationship to protective and risk factors for developing PTSD have not yet been studied thoroughly enough. Given the currently ongoing controversy about the usefulness or potential negative effects of early psychological interventions after trauma, it appears sensible to pause and to try to improve our knowledge about the natural course of the immediate psychological reactions to overwhelming stressors. A better understanding of these processes constitutes a prerequisite for the development of evidence-based rationales for early intervention. Only thereafter can we determine in which cases early intervention is indicated at all and what may be its goals.

The present study, therefore, was aimed at assessing the course and development of psychological disturbances in a sample of accident victims who sustained severe, mostly life-threatening physical trauma. Special emphasis was put on the variety of individual reactions during the course of the first year post-accident. Also, we were interested in the associations between a number of trauma-independent and accident-related variables, and the occurrence of post-traumatic symptomatology over time.

A longitudinal study of severely injured accident victims

Methods

Participants

All participants had sustained accidental injuries that caused a life-threatening or critical condition requiring their referral to the intensive care unit (ICU) of the Traumatology Department at the University Hospital of Zurich (Schnyder et al., 2000, 2001). An Injury Severity Score (ISS; Baker and O'Neill, 1976) of 10 or more, and a Glasgow Coma Scale (GCS; Teasdale and Jennett, 1974) score of 9 or more were required, thus excluding all patients with severe head injuries. Furthermore, patients had to be 18–70 years of age, and capable with regard to both their clinical condition and fluency in German to take part in an extensive interview within 1 month of the accident. Patients suffering from any serious somatic illness or who had been under treatment for any mental disorder immediately prior to the accident, and/or those who showed marked clinical signs or symptoms of mental disorders that were obviously unrelated to the accident, were excluded. This way, 16 patients were excluded due to the presence of pre-existing psychiatric pathology. In addition, all patients who sustained their injuries as a result of a suicide attempt or from a physical attack were excluded from the study.

During a recruitment period of 18 months, all ICU patients were consecutively screened: 135 patients were eligible for the study. After the study was completely described to the subjects, written informed consent was obtained from 121 patients (T1); 14 (10.4%) refused to participate. Follow-up interviews were performed 6 months ±3 weeks (T2), and 12 months±3 weeks after the trauma (T3). Fifteen out of 121 patients (12.4%) were lost during the follow-up period. Thus, the final sample with complete longitudinal data consisted of 106 patients.

The mean age in the sample was 37.9 (SD=13.1) years. The majority were males (79 patients; 74.5%). Road traffic accidents were most frequent (64 patients; 60.4%), followed by severe sports and leisure-time accidents (23; 21.7%), accidents in the workplace (13; 12.3%) and household accidents (6; 5.7%). No significant differences in injury severity (ISS) were found between these four types of accident ($F=0.19$, df$=3,102$, $P=0.90$). According to the surgeons' files, 40 patients (37.7%) suffered from retrograde amnesia; 44 patients (41.5%) sustained a traumatic brain injury, i.e. they had objectively reported loss of consciousness and/or pathological findings in the cranial CT. A significant association was found between retrograde amnesia and traumatic brain injury (Pearson Chi-square$=21.5$, df$=1$, $P<0.001$).

The 14 patients who refused to participate in the study did not differ significantly from the final sample with regard to sex, age, ISS and GCS scores. However, significantly more work-related accidents were found among the refusers (refusers: 7, 50%; sample: 13, 12.3%; Fisher's exact test, $P<0.01$). Therefore, the patients in the sample who had sustained accidents in the workplace (13, 12.3%) were compared to the rest of the sample with regard to PTSD symptomatology (CAPS-2, see below 'Measures'). However, no significant differences were found (CAPS-2 mean total score 24.5 versus 18.1; $t=-1.32$, df$=104$, $P=0.19$). Furthermore, the 15 dropouts did not differ significantly from the final sample with regard to sociodemographic characteristics, accident-related variables or measures of post-accident psychopathology.

Measures

The mean length of stay at the ICU was 5.5 days (SD=5.0, range=1–26). The mean number of days between accident and initial assessment (T1) was 13.4 (SD=6.6, range=3–29). All interviews were conducted by a medical doctor, a clinically experienced internist who had been involved in research for a number of years and was thoroughly trained in the specifics of traumatic stress research. All patients to whom the exclusion criterion 'pre-existing psychiatric pathology' was potentially applicable were discussed in detail between the interviewer and the first author before any decision about inclusion was taken.

Post-traumatic psychological symptoms were assessed using the Clinician-Administered PTSD Scale (CAPS-2; Blake *et al.*, 1990). This instrument allows quantification of the frequency plus intensity of each of the 17 PTSD symptoms according to DSM-III-R. The CAPS-2 has excellent psychometric properties (Blake *et al.*, 1995). Cronbach's alpha for CAPS-2 in this study was 0.71. The patients with retrograde amnesia scored extremely high on item 7 (psychogenic amnesia) of the CAPS-2 scale. Being unable to differentiate organic from psychogenic amnesia, we decided to omit item 7 in all further calculations. This procedure resulted in an increase in Cronbach's alpha from 0.71 to 0.77.

Psychopathological symptoms were further assessed using the Impact of Event Scale (IES; Horowitz *et al.*, 1979) and the Symptom Checklist SCL-90-R (Derogatis, 1986). Information about the patients' social network and recent life events were gathered using a questionnaire compiled from a revised version of the Social Network Index (Berkman and Syme, 1979), an adapted version of the Social Support Questionnaire (Schaefer *et al.*, 1981) and the Inventory for Determining Life-Changing Events (ILE; Siegrist and Dittmann, 1983). Biographical protective and risk factors for the development of psychological and psychosomatic illnesses were determined by using a compilation of scientifically established factors (Egle *et al.*, 1997). Examples of risk factors include psychiatric disorders in a parent and sexual abuse; protective factors include a lasting, good relationship with the person to whom the patient related most closely as a child, and social stimulation in childhood and youth, e.g. through youth groups, etc. The Sense of Coherence questionnaire (SOC; Antonovsky, 1987) is a self-rating questionnaire that measures a person's orientation to life, i.e. the extent to which an individual is likely to construe a stressor as comprehensible and worth overcoming, and the individual's appraisal that he or she will manage to overcome such stressors. Finally, the Freiburg Questionnaire of Coping with Illness (FQCI; Muthny, 1989) was used, a coping questionnaire that includes five satisfactorily independent scales:

- depressive reaction;
- active, problem-orientated coping;
- distraction and enhancing self-esteem;
- religiosity and the search for meaning;
- downplaying and wishful thinking.

Results

Descriptive data

A mean ISS of 21.9 (SD=9.9, range=10–51) indicates that patients were severely injured. Fifteen patients (14.2%) had a GCS score of 9–13, indicating moderate traumatic brain injury; the GCS mean score was 14.4 (SD=1.4, range=9–15).

Figure 10.1 shows individual CAPS-2 total scores over time for all 106 patients. On the one hand, this graph illustrates the decrease in symptomatology in the first half year post-accident (T1–T2). On the other hand, there were quite some patients with low CAPS-2 scores at T1 who developed higher levels of symptomatology at 6 or 12 months follow-up. In other words, the course and development of PTSD symptomatology in this sample of severely injured accident victims was by no means homogeneous. The sample did show a decreasing level of symptomatology, although in several patients we found atypical courses, with a marked increase of PTSD symptoms at 6 or even 12 months post-trauma.

The mean CAPS-2 score of the total sample, unweighted by gender, was 20.5 shortly after the accident (T1), 13.5 at 6 months and 14.8 at 12 months. Analysis of variance over all three measurement points showed a significant main effect of time and a significant gender difference with higher scores in women than in men, but no significant interaction of time and gender. Independent single comparisons revealed a significant decrease of the CAPS-2 mean score between T1 and T2 ($F=16.56$, df$=1,104$, $P<0.001$, $\eta^2=0.14$). The slight increase of the CAPS-2 mean score between T2 and T3 is not significant ($F=1.12$, df$=1,104$, $P>0.05$, $\eta^2=0.01$). CAPS-2 total scores correlated significantly between T1 and T2 (Spearman's correlation coefficient, $r=0.38$, $P<0.001$). An even stronger correlation was found between T2 and T3 CAPS-2 scores ($r=0.69$, $P<0.001$).

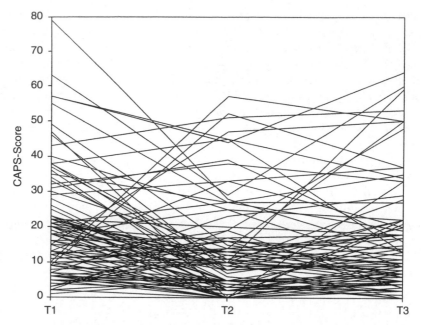

Figure 10.1 Individual total scores on the Clinician-Administered PTSD Scale (CAPS-2) in 106 severely injured accident victims shortly after the accident (T1), and at 6 (T2) and 12 months follow-up (T3).

Shortly after the accident (T1), five patients (4.7%) met all criteria for PTSD with the exception of the time criterion. In accordance with other authors (Blanchard *et al.*, 1995b; Stein *et al.*, 1997), patients were diagnosed with 'subsyndromal PTSD' if they met the symptomatic criteria for criterion B (re-experiencing symptoms), plus either C (avoidance and numbing) or D (hyper-arousal), but not both C and D. Twenty-two patients (20.8%) had subsyndromal PTSD at T1. At 6 months follow-up (T2), four patients (3.8%) had PTSD and 11 (10.4%) had subsyndromal PTSD. At 1-year follow-up (T3), two patients (1.9%) had PTSD and 13 (12.3%) had subsyndromal PTSD. The decrease (T1–T3) in number of patients meeting criteria for subsyndromal or full PTSD was statistically significant (McNemar test, exact $P < 0.05$). None of the five patients who met all criteria for PTSD with the exception of the time criterion shortly after the accident had full PTSD at 1-year follow-up. Nevertheless, a significant association between T1 and T3 was found regarding diagnosis (subsyndromal or full PTSD versus no PTSD; Fisher's exact test, $P < 0.01$).

A total of 36 patients (34.0%) fulfilled the diagnostic criteria for subsyndromal or full-blown PTSD at least once in the first year post-trauma, while 70 patients (66.0%) did not. Fourteen (51.9%) out of 27 women, but only 22 (27.8%) out of 79 men had subsyndromal or full-blown PTSD at least once during the observation period (Pearson $\chi^2 = 4.15$, df$=1$, $P < 0.05$).

Correlations

With regard to pre-traumatic psychosocial variables (independent of the accident), only sex and biographical risk factors correlated significantly with the CAPS-2 total score (see Table 10.1). No correlations were found between the trauma surgeons' objective measures of injury severity, namely ISS and GCS, and the CAPS-2 total score. However, the patients' subjective appraisal of accident severity and the presence of a sense of threat to life during the accident correlated

Table 10.1 Correlations between biographical and accident-related variables assessed at T1, and other psychosocial variables (assessed at all three measurement points) of severely injured accident victims ($n=106$) and post-traumatic stress symptoms, assessed with the Clinician-Administered PTSD Scale (CAPS-2) shortly after the accident (T1), at 6- (T2) and 12-month follow-up (T3). Spearman's correlation coefficients, two-tailed significance

Variables	CAPS-2 T1	CAPS-2 T2	CAPS-2 T3
Variables assessed at T1 only:			
Age	−0.02	0.12	−0.01
Sex (male=1, female=2)	0.18	0.29**	0.21*
Biographical risk factors	0.25**	0.22*	0.26**
Biographical protective factors	−0.18	−0.14	−0.17
ISS	−0.02	−0.13	−0.02
GCS	−0.03	−0.04	−0.05
Subjective appraisal of accident severity	0.27**	0.22*	0.24*
Sense of death threat	0.23*	0.24*	0.42***
Variables assessed at T1, T2, T3:			
Life events (last few months)	0.35***	0.28**	0.43***
Stress due to life events (last few months)	0.47***	0.49***	0.59***
Daily hassles	0.37***	0.38***	0.27**
Social network	−0.12	−0.18	−0.19
SCL–90–R Global Severity Index	0.59***	0.72***	0.69***
IES Intrusion subscale	0.52***	0.58***	0.46***
IES Avoidance subscale	0.40***	0.49***	0.47***
FQCI depressive coping	0.51***	0.62***	0.51***
FQCI problem–oriented coping	0.22*	0.29**	0.18
FQCI distraction	0.19	0.31**	0.42***
FQCI search for meaning	0.21*	0.17	0.07
FQCI wishful thinking	0.17	0.39***	0.30**
SOC total score	−0.36***	−0.44***	−0.36***

ISS: Injury Severity Score; GCS: Glasgow Coma Scale; SOC: Sense of Coherence Questionnaire; FQCI: Freiburg Questionnaire of Coping with Illness; IES: Impact of Event Scale; SCL-90-R: Symptom Checklist.
*$P \leq 0.05$; **$P \leq 0.01$; ***$P \leq 0.001$. n Varies slightly according to the number of patients who completed the self-rating scales.

significantly with the CAPS-2 score. Significant correlations of a mostly moderate degree were also found for life events, stress attributable to life events and daily hassles, but not for the patients' social network. Measures of psychopathology (SCL-90-R, IES) showed mostly high correlations with the CAPS-2 throughout the observation period. Furthermore, most coping sub-scales, depressive coping in particular, correlated significantly with PTSD symptomatology. Finally, the SOC correlated negatively with the CAPS-2 total score.

Overall, correlations of different variables with PTSD symptomatology, as assessed with the Clinician Administered PTSD Scale (CAPS-2), showed a remarkably similar pattern at all three measurement points: we found low correlations for biographical and accident-related variables, moderate correlations for life events, coping, and SOC, and high correlations for all measures of psychopathology.

Discussion

This longitudinal study investigated a sample of accident victims who received severe, mostly life-threatening injuries. Patients were excluded if they showed any signs of prior psychological problems, had attempted suicide or had been exposed to a physical assault, thus ensuring a highest possible homogeneity of the sample.

At first sight, the natural course and development of these patients' early psychological reactions to the traumatic event came up to our expectations, with elevated CAPS-2 scores in the acute aftermath of the accident, a significant decrease in the first half year post-trauma and a stabilization thereafter. It should be emphasized at this point that the decrease in symptomatology in this sample occurred without any formal psychological intervention. However, when taking a closer look, this finding has to be qualified. The degressive course of PTSD symptomatology did apply for the great majority of accident victims; however, a considerable minority of patients showed atypical courses, with high levels of CAPS-2 scores developing only after a certain delay. This indicates that clinically relevant psychological symptoms may occur at a later stage, even in subjects who initially did not report any psychological problems. Therefore, a one-off screening for persons at risk in the immediate aftermath of a traumatic event is maybe not the best way to identify those who will later go on to develop PTSD. Rather, health professionals should be aware throughout the phases of acute treatment and rehabilitation, that trauma-related psychosocial problems that may arise in a certain proportion of patients.

Taking into account the seriousness of the accidents and injuries the patients in this sample had sustained, they scored surprisingly low on the CAPS-2, indicating low levels of post-traumatic stress symptoms. Accordingly, the incidence of subsyndromal or full-blown PTSD at the three measurement points was lower than could have been expected from the literature where PTSD rates of up to 39% have been reported in samples of less severely injured accident victims (Schnyder and Buddeberg, 1996). We think that this difference is at least partly attributable to the strict selection process excluding patients with signs of pre-traumatic psychiatric problems. It may also reflect cultural differences in coping with traumatic experiences: In another European study, only one patient with PTSD was found in a sample of 107 moderately injured accident victims with a mean ISS of 8.6 (Malt, 1988). It must be pointed out, however, that in the Malt study diagnoses were made based on thoroughly conducted clinical interviews and not on a standardized questionnaire such as the CAPS-2. In the USA, too, Breslau and collaborators, reporting data from their 1996 Detroit Area Survey of Trauma, calculated a conditional risk of 2.3% for developing PTSD after serious motor vehicle accidents and concluded that previous studies have over-estimated the conditional risk of PTSD (Breslau et al., 1998).

From a theoretical viewpoint, our findings fit well in Karasek and Theorell's (Karasek and Theorell, 1990) stress concept that integrates the three dimensions of demand, control and support. It is noteworthy that patients in this study were psychologically healthy when they were suddenly and unexpectedly exposed to an overwhelming stressor. During their stay at the ICU, they were provided with the highest possible degree of self-control and with a maximum of professional and personal support. The relatively low level of distress found in these patients might, therefore, be explained by low pre-traumatic vulnerability combined with a maximum amount of post-traumatic control and support.

All the same, it cannot be said that the patients in our sample had no psychological problems at all: when looking at the observation period as a whole, 34% of patients developed subsyndromal or full-blown PTSD at some point in time during the first year after the accident.

Men and women appear to cope differently with serious accidental injuries: 52% of women, but only 28% of men fulfilled the diagnostic criteria for subsyndromal or full-blown PTSD at least once during the observation period. This is in line with the general finding that PTSD is more likely to develop in females than in males after exposure to a traumatic event (Breslau *et al.*, 1991; Norris, 1992; Resnick *et al.*, 1993; Green, 1994; Kessler *et al.*, 1995; Breslau *et al.*, 1997; Solomon and Davidson, 1997). To date, the reason for this gender difference is unclear and cannot be fully explained by different exposure rates or types of trauma (Breslau *et al.*, 1998). The greater susceptibility to post-traumatic psychological problems in females has been demonstrated in studies on accident victims, too: Feinstein and Dolan found more re-experiencing and avoidance symptoms (Feinstein and Dolan, 1991). Malt reported on more adjustment and somatoform disorders (Malt, 1988), whilst Blanchard and collaborators diagnosed more cases of PTSD in women than in men (Blanchard *et al.*, 1995b).

None of the trauma surgeons' objective measures of injury severity correlated with post-traumatic psychopathology. It appears that in life-threatening accidents the occurrence of post-traumatic psychiatric morbidity is unrelated to injury severity. According to the literature, the objective severity of the accident or injury does not necessarily correlate with psychiatric outcome (Malt and Olafsen, 1992; Green *et al.*, 1993). In one study, however, injury severity and perception of a threat to life predicted later development of PTSD (Blanchard *et al.*, 1995a). The missing association between injury severity and psychiatric morbidity in our sample may be at least in part due to a statistically restricted range phenomenon. It is possible that in a study including mild, moderate, and severe injuries, thus covering the full range of ISS values (1–75), the ISS would correlate significantly with psychiatric morbidity. Nevertheless, it is important to recognize that the objective severity of an accidental injury and the patient's subjective perception of the dangerousness of the event are not the same. In fact, in our study, ISS was completely unrelated to the patients' appraisals of accident severity ($r=-0.07$, ns) and their sense of a threat to their life ($r=0.07$, ns). As a consequence, when trying to assess a patient's need for early psychosocial intervention, professionals are well advised to listen to their patient's story, rather than to rely on hard facts such as injury severity exclusively. The significant associations of the patients' subjective appraisal of the accident severity and a sense of threat to their life experienced during the incident with their scores on the CAPS-2 scale lend support to the findings of other authors who found that the subjective appraisal of the trauma was highly predictive for later development of psychological problems including PTSD (Malt and Olafsen, 1992; Dahlmann, 1993; Green *et al.*, 1993; Blanchard *et al.*, 1995a).

Recent life events, stress attributable to these life events and daily hassles correlated significantly with the occurrence of PTSD symptoms. This is a noteworthy finding as it indicates that the pre-traumatic stress load may have an influence in psychologically healthy subjects on their coping with and healing from accidental injuries and their sequelae. As a consequence, trauma surgeons and ICU personnel, as well as health professionals involved in the aftercare of accident victims should pay special attention when recording case histories to the strains and stressors their patients have been and are currently exposed to.

The coping subscales correlated positively with post-traumatic stress symptoms. The highest correlation was found for depressive coping, but active, problem-orientated coping, distraction and wishful thinking correlated significantly, too. Apparently, psychological responses to accidental injuries are related to the patients' current coping patterns. This was also found in other studies on accident victims using different coping questionnaires (Buckelew *et al.*, 1990; Malt, 1992) and in a study on PTSD patients with mixed types of trauma (Amir *et al.*, 1997).

Sense of coherence measures an individual's capacity to respond to stressors with the appropriate application of a variety of coping and other strategies (Antonovsky, 1993). The SOC scale has been used in a large number of studies in mental health (Eriksson and Lundin, 1996; Kushner *et al.*, 1993), psychosomatic medicine (Hawley *et al.*, 1992; Callahan and Pincus, 1995; Sack *et al.*, 1997), public health (Lundberg and Nyström Peck, 1994; Udris *et al.*, 1994) and stress research (Flannery *et al.*, 1994; McSherry and Holm, 1994). It can predict short- or long-term outcome of psychiatric and somatic health problems (Flannery, 1990; Chamberlain *et al.*, 1992; Flannery and Petrie and Brook, 1992). The negative correlation of SOC and CAPS-2 in our study emphasizes the role of sense of coherence as a general measure of resilience in confronting stress. Similarly, Frommberger *et al.* (1998) found significant negative correlations between SOC and post-traumatic stress symptoms in accident victims as did Eriksson and Lundin in a study on survivors of the 'Estonia' ferry disaster (Eriksson and Lundin, 1996).

This study has a number of limitations. First, patients had to be excluded from the study if they did not speak German sufficiently. Proficiency in the official language of a country is a strong determinant of social integration; according to our clinical experience, patients with poor social integration have greater than average difficulties in dealing with the consequences of their accident. Therefore, in future studies, patients whose mother tongue is other than the country's official language should be included using interpreters. Secondly, patients showing pre-traumatic psychiatric symptomatology may also be expected to show increased rates of PTSD and more difficulties in coping with the accident. These two groups of patients should be included in future studies. Furthermore, the study did not include the full spectrum of accident victims, so inferences can only be made about those with very severe accidental injuries. Finally, as patients with work-related accidents more frequently refused participation and tended to show more post-traumatic stress symptoms, they should be studied more thoroughly. The small number of patients with work-related accidents did not allow us to draw any firm conclusions.

In summary, the level of PTSD symptomatology in this sample of severely injured accident victims was surprisingly low. Overall, PTSD symptomatology decreased over time, with a considerable minority of patients showing atypical courses, i.e. high levels of CAPS-2 scores that developed only after a certain delay. Post-traumatic stress symptoms did not correlate with injury severity, but with the patients' subjective appraisal of the accident, with recent life events and general psychopathological symptoms, as well as the patients' current coping pattern, and sense of coherence.

Acknowledgements

This study was supported by the Swiss National Science Foundation (project-no. 32–43640.95).

References

Amir, M., Kaplan, Z., Efroni, R., Levine, Y., Benjamin, J. and Kotler, M. (1997) Coping styles in post-traumatic stress disorder (PTSD) patients. *J Personal Individ Diff* **23**, 399–405.

Antonovsky, A. (1987) *Unraveling the Mystery of Health. How People Manage Stress and Stay Well.* San Francisco: Jossey Bass.

Antonovsky, A. (1993) The structure and properties of the sense of coherence scale. *Soc Sci Med* **36**, 725–33.

APA (1994) *Diagnostic and Statistical Manual of Mental Disorders*, 4th edn. Washington DC: American Psychiatric Association.

Baker, S.P. and O'Neill, B. (1976) The injury severity score: an update. *J Trauma* **16**, 882–5.

Berkman, L.F. and Syme, L. (1979) Social networks, host resistance and mortality: a nine-year follow-up study of Alameda County residents. *Am J Epidemiol* **109**, 186–204.

Blake, D.D., Weathers, F.W., Nagy, L., Kaloupek, D.G., Klauminzer, G., Charney, D.S. and Keane, T.M. (1990) A clinician rating scale for assessing current and lifetime PTSD: the CAPS-1. *Behav Therapist* **18**, 187–8.

Blake, D.D., Weathers, F.W., Nagy, L., Kaloupek, D.G., Gusmann, F.D., Charney, D.S. and Keane, T.M. (1995) The development of a Clinician-Administered PTSD Scale. *J Traum Stress* **8**, 75–90.

Blanchard, E.B., Hickling, E.J., Mitnick, N., Taylor, A.E., Loos, W.R. and Buckley, T.C. (1995a) The impact of severity of physical injury and perception of life threat in the development of post-traumatic stress disorder in motor vehicle accident victims. *Behav Res Ther* **33**, 529–34.

Blanchard, E.B., Hickling, E.J., Taylor, A.E. and Loos, W.R. (1995b) Psychiatric morbidity associated with motor vehicle accidents. *J Nerv Ment Dis* **183**, 495–504.

Breslau, N., Davis, G.C., Andreski, B. and Peterson, E. (1991) Traumatic events and post-traumatic stress disorder in an urban population of young adults. *Arch Gen Psychiat* **48**, 216–22.

Breslau, N., Davis, G.C., Andreski, P., Peterson, E.L. and Schultz, L.R. (1997) Sex differences in post-traumatic stress disorder. *Arch Gen Psychiat* **54**, 1044–8.

Breslau, N., Kessler, R.C., Chilcoat, H.D., Schultz, L.R., Davis, G.C. and Andreski, P. (1998) Trauma and post-traumatic stress disorder in the community—the 1996 Detroit Area Survey of Trauma. *Arch Gen Psychiat* **55**, 626–32.

Brewin, C.R. and Lennard, H. (1999) Effects of mode of writing on emotional narratives. *J Traum Stress* **12**, 355–61.

Brewin, C.R., Andrews, B., Rose, S. and Kirk, M. (1999) Acute stress disorder and post-traumatic stress disorder in victims of violent crime. *Am J Psychiat* **156**, 360–6.

Brewin, C.R., Andrews, B. and Valentine, J.D. (2000) Meta-analysis of risk factors for post-traumatic stress disorder in trauma-exposed adults. *J Consult Clin Psychol* **68**, 748–66.

Bryant, R.A. and Harvey, A.G. (1996) Initial post-traumatic stress responses following motor vehicle accidents. *J Traum Stress* **9**, 223–34.

Bryant, R.A., Harvey, A.G., Dang, S. and Sackville, T. (1998) Assessing acute stress disorder: psychometric properties of a structured clinical interview. *Psycholog Assess* **10**, 215–20.

Buckelew, S.P., Baumstark, K.E., Frank, R.G. and Hewett, J.E. (1990) Adjustment following spinal cord injury. *Rehabil Psychol* **35**, 101–9.

Callahan, L.F. and Pincus, T. (1995) The Sense of Coherence scale in patients with rheumatoid arthritis. *Arthrit Care Res* **8**, 28–35.

Cardena, E. and Spiegel, D. (1993) Dissociative reactions to the San Francisco Bay area earthquake of 1989. *Am J Psychiat* **150**, 474–8.

Chamberlain, K., Petrie, K. and Azariah, R. (1992) The role of optimism and sense of coherence in predicting recovery following surgery. *Psychol Hlth* **7**, 301–10.

Classen, C., Koopman, C., Hales, R. and Spiegel, D. (1998) Acute stress disorder as a predictor of post-traumatic stress symptoms. *Am J Psychiat* **155**, 620–4.

Dahlmann, W. (1993) Psychological sequelae of accidents. Symptoms are seldom recognized. *Fortschr Med* **111**, 234–8.

Dancu, C.V., Riggs, D.S., Hearst-Ikeda, D., Shoyer, B.G. and Foa, E.B. (1996) Dissociative experiences and post-traumatic stress disorder among female victims of criminal assault and rape. *J Traum Stress* **9**, 253–367.

Derogatis, L.R. (1986) *SCL-90-R: administration, scoring and procedure manual-II for the revised version*. Towson: Clinical Psychometric Research.

Egle, U.T., Hoffmann, S.O. and Steffens, M. (1997) Psychosocial risk factors and protective factors in childhood as predisposition to psychic disorders in adulthood. *Curr State Res Nervenarzt* **68**, 683–95.

Eriksson, N.G. and Lundin, T. (1996) Early traumatic stress reactions among Swedish survivors of the m/s Estonia disaster. *Br J Psychiat* **169**, 713–16.

Feinstein, A. (1989) Post-traumatic stress disorder: a descriptive study supporting DSM-III-R criteria. *Am J Psychiat* **146**, 665–6.

Feinstein, A. and Dolan, R. (1991) Predictors of post-traumatic stress disorder following physical trauma: an examination of the stressor criterion. *Psycholog Med* **21**, 85–91.

Flannery, R.B. and Flannery, G.J. (1990) Sense of coherence, life stress and psychological distress: a prospective methodological inquiry. *J Clin Psychol* **46**, 415–20.

Flannery, R.B., Jr, Perry, J.C., Penk, W.E. and Flannery, G.J. (1994) Validating Antonovsky's Sense of Coherence Scale. *J Clin Psychol* **50**, 575–7.

Frommberger, U., Stieglitz, R.D., Nyberg, E., Straub, S. and Berger, M. (1998) Der Einfluss des 'Kohärenzgefühls' auf die Entwicklung post-traumatischer Belastungsstörungen nach Verkehrsunfällen. In Schüffel, W., Brucks, U., Johnen, R., Köllner, V., Lamprecht, F. and Schnyder, U. (eds), *Handbuch der Salutogenese–Konzept und Praxis*. Wiesbaden: Ullstein Medical, pp. 337–40.

Green, B. (1994) Psychosocial research in traumatic stress: an update. *J Traum Stress* **7**, 341–62.

Green, M.M., McFarlane, A.C., Hunter, C.E. and Griggs, W.M. (1993) Undiagnosed post-traumatic stress disorder following motor vehicle accidents. *Med J Aust* **159**, 529–34.

Harvey, A.G. and Bryant, R.A. (1998a) Acute stress disorder after mild traumatic brain injury. *J Nerv Ment Dis* **186**, 333–7.

Harvey, A.G. and Bryant, R.A. (1998b) The relationship between acute stress disorder and post-traumatic stress disorder: a prospective evaluation of motor vehicle accident survivors. *J Consult Clin Psychol* **66**, 507–12.

Harvey, A.G. and Bryant, R.A. (1999) Acute stress disorder across trauma populations. *J Nerv Ment Dis* **187**, 443–6.

Hawley, D.J., Wolfe, F. and Cathey, M.A. (1992) The Sense of Coherence questionnaire in patients with rheumatoid arthritis. *J Rheumatol* **19**, 1912–18.

Horowitz, M.J., Wilner, N. and Alvarez, W. (1979) Impact of Event Scale: a measure of subjective stress. *Psychosom Med* **41**, 209–18.

Karasek, R. and Theorell, T. (1990) *Healthy Work–Stress, Productivity and the Reconstruction of Working Life*. New York: Basic Books.

Kessler, R.C., Sonnega, A., Bromet, E., Hughes, M. and Nelson, C.B. (1995) Post-traumatic stress disorder in the national comorbidity study. *Arch Gen Psychiat* **52**, 1048–60.

Koopman, C., Classen, C. and Spiegel, D. (1994) Predictors of post-traumatic stress symptoms among survivors of the Oakland/Berkeley, Calif., firestorm. *Am J Psychiat* **151**, 888–94.

Kushner, M.G., Riggs, D.S., Foa, E.B. and Miller, S.M. (1993) Perceived controllability and the development of post-traumatic stress disorder (PTSD) in crime victims. *Behav Res Ther* **31**, 105–10.

Lundberg, O. and Nyström Peck, M. (1994) Sense of coherence, social structure and health. Evidence from a population survey in Sweden. *Eur J Publ Hlth*, **4**, 252–7.

Malt, U. (1988) The long-term psychiatric consequences of accidental injury. A longitudinal study of 107 adults. *Br J Psychiat* **153**, 810–18.

Malt, U.F. (1992) Coping with accidental injury. *Psychiat Med* **10**, 135–47.

Malt, U.F. and Olafsen, O.M. (1992) Psychological appraisal and emotional response to physical injury: a clinical, phenomenological study of 109 adults. *Psychiat Med* **10**, 117–34.

McSherry, W.C. and Holm, J.E. (1994) Sense of Coherence: its effects on psychological and physiological processes prior to, during and after a stressful situation. *J Clin Psychol* **50**, 476–87.

Muthny, F.A. (1989) *Freiburger Fragebogen zur Krankheitsverarbeitung*, Manual. Weinheim: Beltz.

Norris, F.H. (1992) Epidemiology of trauma: frequency and impact of different potentially traumatic events on different demographic groups. *J Consult Clin Psychol* **60**, 409–18.

Petrie, K. and Brook, R. (1992) Sense of coherence, self-esteem, depression and hopelessness as correlates of reattempting suicide. *Br J Clin Psychol* **31**, 293–300.

Resnick, H.S., Kilpatrick, D.G., Dansky, B.S., Saunders, B.E. and Best, C.L. (1993) Prevalence of civilian trauma and post-traumatic stress disorder in a representative national sample of women. *J Consult Clin Psychol* **61**, 984–91.

Rothbaum, B.O., Foa, E.B., Riggs, D.S., Murdock, T. and Walsh, W. (1992) A prospective evaluation of post-traumatic stress disorder in rape victims. *J Traum Stress* **5**, 455–75.

Sack, M., Künsebeck, H.W. and Lamprecht, F. (1997) Sense of Coherence and psychosomatic outcome: an empirical investigation on salutogenesis. *Psychother Psychosom Med Psychol* **47**, 149–55.

Schaefer, C., Coyne, J.C. and Lazarus, R.S. (1981) The health-related functions of social support. *J Behavior Med* **4**, 381–402.

Schnyder, U. and Buddeberg, C. (1996) Psychosocial aspects of accidental injuries–an overview. *Langenbecks Arch Chir* **381**, 125–31.

Schnyder, U. and Malt, U.F. (1998) Acute stress response patterns to accidental injuries. *J Psychosom Res* **45**, 419–24.

Schnyder, U., Mörgeli, H.P., Nigg, C., Klaghofer, R., Renner, N., Trentz, O. and Buddeberg, C. (2000) Early psychological reactions to severe injuries. *Crit Care Med* **28**, 86–92.

Schnyder, U., Mörgeli, H., Klaghofer, R. and Buddeberg, C. (2001) Incidence and prediction of PTSD symptoms in severely injured accident victims. *Am J Psychiat* **158**, 594–599.

Shalev, A.Y., Peri, T., Canetti, L. and Schreiber, S. (1996) Predictors of PTSD in injured trauma survivors: a prospective study. *Am J Psychiat* **153**, 219–25.

Siegrist, J. and Dittmann, K.H. (1983) *Inventar zur Erfassung lebensverändernder Ereignisse (ILE) ZUMA—Handbuch sozialwissenschaftlicher Skalen.* Bonn: Informationszentrum Sozialwissenschaften.

Sloan, P. (1988) Post-traumatic stress in survivors of an airplane crash-landing: a clinical and exploratory research intervention. *J Traum Stress* **1**, 211–29.

Solomon, S.D. and Davidson, J.R. (1997) Trauma: prevalence, impairment, service use and cost. *J Clin Psychiat* **9**, 5–11.

Staab, J.P., Grieger, T.A., Fullerton, C.S. and Ursano, R.J. (1996) Acute stress disorder, subsequent post-traumatic stress disorder and depression after a series of typhoons. *Anxiety* **2**, 219–25.

Stein, M.B., Walker, J.R., Hazen, A.L. and Forde, D.R. (1997) Full and partial post-traumatic stress disorder: findings from a community survey. *Am J Psychiat* **154**, 1114–19.

Teasdale, G. and Jennett, B. (1974) Assessment of coma and impaired consciousness: a practical scale. *Lancet* **2**, 81.

Udris, I., Kraft, U. and Mussmann, C. (1994) Personal and organisational resources of salutogenesis. J.-P. Dauwalder (ed.): Hogrefe & Huber, *Psychology and Promotion of Health.* Seattle, pp. 3–7.

Yehuda, R. (1999) Risk factors for post-traumatic stress disorder. In Spiegel, D. (ed.) *Progress in Psychiatry.* Washington, DC: American Psychiatric Press.

Yehuda, R. and McFarlane, A.C. (1995) Conflict between current knowledge about post-traumatic stress disorder and its original conceptual basis. *Am J Psychiat* **152**, 1705–13.

Yehuda, R., McFarlane, A.C. and Shalev, A.Y. (1998) Predicting the development of post-traumatic stress disorder from the acute response to a traumatic event. *Biolog Psychiat* **44**, 1305–13.

11 Mapping the multidimensional picture of acute responses to traumatic stress

Arieh Y. Shalev and Robert J. Ursano

Introduction

Recent years have seen a growing interest in the immediate responses evoked by traumatic stressors. This renewed interest has several sources, not the least of which is the desire to prevent the occurrence of prolonged stress disorders among survivors. Accordingly, the mapping of the early responses to traumatic events has recently focused on the challenge of identifying risk factors for developing prolonged stress disorders and, in particular, post-traumatic stress disorder (PTSD; for review see Brewin *et al.*, 2000). Early therapeutic interventions have equally been evaluated and sanctioned by their preventive long-term effects (Wessely *et al.*, 2000).

Yet, the attempts to identify predictors of PTSD and to implement early preventive interventions have so far yielded limited results (see other chapters of this book). One reason for such shortcoming might be an inappropriate shift of the field of observation from examining the obvious (i.e. the inherent reasons for reacting one way or another) to exploring and manipulating elusive risk factors, such as symptoms that may be predictive of PTSD. At this point in time, therefore, there is a need and a reason to re-evaluate the early responses to traumatic events in their proper context.

Examining the early responses can be done at different levels. Aiming to instruct potential helpers, this chapter is both descriptive and explanatory. It assumes that given the heterogeneity of traumatic situations and post-traumatic responses, description is not enough, and one must resort to generalizations and theory. The text is guided by several ideas. First, it tries to avoid the confusion between symptoms (i.e. manifestations of diseases) and emitted behaviour. Because most trauma survivors are not diseased it makes no sense to read their behaviour as being 'symptomatic'.

Secondly, the chapter does not follow the current trend of preferring the reliability of observation and neglecting the validity of underlying mental processes. It posits that comprehending the psychological tasks related to surviving adversity is essential for organizing one's observation, and hence for a proper practice of rescue and support.

Thirdly, the early responses to traumatic events are construed as primarily adaptive. Accordingly, all the early responses are, in essence, survival-driven. Survival, here, includes short- (e.g. avoiding harm, recruiting support) and long-term (e.g. learning) goals.

This is not to say that the early responses are always and invariably adaptive. Indeed, they may either succeed or fail. A mismatch between situational demands, personal resources and survival mechanism is one reason for failure (e.g. when withdrawal is used as a survival mechanism in situations from which one can escape or vice versa, when scarce resources are wasted in fighting against uncontrollable dimensions of a stressor). Additionally, the effectiveness of the early responses, and ultimately their outcome depend on human interactions that are entered into at the time. Vignettes 1 and 2 illustrate a happy, yet totally fortuitous success in coping with severe trauma and a happy match between survivor and helper.

Vignette 1

This lady reacted to a bomb attack, in which she was slightly wounded, by immediately looking for a young relative, blown away by the blast of the explosion. She had to overcome pain and physical limitations, yet succeeded in finding her relative alive and pull him out of danger. In her mind, saving her relative revealed her strength of character and determination. Had she found him dead or disfigured, this 'success' might have turned into agony.

Vignette 2

Brought to a hospital, a wounded survivor of a mass casualty event was extremely distressed by the idea that the news of her being in an incident might reach her unprepared family. Being in a bed she could not easily reach a telephone, yet on her way to the X-ray Department an attentive aid brought her to a public phone, from which she could call home, still lying in bed. She describes this incident as 'the moment in which she took control' and following which she knew that things were going to be fine.

Finally, as assiduous observer of human reactions to traumata, the authors of this chapter are repeatedly humbled by the bravery and the sophistication with which survivors cope with their misfortune. This chapter, therefore, is a tribute to human resourcefulness and resilience. It does not deny the painfulness of traumatic experiences. It simply avoids the pitfall of perceiving survivors as passive receivers of adversity, as often depicted by sensational dramatizations. The latter clearly betray and disrespect the human way of surviving adversity.

Limitations of current views

Symptoms are not enough

The morphology (i.e. the overt expression) of early responses to traumatic events has been repeatedly described (e.g. Solomon, 1993). Yet there seems to be little agreement about the nature of these responses. For example, the early distressful responses to traumatic events have been construed as both 'pathogenic' and 'normal' in the sense of being a risk factor for developing of PTSD and, at the same time, a necessary step towards recovery.

To make the problem worse, specific symptoms, such as dissociation, intrusive recall of the event and early depression have been conceived as 'pathogenic' (Marmar *et al.*, 1994; Shalev *et al.*, 1998b; Freedman *et al.*, 1999). All the same, almost everyone is perturbed during the aftermath of a trauma, and everyone experiences a degree of intrusive recall and sadness.

Alternatively, better understanding might be gained from looking at the adaptive role of behaviour emitted at the aftermath of traumatic events. The following enclosure offers a short formulation of this approach, specifically addressing the adaptive value of early PTSD 'symptoms'.

An important function of the early response is communication. Outcry is universally emitted in situations of pain, forced separation and distress. Recruiting support from co-species, signalling

In their progression towards recovery, trauma survivors express common responses that may enhance communication with others (e.g. by telling their story time and again), recruit support (e.g. by emitting a 'cry for help') and effectively initiate a process of learning and reappraisal (by going back to memories of the traumatic event and associating them with other experiences).

The same expressions may, in some cases, prevent communication (e.g. when telling the story is fearfully avoided), reduce the helping responses of others (who might be burdened themselves) and consolidate the link between traumatic memories and negative emotions.

Consequently, the effectiveness of expressed behaviour at this stage is as important as its overt expression.

one's position upon forced separation and, in general, communicating distress to helping others are extremely useful survival-related behaviour. Yet, like most emitted signals, the ultimate outcome of such behaviour depends on its ability to elicit appropriate responses from others and make use of such responses. Continuous expressions of distress may, therefore, reflect either a failure to elicit proper responses or a failure to use it appropriately. This is illustrated by Vignette 3.

Vignette 3

Upon admission to a hospital, following a road accident in which she incurred slight wounds, the survivor felt that she could not possibly trust the nursing staff. Her husband came to see her, but he was also 'remote' 'cruel' and 'cold'. She developed PTSD. An exploration of her life history revealed two previous instances of traumatization—sexual abuse by a 'friend of the family' and prolonged physical abuse by her mother (Shalev et al., 1992).

The multiple dimensions of a 'trauma'

Another problematic point is the erroneous assertion that traumatic stressors are distinguished by the presence of a threat, as exemplified by the current definition of a traumatic event by DSM IV (American Psychiatric Association, 2000) '… event or events that involve actual or threatened death or serious injury, or a threat to the physical integrity of self or others'. This widely publicized injunction does not capture the essential nature of human traumatization. For example, studies of traumatic stress disorders among body handlers (e.g. McCaroll et al., 1995) show that concrete threat is not a necessary condition for being traumatized. Extreme events often involve several traumatizing elements, some of which are depicted in Table 11.1.

Few of these terms require detailed explanation, yet they significantly shape the early responses. *Loss* can be concrete or symbolic (beliefs and expectations). Loss may also involve social networks, community structures, financial and personal resources (Hobfoll, 1989). *Relocation* is an assault on a deeply embedded territorial habit of humans. It uproots people from cherished land, familiar environment, dear objects and reassuring life routines. *Isolation* (e.g. during captivity) violates a profound need of humans to share the company of others. Importantly, mental isolation may occur even when others are present. Feeling disconnected, detached and unable to resonate with others is a salient description of many traumatized survivors (e.g. Dasberg, 1976; Shalev and Munitz, 1989). *Dehumanization and degradation* (e.g. as prisoner or war, during sexual assault or group rape) leave severe psychological scars beyond those engendered by threat.

Table 11.1 Traumatizing elements of extreme events

Threat
Physiological strain (pain, starvation, dehydration)
Exhaustion
Surrender
Separation
Relocation
Loss
Isolation
Dehumanization
Uncertainty
Incongruent experience
Exposure to the grotesque

This is particularly true when surrender and obedience are enforced. *Uncertainty* during traumatic events (e.g. as to the duration or the source of adversity) is often depicted as extremely distressful.

Finally, *incongruence*, i.e. the absolute novelty of an experience and its salient contrast with what had been believed in, known, expected or experienced beforehand is probably the most difficult part of the trauma for many survivors. Examples of the above include:

- the responses of trained rescue workers to being exposed to body parts of young children;
- of a survivor of sadistic rape who reported having been faced with evil;
- of a wounded soldier who, during air-evacuation was exposed to the agonizing screams of a friend and, ultimately, to his death.

Holocaust survivors coined the name 'the other planet' to describe Auschwitz. Scholars of the Vietnam War spoke of a psychological 'trauma membrane', separating what had been experienced 'there' from the rest of their lives (Lindy, 1985). These terms epitomize the idea of incongruent experiences and properly place them at the core of mental traumatization.

Responses are 'polymorphous and labile'

Given the variety of traumatic experiences, it is clear that, according to circumstances, survivors' responses may involve apprehension, anger, bewilderment, grief, regret, yearning, attempts to retrieve and repair, efforts to control emotions, attempt to forget, and attempts to re-appraise and make sense of what has just happened. Empirical studies of the early responses reveal these to be polymorphous and labile. That is; they change rapidly and include a mixture of anxiety, depression, agitation, stupor, numbing and irritability. Grinker and Spiegel (1945) describe the early 'neurotic' response as consisting of 'a passing parade of every type of psychological and psychosomatic symptom'.

Whilst the 'heterogeneity' or 'polymorphism' can baffle researchers, the experience of those who rescue trauma survivors is very different. Rather than being erratic and incomprehensible to the intimate observer, early responses are eminently and intuitively understandable. They are also very communicative, and readily evoke intense emotional responses and enduring impressions in helpers. Indeed, they rapidly create intense and mutual bonding between rescuer and survivors (Shalev *et al.*, 1993).

In their proper context, therefore, the early responses are clearly understandable, especially when one is ready to read human faces and respond to human emotion. Emotional reading, a deeply embedded function of the human brain offers one of the best approaches to 'mapping the multidimensional picture' of the acute response to traumatic events.

Along the same line, the 'lability' of the early responses is also understandable. Intuitively we know that the response to traumatic should change with time, from an initial 'outcry' to the subsequent phases of mourning and elaboration. Yet, the proper time unit here is 'psychological time', and the latter may differ from one individual to another. Moreover, the sequence of responses may be different in different individuals, with some being initially shut down and unexpressive, and opening up later, and others reacting in very expressive ways, to be soothed with time. When one evaluates groups of survivors, the differences in personal timing, inner experiences, personal and cultural style almost invariably yields a 'labile and polymorphous' picture. Much better understanding may be gained from following individual paths. Indeed, a single observation can hardly inform us about the quality and complexities of an individual's response.

Finally, the period that follows a traumatic event is not uneventful. Secondary stressors (e.g. relocation; disclosing rape experience, enduring surgical operations) tend to follow the primary ones. These new stressors evoke new responses and, as will be argued below, send the survivor, who may already be in a phase of learning and re-appraisal, back to fighting for survival.

Can one generalize?

The question, therefore, is can one can make any generalizations without being too schematic? Can one reduce the variety of observable responses, while leaving enough room for the specifics of each event, individual and group? We offer the following as a 'productive reduction'. First, we describe a temporal sequence of the responses to traumatic events, dividing them to four phases: impact phase, rescue, recovery, and return to life. Secondly, we outline the psychological tasks related to each phase and the typical expressions of distress. Finally, we use Pearlin and Schooler's (1978) coping model to organize clinical observations by focusing on the effectiveness of emitted behaviour, rather than on its morphology. A failure to cope may occur at each stage of the response to traumatic events, and such failures are likely to generate similar and easily identifiable behaviour patterns. We recommend, therefore, that observers first identify the stage (or overlapping stages) in which they find the survivor. Then they should evaluate external and internal stressors. Finally, they can identify behaviour patterns related to either successful or unsuccessful coping with these stressors. Manifestations of distress will consequently be examined within their proper context, and this in turn may make more sense and lead to more adaptive responses.

Succession of responses

Table 11.2 summarizes a succession of stages of and responses to traumatic events. It addresses the above-mentioned four different stages, specifying for each the principal stressor, concrete goals of behaviour, salient responses and concurrent roles of helpers. The table is meant to be read vertically first to give a summary of the stages and outline their inherent complexity. When read horizontally the table illustrates the extent to which survivors may have different experiences and needs at different stages. Importantly, the table is not meant to suggest a strict temporal progression from

Table 11.2 Successive and overlapping stages of the response to traumatic events

	Impact phase	Rescue	Recovery	Return to life
Principal stressor	Threat, separation, exposure, incongruence, etc	New external and internal realities	Learning about the consequences of the event	Incongruence between inner experience or resources and external demands
Concrete goals of behaviour	Survival	Adjustment to new realities	Appraisal and planning	Re-integration
Psychological tasks	Primary stress responses	Accommodation	Assimilation	Practicing and implementing change
Salient behaviour pattern	Fight/flight, freezing, surrender, etc.	Resilience versus exhaustion	Grief, re-appraisal, intrusive memories, narrative formation	Adjustment versus phobias, avoidance, depression and PTSD
Role of all helpers	Rescue and protection	Orientation, provision for needs	Presence, responsiveness and sensitive interaction	Continuity of concrete and symbolic assistance
Role of professional helpers	Organizer	Holder	Interlocutor	Diagnostician and therapist

one stage to the other. Most often these schematic stages will overlap in reality (Fig. 11.1). For example, a survivor (e.g. of a car accident) may already be adapting to a new reality (e.g. of being injured and hospitalized) when another threat presents itself (e.g. a medical complication), sending him or her back to fighting for survival. Indeed, many survivors will be found simultaneously in more than one stage and therefore have overlapping needs. Finally, because the phase of 'return to life' is not part of the 'immediate responses', it will not be elaborated in this chapter.

The impact phase

The impact phase of a traumatic event is characterized by actual presence of adversity. Despite the use of the word 'impact', this period can be of various duration. The various types of traumatic adversities that have been described in Table 11.1 are present and often co-occur (e.g. threat, separation, isolation, etc.). The survivor's very concrete tasks during this phase are survival, and reduction of harm to self and significant others. Yet other goals are also present, such as preserving one's dignity, remaining in contact with others and helping others. Issues of altruism and risk-taking by survivors and rescuers are beyond the scope of this chapter. Suffice it to say that these are frequently observed, reminding us of Fredrick Manning's (1990) intuitive reference to an 'inalienable sympathy of one man to another' as a motivating force of soldiers during the carnage of World War I. Simply assuming human sympathy, however, seems quite odd at the present time. For sceptics, therefore, let it be said that rescuing others has evolutionary advantage.

Importantly, primary stress responses are seen at this stage (e.g. fear, surrender, fight, etc.), and these responses are often very powerful, unexpected and take control of a person's behaviour.

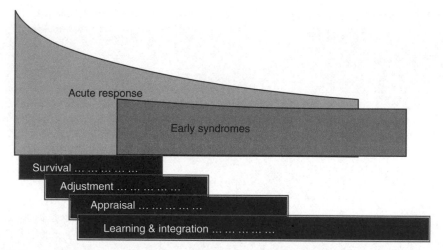

Figure 11.1 Successive and overlapping stages of the response to traumatic events.

Survivors, therefore, often find themselves acting in ways that they did not expect and had no previous experience of. For example, threatened by likely death, a rape victim may surrender her body. A young father may escape from a burning house, leaving a child behind. A soldier may find himself paralysed by fear, while others launch an attack. To the extent that these acts are 'out of character' or 'out of one's repertoire' these very early responses will be revisited later during the phase of re-appraisal when self-criticism may be harsh and condemning (see vignette 4).

Vignette 4

A policeman who had specialized in diffusing explosives, developed severe PTSD following an incident in which he found himself paralysed for what seemed like a long time, but was in fact only seconds, whilst he tried to detonate a bomb in one of Jerusalem's public places. First, he did not believe that the object that he examined could be a bomb. Then he realized that it was, and also that he did not have the equipment at hand needed for this job and that it was too late to make use of a bomb-detonating robot. He had to go back to safety, fetch his tools and, then, knowing that the object was a bomb, return to the explosive and dismantle it. He froze at about 1 m from the bomb with thoughts running through his head about his life and that of others around him. He proceeded to dismantle the bomb, yet could never recover from the instants of 'freezing', the thoughts of which undermined his sense of competence and self–worth.

During the impact phase survivors primarily require protection from adversity. This, however, may not always be possible because the adverse effect of some events continue (e.g. when one's child is missing following a disaster). Even during prolonged adversities to is possible for, adequate help to reduce the randomness of the situation as well as the survivor's helplessness and loneliness. The main role of helpers at this stage can be equated with that of a 'primary organizer', that is, a person who, by his or her stable presence reduces the randomness of both external and internal realities.

The immediate post-impact phase (Rescue phase)

At this point in time, survivors have typically been rescued from the primary stressor and may have been moved to a place of relative safety. However, they now face a new reality. For instance, evacuees find themselves in a shelter; injured survivors in hospital; released hostages may be on their way home. Importantly, the new reality is also psychological. Having survived a sadistic assault a person's internal reality is very different, but not yet shaped in any specific way.

Typically, at this stage, one has to face the new reality without having changed internally. Hence, it is the old self that struggles with a new reality; often with a great amount of confusion and bewilderment. This process is referred to as 'accommodation', in the sense that existing resources are used and extended to cope with novelty. The prevalent feeling is that the world is not the same. Yet the intensity and the pervasiveness of the experience differ between survivors. Importantly, this feeling of alienation and of major (and negative) change may remain with the survivor, and become part of his or her prolonged response to the trauma. The role of helpers at this stage is to mitigate the novelty of the situation such that survivors are not totally estranged and alienated. In other words, the presence and the warmth of helpers, as well as their somewhat better capacity to endure emotions, provide the necessary 'holding' for distraught survivors. Indeed, this is the stage where people are often observed to hug one another. It is also important to acknowledge that helpers can function as effective 'holders' to the extent that they are assisted and supported themselves for instance by being part of a team (e.g. Shalev et al., 1993).

The early recovery phase

Overlapping with the previous phase, recovery includes two contrasting mental efforts: to distance oneself from the traumatic event and to re-evaluate the traumatic experience. Few survivors do well with just distancing themselves from what has happened. Most will repeatedly, vividly and involuntarily recall the traumatic event through intrusive thoughts and images, nightmares and flashbacks. Many will share these experiences with others, for instance, by repeating their story again and again. Others may think that they are going mad because of the unusualness of the intrusive and vivid images and memories. Negative appraisal of one's early symptoms increases the likelihood of subsequent PTSD (Ehlers and Steil, 1995; Ehlers et al., 1998).

At this phase survivors are psychologically assimilating their recent experiences, try to understand its meaning, and examine key learning points relevant taking account of previous life experiences and future expectations. This is properly the 'post-traumatic' period, during which the concrete event becomes a mental event. Optimally, the new experience can be assimilated and this is likely to be reflected in subtle yet consistent changes in the survivor's appraisal the circumstances of the event, and of his or her feelings and actions. Dreams become more detailed with elements from one's past appearing alongside representations of the traumatic event. The telling of the story becomes a conversation. Other pieces of information (e.g. observations made by others, references to options and choices, links with past experiences) can be brought in and accepted. The traumatic event can thereby become a formative event. There is a sense of being changed, but not of being torn apart.

Survivors differ in the extent to which they tolerate the necessary phase of intrusive recall. For some, nightmares are a dreadful experience and recall is fearfully avoided. The story is never told, may be truncated, reduced or even 'schematized', and repeated without change. Importantly, nothing changes with time. The event is not compared with previous experiences. Conversations about the traumatic event is avoided because 'no one can understand', including oneself. Memories remain fragmented, iconic, poorly verbalized. Negative perception of self and others generalize and extend to other events and people. A sense of radical unwelcome transformations prevails. The traumatic event becomes destructive life experience.

It is during this period that a stable narrative of the traumatic events and of one's own responses to it are formed and consolidated (Shalev *et al.*, 1998a). Holloway and Ursano (1984) suggested that both the past, as well as the present and a person's view of the future mould the emergent narrative and conscious recall of what has happened. The narrative, however, is never purely an individual creation, but rather includes elements of what has been said by others and of the larger social appraisal of the event (e.g. a heroic act, a shameful blunder, etc.). The resulting mixture of personal experience and adopted facts may consolidate into a set of memories that will later be remembered as 'authentic' and 'accurate' (e.g. Loftus, 1979).

The roles of helpers differ from that of 'holders' seen in the previous phase. Helpers, at this phase must be available for conversations and talking about what has happened, and its aftermath so far. They should also be able to foresee and tolerate the repetitiveness and vividness of intrusive experiences, and also share their knowledge with survivors and with other helpers. They must also be able to respond emotionally without themselves being flooded or frustrated. Finally, they should be able to recognize, on the basis of repeated observations, when things are going badly, (i.e. when isolation, poorly modulated states of mind and aversive emotions increase with time). A sign of particular importance during this period is the degree to which the survivor is constantly distressed; in contrast to his or her fluctuating back and forth from well modulated to poorly modulated states of affect. The latter is generally a more reassuring presentation. This is a time in which verbalization is the key element, hence the role of professional helpers as interlocutors. Specifically, they should help putting experiences into words and encourage the sharing of these narratives. It might be unwise to 'intervene' or otherwise 'treat' the subject since priority should be given to smoothing a natural healing path. However, excessive anxiety, episodes of dissociation, intolerable insomnia, daily agitation and uncontrollable pain must be treated.

The construct of coping

'Coping' is the psychological and behavioural correlate of the bodily efforts to maintain its inner milieu within viable (or homeostatic) boundaries despite excessive demands. By analogy, coping with stress is an effort to maintain psychological balance and functioning despite excessive demands. Coping theorists describe a broad range of mechanisms designed to 'increase the gap between stress and distress'. Such 'coping strategies' are generally divided into 'problem-focused', 'emotional-focused' and 'appraisal-related' (e.g. Haan, 1969; Lazarus and Folkman, 1984). Individuals are said to have specific 'coping styles'. That is, they engage in a typical mixture of tactics when faced with stress. Some individuals tend to prefer action to reflection; others are preferentially help-seekers, yet others tend to be emotional and expressive.

Studies of trauma survivors have mainly addressed the effectiveness of particular coping strategies. Among combat veterans, Solomon *et al.* (1991), for example, found the use of emotion-focused and blunting coping strategies to be associated with higher levels of psychiatric symptoms whereas problem-focused strategies lead to a decrease in symptoms. In body handlers, in contrast, McCaroll *et al.* (1993) found an advantage to accrue from avoidance, denial and receiving group support. Spurrell and McFarlane (1993) found no clear advantage of any coping strategy.

These conflicting results should not surprise us, because it might be true that achieving effective coping is more important than any particular strategy. In order to succeed one's coping must match the circumstances of the event and the survivor's resources. These, in turn, differ between events, within events (e.g. at different stages) and between individuals. Surrender, stoic acceptance and cognitive re-framing may be more appropriate to situations in which the stressor is uncontrollable (e.g. captivity), whereas action to reduce the stressor or help seeking are more appropriate in other circumstances.

The idea of evaluating coping efficacy has distinct advantages for understanding the early responses to traumatic events. Regardless of the type of trauma, the stage of the response sequence a person is in or the task to be accomplished successful coping will affect the survivor in a very typical way. Pearlin and Schooler (1978) suggested four observable consequences of effective coping:

- relief of distress;
- sense of personal worth;
- ability to enjoy rewarding interpersonal contacts;
- sustained task performance.

Ineffective coping will lead to impaired task performance, uncontrollable emotions, self-blame (or worthlessness) and inability to enjoy the presence of others (Table 11.3).

Early responses to traumatic events can also be evaluated using these four areas. A survivor is coping better when he or she experiences relatively controllable emotions, can continue the task at hand (e.g. seeking shelter, reviewing his or her nightmares), keeps a sense of self-worth and, most importantly, engages in rewarding communication. Traumatic events certainly disrupt a person's sense of coping and, therefore, lead to temporary periods in which individuals may be flooded by distress, feelings of worthlessness and may be unable to make use of help offered. This is not by any means true for all survivors nor for all stages of the response. For some survivors the impact phase may involve paralysing fear, disrupted behaviour and a sense of total chaos. For others, however, the rescue period can be extremely difficult despite having coped well during the impact phase (e.g. when bad news is brought). Finally, and most importantly, the long-term effect of traumatic events is significantly affected by the way in which survivors cope with the particular tasks of the reappraisal and recovery phases. At each of the phases listed in Table 11.3 the 'signs and symptoms' of ineffective coping are likely to be very similar.

Importantly, effective coping should not and does not lead to a 'victory'. Nor is it always directed towards the most important stressor. Instead, coping may involve contingent (yet more controllable) stressors, as well as one's own responses. In a study of survivors of a terrorist attack, Shalev et al. (1993) described various coping efforts used during the impact phase. These included actively rescuing other survivors, sharing important information with the rescuers, preserving one's dignity by covering one's body or controlling the disclosure of information about the event to one's relatives. Successfully achieving such individual goals increased the survivors' sense of control and reduced their distress.

Table 11.3 Signs of effective coping

Effective coping	Failure to cope
Sustained task performance	Impaired task performance
Reduction of distress	Distress, uncontrollable emotions
Sustained ability for rewarding human contacts	Inability to make use of the presence of others
Ability to maintain a sense of personal worth	Self-blame, worthlessness

Comment

Practically, what one sees during the aftermath of traumatic events is a combination of primary and secondary stressors, a mixture of overlapping stages of response to what has happened and various degrees of coping with each. This chapter does not discuss the various ways in which a failure to cope may induce permanent negative changes such as a permanent reduction in one's ability to tolerate anxiety or a permanent shift in the central nervous system's response to stimuli (Shalev et al., 2000). These allostatic changes, and their leading causes are not well understood at this point. Indeed, some of the causes for permanent changes may precede the traumatic event (e.g. prior traumata, prior mental disorders, adverse rearing environment; Brewin et al., 2000). It is important to recognise that to clearly discern the expression of such factors is beyond the capacity of those involved in attending to survivors' needs during the early aftermath of traumatic events.

The model proposed here posits, therefore, that, in general, human traumatization engages powerful adaptive mechanisms, of which all helpers should be aware. The survivor therefore is not a passive 'receiver' of a 'package' of care, but is more usefully viewed as the helper's active guide. Identifying and managing obstacles to self-regulation and recovery becomes the 'therapeutic' endeavour. The same active attributes extend to families and communities whenever this is reasonable as they persist in their endeavours to regain equilibrium.

Hence, rather than bursting on to the dynamic scene of a recent trauma with pre-fabricated ideas and techniques the professional helper will do well to follow the advice of Marshall (1944) to 'conduct himself as a student, rather than as a teacher'. He or she is riding a horse, rather than driving a car. Natural forces operate at all stages, and he or she should be able to recognize these as they occur and assist in their successful resolution. Ignorance of such adaptive forces and failure to engage them might have been the worse systematic error of early interventions programmes devised so far. As argued in this chapter the main *a priori* wisdom of helpers is to be found in their knowledge of generic processes and their progression. Helpers' skills should first be expressed as a capacity to identify the specific motion, the typical rhythm and the salient trend of survivors' progression, as well as the underlying contingencies. Secondly, and most importantly, helpers should be able to join forces with survivors and, in turn, help each of optimize his or her early responses.

References

American Psychiatric Association (2000) *Diagnostic and statistical manual of mental disorders*, 4th edn (DSM-IV-TR) Washington DC: American Psychiatric Press.

Brewin, C.R., Andrews, B. and Valentine, J.D. (2000) Meta analysis of risk factors for posttraumatic stress disorder. *J Consult Clin Psychol* **68**, 784–66.

Dasberg, H. (1976) Belonging and loneliness in relation to mental breakdown in battle. *Isr Ann Psychiat Relate Sci* **14**, 307–21.

Ehlers, A. and Steil, R. (1995) Maintenance of intrusive memories in Posttraumatic Stress Disorder: a cognitive approach. *Behaviour Cognit Psychother* **23**, 217–49.

Ehlers, A., Mayou, R.A. and Bryant, B. (1998) Psychological predictors of chronic posttraumatic stress disorder after motor vehicle accidents. *J Abnorm Psychol* **107**, 508–19.

Freedman, S.A., Peri, T., Brandes, D. and Shalev, A.Y. (1999) Predictors of chronic PTSD: A prospective study. *Br J Psychiat* **174**, 353–9.

Grinker, R.R. and Spiegel, J.P. (1945) The neurotic reactions to severe combat stress. In *Men Under Stress*. Philadelphia: Blackiston, pp. 82–4.

Haan, N. (1969) A tripartite model of ego functioning: value and clinical research application. *J Nerv Ment Dis* **148**, 14–30.

Hobfoll, S.E. (1989) Conservation of resources. A new attempt at conceptualizing stress. *Am Psycholog* **44**, 513–24.

Holloway, H.C. and Ursano R.J. (1984) The Vietnam veteran: memory, social context, and metaphor. *Psychiatry* **47**, 103–8.

Lazarus, R.S. and Folkman, S. (1984) *Stress, Appraisal and Coping*. New York: Springer.

Lindy, J.D. (1985) The trauma membrane and other clinical concepts derived from psychotherapeutic work with survivors of natural disasters. *Psychiat Annl* **15**, 153–60.

Loftus, E.F. (1979) *Eyewitness Testimony*. Cambridge: Harvard University Press.

Manning, F. (1990) *The Middle Part of Fortune*. London: Penguin Books.

Marmar, C.R., Weiss, D.S., Schlenger, W.E., Fairbank, J.A., Jordan, B.K. and Kulka, R.A. (1994) Peritraumatic dissociation and posttraumatic stress in male Vietnam theater veterans. *Am J Psychiat* **151**, 902–7.

Marshall, S.L.A. (1944) *Island Victory*. New York: Penguin Books.

McCarroll, J.E., Ursano, R.J., Wright, K.M. and Fullerton, C.S. (1993) Handling bodies after violent death: strategies for coping. *Am J Orthopsychiat* **63**, 209–14.

McCarroll, J.E., Ursano, R.J. and Fullerton, C.S. (1995) Symptoms of PTSD following recovery of war dead: 13–15-month follow-up. *Am J Psychiat* **152**, 939–41.

Pearlin, L.I. and Schooler, C. (1978) The structure of coping. *J Hlth Soc Behav* **22**, 337–56.

Shalev, A.Y. and Munitz, H. (1989) Combat stress reaction in Ries N.D. In Dolev, E. (ed.), *Manual of Disaster Medicine*. Berlin: Springer Verlag, pp. 169–82.

Shalev, A., Orr, S.P. and Pitman, R.K. (1992) Psychophysiologic response during script driven imagery as an outcome measure in post-traumatic stress disorder. *J Clin Psychiat* **53**, 324–6.

Shalev, A.Y., Galai, T. and Eth, S. (1993) Levels of trauma: multidimensional approach to the psychotherapy of PTSD. *Psychiatry* **56**, 166–77.

Shalev, A.Y., Peri, T., Rogel-Fuchs, Y., Ursano, R.J. and Marlowe, D. (1998a) Historical group debriefing following exposure to combat stress. *Military Med* **163**, 494–8.

Shalev, A.Y.S., Freedman, T., Peri, D., Brandes, T., Sahar, S.P., Orr. and Pitman, R.K. (1998b) Prospective study of posttraumatic stress disorder and depression following trauma. *Am J Psychiat* **155**, 630–7.

Shalev, A.Y., Pitman, R.K., Orr, S.P., Peri, T. and Brandes, D. (2000) Auditory Startle in trauma survivors with PTSD: a prospective study. *Am J Psychiat* **157**, 255–61.

Solomon, Z. (1993) *Combat Stress Reaction*. New York: Plenum.

Solomon, Z., Mikulincer, M. and Arad, R. (1991) Monitoring and blunting: implications for combat-related post-traumatic stress disorder. *J Traum Stress* **4**, 209–21.

Spurrell, M.T. and McFarlane, A.C. (1993) Post-traumatic stress disorder and coping after a natural disaster. *Soc Psychiat Psychiatric Epidemiol* **28**, 194–200.

Wessely, S., Rose, S. and Bisson, J. (2000) Brief psychological interventions ('debriefing') for trauma-related symptoms and the prevention of post-traumatic stress disorder. *Cochrane Database Syst Rev* 2, CD000560.

12 Screening to identify individuals at risk after exposure to trauma

Chris R. Brewin, Suzanna Rose, and Bernice Andrews

Introduction

Studies of psychological debriefing as a brief early intervention following exposure to trauma have not, to date, yielded evidence for the effectiveness of the procedure (e.g. Rose and Bisson, 1998; Wessely *et al.*, 1998). Following our own study of psychological debriefing for victims of violent crime (Rose *et al.*, 1999) we therefore proposed that clinicians should refrain from focused, symptom-orientated early intervention in favour of monitoring survivors for psychological disorder, particularly post-traumatic stress disorder (PTSD), and intervening more intensively should a diagnosable condition develop. However, although awareness of PTSD is increasing, health care providers may not be sufficiently trained to identify the disorder when it occurs and to refer the patient for treatment. This problem is likely to apply in primary health care, in secondary medical settings, such as intensive care units, and among aid workers dealing with victims of accidents and disasters. The successful management of post-disaster psychopathology would therefore benefit greatly from screening instruments that could be used by non-specialists to identify people who are likely to be suffering from PTSD and who need more detailed assessment.

This chapter discusses the qualities that are desirable in screening instruments, reviews the current evidence on their effectiveness and presents some recent research on the development of a new, brief instrument. Although there is a wide range of possible adverse psychological reactions following trauma, in practice evidence is only available on instruments that screen for PTSD. Current estimates of the prevalence of PTSD in trauma populations are highly diverse, but confirm that it is a relatively common response. Some illustrative figures range from 47% in rape victims twelve weeks post-assault, to 12% in road traffic accident victims, to between 5 and 8% among victims of some natural disasters (Resick, 2001). Another limitation of the literature is that screening studies have been carried out at widely differing times post-trauma, but the findings are still likely to be relevant to the context of early intervention.

To be useful, screening instruments should ideally be short and contain the minimum number of items necessary for accurate case identification. They should be simple and should preferably not require respondents to ponder over large numbers of alternative scale points. They should be written in language that is easy to understand. Their purpose should be plain and acceptable to respondents. For ease of administration self-report questionnaires would appear to be the most flexible solution. If they are to be scored by non-specialists, which would widen their applicability, simple decision rules for determining who passes and fails the screen would be at a premium. Also highly desirable for successful instruments is that they be accurate at detecting both current

PTSD and the risk of future PTSD, and that they should be applicable to populations experiencing different traumas and with a varying prevalence of PTSD.

Over and above these considerations, the instrument must be effective in ruling in respondents who are cases and ruling out respondents who are not. The performance of a screening instrument such as a diagnostic test for PTSD is generally assessed by reference to several criteria of which two are most commonly encountered:

- sensitivity, i.e. the probability that someone with a PTSD diagnosis will have tested positive;
- specificity, i.e. the probability that someone without a PTSD diagnosis will have tested negative.

The definitions of these criteria in terms of the relation between a diagnosis and a test result are shown in Table 12.1. A good test will have a reasonable balance of sensitivity and specificity. For example, a test for PTSD can be made highly sensitive by setting a very low threshold, e.g. two re-experiencing symptoms present at any time in the past month, with the result that almost everyone with a PTSD diagnosis will exceed this threshold. However, many people will exceed this threshold even though they do not have the disorder, with the result that the specificity of the test will be correspondingly low. In the same way, a test for PTSD can be made highly specific by setting a very high threshold, e.g. five avoidance or numbing symptoms present during the past week, with the result that almost none without a PTSD diagnosis will exceed this threshold. However, many people will fall short of this threshold even though they do have the disorder, with the result that the sensitivity of the test will be correspondingly low.

Other criteria for evaluating screening tests are relevant to two slightly different, but highly practical questions: what is the probability that someone with a positive test result will report a diagnosis of PTSD, and what is the probability that someone with a negative test result will not receive a PTSD diagnosis? The answer to the first question, as shown in Table 12.1, is given by the positive predictive power of the screening test and the answer to the latter by the negative predictive power of the test. Finally, the performance of a test can also be expressed in terms of the percentage of cases correctly classified by the test as having or not having PTSD, which is referred to as its overall efficiency.

Whereas sensitivity and specificity are independent of the prevalence of the disorder in the population, and so can readily be compared across studies, positive and negative predictive power *are* sensitive to population prevalence. If there are very few cases to detect, the positive predictive power of the test will suffer, whereas if the vast majority of the population are cases, its negative predictive power will be correspondingly limited (Baldessarini *et al.*, 1983). In other words, at low prevalences a negative test result is more likely to be correct, whereas at high prevalences a positive result is more likely to be correct.

Table 12.1 Classification of subjects by diagnosis and test result, and definitions of performance criteria for screening tests

Test result	Diagnostic result		Total
	Positive	Negative	
Positive	a	b	a+b
Negative	c	d	c+d
Total	a+c	b+d	n

Note: sensitivity=a/(a+c); specificity=d/(b+d); positive predictive power=a/(a+b); negative predictive power=d/(c+d); overall efficiency=(a+d)/n.

Although these criteria address slightly different aspects of performance, sensitivity tends to co-vary with negative predictive power. This is because if sensitivity is high most people who receive the diagnosis will have a positive test result (and there will be few false negatives), so a negative test result will give a relatively better indication that the person does not suffer from the condition. Conversely, specificity tends to co-vary with positive predictive power. This is because if specificity is high most people who do not suffer from the condition will have a negative test result (and there will be few false positives), so a positive test result will give a relatively better indication that the person should receive the diagnosis.

Baldessarini *et al.* (1983) comment that highly specific tests (those having a low rate of false positives), even with moderate sensitivity, are particularly useful when test results are positive and when the prevalence of the condition is high. These conditions might obtain in a specialist service, or in screening a sample exposed to a severe stressor involving high levels of injury and death. In such conditions, highly specific tests should help to identify individuals requiring more intensive assessment. Conversely, highly sensitive tests (those having a low false negative rate), even with moderate specificity, are particularly useful when test results are negative and when the prevalence of the condition is low. These conditions might obtain in screening a population following a less severe stressor in which there was little injury and death. In such conditions, highly sensitive tests should be useful in excluding individuals from further assessment.

In practice, what levels of test performance is it realistic to expect? One guide to an upper limit of performance can be derived from a comparison of diagnoses yielded by the two most highly regarded interview assessments currently available, the Structured Clinical Interview for DSM-IV (SCID) PTSD module and the Clinician Administered PTSD Scale (CAPS). In a sample of 123 combat veterans, a CAPS total score of 65 was found to have a sensitivity of 0.84 and a specificity of 0.95 relative to a SCID diagnosis (Blake *et al.*, 1995).

Another approach is to examine the performance of individual items from a structured interview to determine whether a smaller set of items successfully identifies people with the diagnosis. For example, North *et al.* (1999) studied survivors of the Oklahoma City bombing using the Diagnostic Interview Schedule and found that 34% had PTSD. They reported that simply meeting the DSM-IV criterion of at least three avoidance or numbing symptoms identified individuals suffering from PTSD with a high degree of accuracy (positive predictive power 94%). Breslau *et al.* (1999) recently reported a short seven-item screening scale for detecting lifetime PTSD. The scale was derived from the longer diagnostic interviews used in the Detroit Area Survey of Trauma and based on analysis of the 17 criterion symptoms of PTSD identified in the DSM-IV [American Psychiatric Association (APA), 1994]. The sample size was 1830, of whom just under 8% were diagnosed with PTSD. Setting a threshold of four or more symptoms resulted in a sensitivity of 0.80, specificity of 0.97, positive predictive value of 0.71, and negative predictive value of 0.98. Five of the symptoms making up the scale were from the avoidance and numbing group, including all four numbing symptoms, and the remaining two were arousal symptoms.

In the remainder of the chapter we review currently available screening instruments for use with children and adolescents, and with adults. We report instruments that have been validated in civilian samples against structured interviews for PTSD and that have published information about their diagnostic utility. Where possible, we distinguish instruments that enquire about the full range of PTSD symptoms and briefer measures that focus on key symptoms. To enable the reader to evaluate the available information, we include details of the prevalence of PTSD in the original sample studied and whether the instrument has been validated on an independent sample. This is particularly critical in those cases where an optimum cut-off score has been determined *post hoc* from the existing dataset, thus potentially inflating the diagnostic utility of the instrument. Where appropriate, we also draw attention to those instruments that have been evaluated within the first year post-trauma and that are therefore particularly relevant to the context of early intervention. In the final section, we report progress on the development of a new brief screening measure for PTSD that has been investigated shortly after exposure to trauma in two groups of civilian trauma victims.

Screening of children and adolescents

In one of the earliest studies of children involved in a traumatic incident, the sinking of the cruise ship Jupiter, Yule and Udwin (1991) proposed a screening battery for PTSD consisting of the Impact of Event Scale (IES; Horowitz *et al.*, 1979), the Birleson Depression Inventory (Birleson, 1981), and the Revised Children's Manifest Anxiety Scale (R-CMAS: Reynolds and Richmond, 1978). A cut-off score of 30 has been suggested when the original 15-item IES is used to detect PTSD in children (Yule, 1997). However, because of evidence that younger children might misinterpret some of the IES items, Yule developed an abbreviated eight-item version of the IES for use with children aged 8 and above.

Stallard *et al.* (1999) examined the ability of Yule and Udwin's screening battery to detect PTSD as measured by the CAPS-C (Nader *et al.*, 1994) in 170 children who had been involved in road traffic or sporting accidents approximately 6 weeks earlier. The average age of the sample was 14 years, and the rate of PTSD was 23% according to the CAPS-C structured interview. Stallard *et al.* (1999) compared the performance of the IES-15 and the IES-8, and studied the effects of combining the different elements of the battery. Of the three measures, the IES (in either version) was by far the most accurate in detecting PTSD, followed by the R-CMAS. They reported that the performance of the IES-8 (sensitivity 0.69, specificity 0.83, positive predictive value 0.55, negative predictive value 0.90, overall efficiency 0.80) was similar, but did not quite match up to the IES-15 (sensitivity 0.74, specificity 0.87, positive predictive value 0.63, negative predictive value 0.92, overall efficiency 0.84). Identification of PTSD was slightly improved when IES scores were added to scores on the other measures. A summed score of 45 (determined *post hoc*) on the IES-15, the R-CMAS and the Birleson measure, yielded a sensitivity 0.85, specificity 0.85, positive predictive value 0.62, negative predictive value 0.95 and overall efficiency 0.85. The relative performance of these various measures was the same in predicting PTSD 8 months post-accident.

Muris *et al.* (2000) reported preliminary data on a new instrument, Birmaher *et al.*'s (1997) Screen for Child Anxiety Related Emotional Disorders (SCARED). The SCARED contains a Traumatic Stress Disorder subscale consisting of four items. In Muris *et al.*'s study, the 43 children who answered 'often' or 'always' on a 4-point scale to all these four items were compared with 43 children who failed to indicate traumatic symptoms. The 86 children were interviewed and completed a self-report measure of trauma symptoms, the PTSD Reaction Index (PTSD-RI). The PTSD-RI was originally devised as an interview to assess PTSD symptoms in children (Pynoos *et al.*, 1987), and was subsequently adapted as a self-report measure by Shannon *et al.* (1994). Only three children appeared to meet DSM criteria for PTSD, as assessed by the PTSD-RI. Therefore, although the SCARED correctly identified all three of these children (sensitivity 100%), the measure was effectively unable to identify children not suffering from PTSD (specificity 52%).

Summary

There are few screening instruments currently available for children and adolescents. At present, the instrument with the most empirical support would appear to be the Impact of Event Scale, using a cut-off score of 30, which has demonstrated reasonably good performance in the early identification of PTSD. However, there is no generally accepted cut-off score for detecting PTSD using the IES. Some authors have used Horowitz's (1982) suggestion that a total score of 19 indicates high levels of stress, but this has sometimes produced disappointing results (e.g. Sack *et al.*, 1998). For younger children, the briefer IES-8 may be more appropriate. The data of Stallard *et al.* (1999) suggest that the sensitivity of the IES with a cut-off score of 30 may be improved by including additional measures of anxiety and depression, without any consequent loss of specificity.

Screening of adults

A few studies have adopted general measures of psychopathology such as the General Health Questionnaire and the Millon Clinical Multi-axial Inventory to screen for PTSD (Craig and Olson, 1997; Darves-Bornoz *et al.*, 1998). In the main, however, researchers have utilized measures that specifically target trauma symptoms and these are the focus of this section. Details of sensitivity, specificity, etc., for each instrument are shown in Table 12.2. We consider first measurement instruments that include a wide range of trauma symptoms and, secondly, very brief instruments suitable for screening.

PTSD-specific screening questionnaires

PTSD checklist (PCL)

This measure, developed by Weathers *et al.* (1991, 1993), requires respondents to indicate the degree to which they have been bothered during the past month by the 17 PTSD symptoms contained in the DSM-IV. Symptoms are related to a particular traumatic event, and respondents answer the 17 items on a scale ranging from 1 ('not at all') to 5 ('extremely'). A diagnosis of PTSD can be based on endorsement (a symptom rating of at least 3) of at least one re-experiencing symptom, three avoidance symptoms and two arousal symptoms. Alternatively, a cut-off score of 50 was proposed to suggest a PTSD diagnosis (Weathers *et al.*, 1993).

Blanchard *et al.* (1996) examined the diagnostic efficiency of the PCL in a largely female sample of 40 adults who had been involved in accidents or sexual assaults. The prevalence of PTSD in this sample, as assessed with the CAPS, was 45%. Using the cut-off score of 50 the performance of the PCL was good, but reducing the cut-off to 44 resulted in still better performance (see Table 12.2 for details). Andrykowski *et al.* (1998) reported a similar study of 82 women with breast cancer, using the cut-off score of 50. The prevalence of PTSD as determined by the SCID was 6%, which reduced the positive predictive power somewhat, but negative predictive power and overall efficiency were high.

Post-traumatic Diagnostic Scale (PDS)

This measure is a development of the earlier PTSD Symptom Scale—Self Report (PSS-SR: Foa *et al.*, 1993). A version of the PSS-SR, modified to include severity, as well as frequency ratings, was used to screen for PTSD in a substance abuse sample (Coffey *et al.*, 1998). Foa *et al.* (1997) revised the PSS-SR in accordance with DSM-IV. The PDS consists of 12 items inquiring about the occurrence of specific traumatic experiences. After nominating the event that has disturbed them most in the past month, respondents answer four questions about the nature of the stressor, corresponding to Criterion A. They then answer 17 questions about the frequency in the past month of the symptoms mentioned in Criteria B, C and D, using a 4-point scale ranging from 0 ('not at all or only one time') to 3 ('five or more times a week/almost always'). Finally, nine items assess impairment. A diagnosis of PTSD is based on the presence of a trauma satisfying

Table 12.2 Sensitivity, specificity and power to predict PTSD in adults of different screening instruments

Authors	Instrument	Prevalence of PTSD	Sensitivity	Specificity	Positive predictive power	Negative predictive power	Overall efficiency
Blanchard et al. (1996)	PCL/cut-off 50	45%	0.78	0.86	0.82	0.83	0.82
Blanchard et al. (1996)	PCL/cut-off 44	45%	0.94	0.86	0.85	0.95	0.90
Andrykowski et al. (1998)	PCL/cut-off 50	6%	0.60	0.99	0.75	0.97	0.96
Foa et al. (1997)	PDS	52%	0.89	0.75	–	–	0.82
Davidson et al. (1997a)	DTS	52%	0.69	0.95	0.92	0.79	0.83
Mollica et al. (1992)	HTQ/cut-off 2.5	70%	0.78	0.65	0.85	0.55	0.75
Smith Fawsi et al. (1997)	HTQ/cut-off 1.17	86%	0.98	1.0	–	–	–
Smith Fawsi et al. (1997)	HTQ/cut-off 2.5	86%	0.16	1.0	–	–	–
Fullerton et al. (2000)	DSMPTSD-IV	15%	0.73	0.88	0.55	0.94	0.86
Fullerton et al. (2000)	DSMPTSD-IV	50%	0.64	0.92	0.89	0.72	0.78
Meltzer-Brody et al. (2000)	SPAN	50%	0.77	0.82	0.81	0.78	0.80
Fullerton et al. (2000)	BPTSD-6	–	0.77	0.87	0.75	0.88	0.84

Criterion A, endorsement (rating of 1 or higher) of at least one re-experiencing symptom, three avoidance symptoms and two arousal symptoms, duration of at least 1 month, and impairment in at least one area of functioning. Foa *et al.* (1997) reported a validation study of a PDS-based diagnosis against a SCID (interview-based) diagnosis in 248 mixed trauma victims. The prevalence of PTSD in this sample was 52%. The sensitivity of the PDS was 0.89, specificity was 0.75 and the overall efficiency was 0.82.

Davidson Trauma Scale (DTS)

Davidson *et al.* (1997a) report the development of this PTSD symptom scale based on DSM-IV. The DTS consists of 17 items corresponding to each of the DSM-IV symptoms. For each item, respondents rate both frequency and severity during the previous week on 0–4 scales, yielding a total score of 136. Davidson *et al.* (1997a) report a validation study of the DTS against SCID diagnoses. The sample consisted of 129 mixed trauma victims and the prevalence of PTSD was 52%. Using a cut-off score of 40 determined *post hoc*, the DTS demonstrated high specificity and positive predictive power, with rather lower sensitivity and negative predictive power.

Harvard Trauma Questionnaire (HTQ)

This measure was developed by Mollica *et al.* (1992) to assess traumatic events and symptoms among refugee populations. The trauma symptoms section of the HTQ consists of 16 trauma symptom items based on the DSM framework, together with 14 additional 'refugee' items. Items are scored on a 4-point scale ranging from 1 ('not at all') to 4 ('extremely'), reflecting the severity of symptoms during the past week and the overall score is expressed as the mean of the individual items. Mollica *et al.* (1992) initially validated the HTQ among 91 South-East Asian refugee outpatients, against a criterion of PTSD diagnosed according to DSM-III-R by teams of bicultural staff and psychiatrists. The prevalence of PTSD in this sample was 70%. Using a cut-off score of 2.5, the HTQ demonstrated average screening performance with overall efficiency 75%. More recently, Smith Fawsi *et al.* (1997) conducted a further validation among 51 former Vietnamese political prisoners. The prevalence of PTSD in this sample, as determined by the Structured Clinical Interview for DSM-III-R (SCID) was 86%. Against a cut-off score of 1.17, determined *post hoc* in this sample, sensitivity and specificity were very high, but if the former cut-off score of 2.5 was used sensitivity was only 0.16.

DSMPTSD-III-R and DSMPTSD-IV

The DSMPTSD-III-R (Ursano *et al.*, 1995) and the DSMPTSD-IV (Fullerton *et al.*, 2000) are based on the Impact of Event Scale (Horowitz *et al.*, 1979) and the Symptom Checklist (SCL-90-R: Derogatis, 1983) as core instruments, supplemented by 12 PTSD-specific items. These 12 items are scored in accordance with the SCL-90-R on a 5-point scale ranging from 0 ('not at all') to 4 ('extremely'). Both they and an additional 31 PTSD-relevant SCL-90-R items are grouped in accordance with DSM-III-R or DSM-IV criteria B, C and D. Respondents are classified as probable PTSD if they score more than 19 on the IES and meet PTSD symptom distribution criteria on the remaining 43 items (symptoms rated at least 2 counted as present).

Fullerton *et al.* (2000) reported on the performance of these scales (which were both very similar) at predicting SCID diagnoses of PTSD in a sample of road traffic accident victims, assuming varying PTSD prevalence rates of 15, 50 and 75%. For acute PTSD 1 month post-trauma present in 15% of the sample, the sensitivity of the DSMPTSD-IV was 0.73 and specificity 0.88, with overall efficiency 0.86. If acute PTSD was assumed to be present at a rate of 50%, the sensitivity and overall efficiency of the DSMPTSD-IV fell slightly, while specificity improved. Fullerton *et al.* provide other figures for the ability of both instruments to detect chronic PTSD.

Summary

On average, the overall efficiency of this group of instruments was around 80%, although a higher figure was sometimes achieved by changing cut-off scores *post hoc* or by having a very low prevalence rate. The instrument with the most empirical support to date is the PTSD Checklist (PCL), which has been tested across several different trauma groups and with several different prevalence rates. The DSMPTSD-IV also appears to work well, particularly with lower prevalence rates, but is much longer, requiring that the IES and SCL-90-R are administered. On the other hand, it is the only instrument in this group to have been investigated soon after the occurrence of trauma. Other promising, but little researched instruments include the DTS and the PDS. The former has good specificity, but weaker sensitivity, whereas for the latter the opposite is the case. This may be because the PDS incorporates a low threshold for counting a symptom as present.

Brief PTSD-specific screening questionnaires

Post-traumatic Symptom Scale (PTSS-10)

The first brief measure employed was this 10-item scale developed in Norway (Holen *et al.*, 1983; Weisaeth, 1989). Questions are answered using a Yes/No response format. In his study of a tortured Norwegian ship's crew, Weisaeth (1989) reported that there was no overlap in the PTSS-10 scores of the seven seamen clinically diagnosed with PTSD and the six seamen without PTSD. Subsequent studies have used the PTSS-10 in its original or an adapted form (e.g. Eriksson and Lundin, 1996; Thulesius and Håkansson, 1999), but its performance has not yet been systematically compared with diagnoses yielded by a structured interview.

SPAN scale

This four-item measure was derived from the Davidson Trauma Scale (see above) by Meltzer-Brody *et al.* (1999). A mixed group of 243 patients completed the DTS and was administered a structured diagnostic interview, either the SCID or the Structured Interview PTSD measure (SIP: Davidson *et al.*, 1997b). The sample was divided into two, so that results from the first subsample could be replicated on the second. The prevalence of PTSD was approximately 50% in both subsamples. Good discrimination was obtained using severity scores from the items measuring startle, physiological arousal to trauma cues, anger and numbness (from which the name of the scale was derived). In the replication sample, using a severity score of 5 as a cut-off, screening performance compared favourably with the longer instruments reviewed above. Similar results were obtained when a PTSD prevalence of 10% was assumed.

Brief DSMPTSD-III-R and DSMPTSD-IV

As noted above, 12 PTSD-specific items were developed to supplement the IES and the SCL-90-R in the development of the DSMPTSD-III-R and DSMPTSD-IV. Fullerton *et al.* (2000) reported on the use of these 12 items alone in screening for PTSD. Both 12-item (BPTSD-12) and six-item (BPTSD-6) versions were used, with similar results. Fullerton *et al.* (2000) reported the performance of these brief measures with a number of alternative cut-off scores. For example, using a cut-off score of at least 4 on the BPTSD-6 yielded an overall efficiency of 84%.

Summary

Table 12.2 shows that two new brief screening measures have shown promising results comparable to longer instruments. The four-item SPAN has demonstrated acceptable performance in a replication sample and with varying prevalence rates. The performance of the BPTSD-12 and BPTSD-6 was slightly better than the SPAN, but the former have not been tested as thoroughly.

Development of the Trauma Screening Questionnaire

As part of a randomized controlled trial of psychological debriefing, we interviewed 157 victims of violent crime within 1 month of their assault (Rose *et al.*, 1999). Diagnoses of PTSD corresponding to DSM-III-R (except for the duration criterion) were derived from the PSS-Self Report version. When we counted any symptom scoring at least 1 on the PSS scale (once per week or less/a little bit/once in a while) as present, as recommended by Foa *et al.* (1993), some participants received PTSD diagnoses even though the total PSS score was as low as 9. In order to eliminate low scorers and to conform more exactly to the DSM-III-R requirement for symptoms to be persistent, PSS items were therefore only counted towards a PTSD diagnosis if they were scored 2 or more on the PSS scale (2–4 times per week/somewhat/half the time). This yielded total PSS scores and a rate of PTSD (26.8%) that were comparable with previous studies of crime victims.

The diagnostic utility for detecting concurrent PTSD of endorsing varying numbers of symptoms in the different symptom clusters is shown in Table 12.3. This illustrates, among other things, the more general point that if symptom thresholds are set very low, the sensitivity and negative predictive power of a test will be high, whereas if thresholds are set high, there will be a corresponding increase in specificity and positive predictive power. From Table 12.3 it is evident that the overall efficiency of each symptom cluster peaks at around three or four symptoms. In other words, setting a cut-off of a minimum of three or four symptoms in any of the symptom clusters is the most efficient marker of the presence or absence of PTSD. In the case of the avoidance cluster, of course, three symptoms is a requirement to receive the diagnosis, thereby inflating the figures somewhat. However, this artefact does not affect the other symptom clusters, which perform at virtually the same level and as well as much longer instruments. The sensitivity yielded by using three arousal symptoms is equivalent to figures quoted above for the CAPS structured interview, and likewise the specificity yielded by using three arousal or re-experiencing symptoms matches the CAPS.

What is the utility of using similar thresholds to predict PTSD 6 months later? We followed up our sample after this period and re-administered the PSS to 138 respondents. A complete table similar to Table 12.3 has been published in a previous report (Brewin *et al.*, 1999). Because the focus of the report was on acute stress disorder, figures were provided for avoidance and dissociative symptoms separately. Once again, thresholds of three re-experiencing symptoms (sensitivity 0.71, specificity 0.85, positive predictive value 0.55, negative predictive value 0.92 and overall efficiency 0.83) or three arousal symptoms (sensitivity 0.71, specificity 0.81, positive predictive value 0.49, negative predictive value 0.92 and overall efficiency 0.79) measured after 1 month were efficient at predicting the presence or absence of disorder 6 months later. Analysing the seven PTSD avoidance symptoms, as was done above for concurrent PTSD, would yield similar figures for sensitivity (0.71) and negative predictive value (0.92), but rather poorer results for specificity (0.75), positive predictive value (0.44) and overall efficiency (0.75).

Given the superior performance of the re-experiencing and arousal symptoms at predicting later PTSD, as well as the fact that there were fewer of these symptoms and, hence, a screening instrument could be shorter, we decided to validate the use of these symptoms as a screening tool in an independent sample of trauma victims. Survivors of the Ladbroke Grove train crash were therefore administered a short questionnaire between 7 and 11 months post-trauma, and were asked to indicate whether or not they had experienced each of the five re-experiencing and arousal symptoms at least twice in the past week, using a simple Yes/No response format. Their responses were related to a diagnostic assessment of PTSD using the CAPS, which was administered on

Table 12.3 Sensitivity, specificity and power to predict PTSD of varying numbers of re-experiencing, avoidance and arousal symptoms

PTSD criteria and number of symptoms	Sensitivity	Specificity	Positive predictive power	Negative predictive power	Overall efficiency
B. Re-experiencing					
At least 1 symptom	1.00*	0.64	0.51	1.00*	0.74
At least 2 symptoms	0.90	0.83	0.66	0.96	0.85
At least 3 symptoms	0.74	0.93	0.79	0.91	0.88
At least 4 symptoms	0.50	0.97	0.87	0.84	0.85
At least 5 symptoms	0.14	0.99	0.86	0.76	0.76
C. Avoidance					
At least 1 symptom	1.00*	0.56	0.46	1.00*	0.68
At least 2 symptoms	1.00*	0.71	0.56	1.00*	0.79
At least 3 symptoms	1.00*	0.90	0.79	1.00*	0.93
At least 4 symptoms	0.74	0.97	0.91	0.91	0.91
At least 5 symptoms	0.43	0.98	0.90	0.82	0.83
At least 6 symptoms	0.29	0.98	0.86	0.79	0.80
At least 7 symptoms	0.05	1.00	1.00	0.74	0.75
D. Arousal					
At least 1 symptom	1.00*	0.48	0.41	1.00*	0.62
At least 2 symptoms	1.00*	0.71	0.56	1.00*	0.79
At least 3 symptoms	0.86	0.93	0.82	0.95	0.91
At least 4 symptoms	0.79	0.97	0.89	0.92	0.92
At least 5 symptoms	0.48	0.98	0.91	0.84	0.85

*Values reflect the diagnostic criteria for PTSD laid down in the DSM.

average 1 week later (Brewin *et al.*, 2002). Of the 41 survivors we interviewed, 14 had diagnosed PTSD (prevalence 34%). The criterion of endorsing at least three re-experiencing or arousal symptoms has demonstrated good performance comparable to the other measures reviewed above. However, even better performance (sensitivity 0.86, specificity 0.93, positive predictive value 0.86, negative predictive value 0.93 and overall efficiency 0.90) was achieved by requiring respondents to endorse at least six re-experiencing or arousal symptoms, in any combination. This level of performance is equivalent to that obtained by comparing the CAPS with the SCID (Blake *et al.*, 1995). A similar criterion worked equally well when we re-analysed our data on victims of violent crime. To date, therefore, endorsing at least six re-experiencing or arousal symptoms, in any combination, appears to be an excellent cut-off for detecting PTSD across different time frames, trauma populations and prevalence rates.

Conclusions

To date the Trauma Screening Questionnaire (Brewin *et al.*, 2002) best meets the criteria put forward at the beginning of this chapter. Nevertheless, the knowledge base is steadily growing and it is likely that the next few years will see the development of other instruments that offer good predictive power across a range of other civilian trauma populations and prevalence rates. Already questionnaire measures such as the PTSD Checklist are offering reasonable all-round performance. The evidence reviewed is encouraging in as much as brief questionnaire instruments with 10 items or fewer appear to perform at a similar level to much longer instruments. As such instruments are generally easier to understand, complete and score, this should bring considerable benefits. The finding that a threshold of at least six re-experiencing or arousal symptoms (all at moderate intensity, but in any combination) constitutes an efficient marker of PTSD promises to be extremely useful in helping to monitor victims in the early months post-trauma and identifying who requires more intensive intervention. A simple screening tool of this kind promises to improve the recognition of the disorder in a variety of non-specialist settings. To give just one example, it would facilitate the development in the near future of computer-based screening in GP surgeries, with links to self-help materials and internet-based treatment packages.

References

American Psychiatric Association (1994) *Diagnostic and Statistical Manual of Mental Disorders*, 4th edn. Washington DC: APA.

Andrykowski, M.A., Cordova, M.J., Studts, J.L. and Miller, T.W. (1998) Posttraumatic stress disorder after treatment for breast cancer: prevalence of diagnosis and use of the PTSD Checklist—Civilian version (PCL-C) as a screening instrument. *J Consult Clin Psychol* **66**, 586–90.

Baldessarini, R.J., Finklestein, S. and Arana, G.W. (1983) The predictive power of diagnostic tests and the effect of prevalence of illness. *Arch Gen Psychiat* **40**, 569–73.

Birleson, P. (1981) The validity of depressive disorder in childhood and the development of a self-rating scale. *J Child Psychol Psychiat* **22**, 73–88.

Birmaher, B., Khetarpal, S., Brent, D., Cully, M., Balach, L., Kaufman, J. and McKenzie Neer, S. (1997) The screen for child anxiety related emotional disorders (SCARED): scale construction and psychometric characteristics. *J Am Acad Child Adolesc Psychiat* **36**, 545–53.

Blake, D.D., Weathers, F.W., Nagy, L.M., Kaloupek, D.G., Gusman, F.D., Charney, D.S. and Keane, T.M. (1995) The development of a clinician-administered PTSD scale. *J Traum Stress* **8**, 75–90.

Blanchard, E.B., Jones-Alexander, J., Buckley, T.C. and Forneris, C.A. (1996) Psychometric properties of the PTSD Checklist (PCL). *Behav Res Ther* **34**, 669–73.

Breslau, N., Peterson, E.L., Kessler, R.C. and Schultz, L.R., (1999) Short screening scale for DSM-IV posttraumatic stress disorder. *Am J Psychiat* **156**, 908–11.

Brewin, C.R., Andrews, B., Rose, S. and Kirk, M. (1999) Acute stress disorder and posttraumatic stress disorder in victims of violent crime. *Am J Psychiat* **156**, 360–6.

Brewin, C.R., Rose, S., Andrews, B., Green, J., Tata, P., McEvedy, C., Turner, S. and Foa, E.B. (2002) Brief screening instrument for post-traumatic stress disorder. *Brit J Psychiat* **181**, 158–62.

Coffey, S.F., Dansky, B.S., Falsetti, S.A., Saladin, M.E. and Brady, K.T. (1998) Screening for PTSD in a substance abuse sample: psychometric properties of a modified version of the PTSD Symptom Scale Self-Report. *J Traum Stress* **11**, 393–9.

Craig, R.J. and Olson, R. (1997) Assessing PTSD with the Millon Clinical Multiaxial Inventory-III. *J Clin Psychol* **53**, 943–52.

Darves-Bornoz, J.M., Pierre, F., Lepine, J.P., Degiovanni, A. and Gaillard, P. (1998) Screening for psychologically traumatized rape victims. *Eur J Obstet Gynaecol Reprod Biol* **77**, 71–5.

Davidson, J.R.T., Book, S.W., Colket, J.T., Tupler, L.A., Roth, S., Hertzberg, M., Mellman, T., Beckham, J.C., Smith, R.D., Davidson, R.M., Katz, R. and Feldman, M.E. (1997a) Assessment of a new self-rating scale for post-traumatic stress disorder. *Psychol Med* **27**, 143–60.

Davidson, J.R.T., Malik, M.A. and Travers, J. (1997b) Structured Interview for PTSD (SIP): psychometric validation for DSM-IV criteria. *Depress Anxiety* **5**, 127–9.

Derogatis, L.R. (1983) *SCL-90-R Administration, Scoring and Procedures Manual-II for the Revised Version*, 2nd edn. Towson: Clinical Psychometric Research.

Eriksson, N-G. and Lundin, T. (1996) Early traumatic stress reactions among Swedish survivors of the m/s Estonia disaster. *Br J Psychiat* **169**, 713–16.

Foa, E.B., Riggs, D.S., Dancu, C.V. and Rothbaum, B.O. (1993) Reliability and validity of a brief instrument for assessing post-traumatic stress disorder. *J Traum Stress* **6**, 459–73.

Foa, E.B., Cashman, L., Jaycox, L. and Perry, K. (1997) The validation of a self-report measure of posttraumatic stress disorder: the Posttraumatic Diagnostic Scale. *Psycholog Assess* **9**, 445–51.

Fullerton, C.S., Ursano, R.J., Epstein, R.S., Crowley, B., Vance, K.L., Craig, K.J. and Baum, A. (2000) Measurement of posttraumatic stress disorder in community samples. *Nordic J Psychiat* **54**, 5–12.

Holen, A., Sund, A. and Weisaeth, L. (1983) *The Alexander Kielland Disaster March 27th 1980: psychological reactions among the survivors*. Oslo: Division of Disaster Psychiatry, University of Oslo.

Horowitz, M.J. (1982) Stress response syndromes and their treatment. In Goldberger, L. and Breznitz, S. (ed) *Handbook of Stress: clinical and theoretical aspects*. New York: Free Press, pp. 711–32.

Horowitz, M.J., Wilner, N. and Alvarez, W. (1979) Impact of Event Scale: a measure of subjective stress. *Psychosom Med* **41**, 209–18.

Meltzer-Brody, S., Churchill, E. and Davidson, J.R.T. (1999) Derivation of the SPAN, a brief diagnostic screening test for post-traumatic stress disorder. *Psychiat Res* **88**, 63–70.

Mollica, R.F., Caspi-Yavin, Y., Bollini, P., Truong, T., Tor, S. and Lavelle, J. (1992) Validating a cross-cultural instrument for measuring torture, trauma, and post-traumatic stress disorder in Indochinese refugees. *J Nerv Ment Dis* **180**, 110–15.

Muris, P., Merckelbach, H., Körver, P. and Meesters, C. (2000) Screening for trauma in children and adolescents: the validity of the Traumatic Stress Disorder Scale of the Screen for Child Anxiety Related Emotional Disorders. *J Clin Child Psychol* **29**, 406–13.

Nader, K.O., Kriegler, J.A., Blake, D.D. and Pynoos, R.S. (1994) *Clinician Administered PTSD Scale for Children (CAPS-C)*. Boston: National Center for PTSD.

North, C.S., Nixon, S.J., Shariat, S., Mallonec, S., McMillen, J.C., Spitznagel, E.L. and Smith, E.M. (1999) Psychiatric disorders among survivors of the Oklahoma City bombing. *J Am Med Ass* **282**, 755–62.

Pynoos, R.S., Frederick, C., Nader, K., Arroyo, W., Steinberg, A., Eth, S., Nunez, F. and Fairbanks, L. (1987) Life threat and posttraumatic stress in school-age children. *Arch Gen Psychiat* **44**, 1057–63.

Resick, P.A. (2001) *Stress and Trauma*. Hove: Psychology Press.

Reynolds, C.R. and Richmond, B.O. (1978) What I think and feel: a revised measure of children's manifest anxiety. *J Abnorm Child Psychol* **6**, 271–80.

Rose, S. and Bisson, J.I. (1998) Brief early psychological interventions following trauma: a systematic review of the literature. *J Traum Stress* **11**, 697–710.

Rose, S., Brewin, C.R., Andrews, B. and Kirk, M. (1999) A randomised trial of psychological debriefing for victims of violent crime. *Psycholog Med* **29**, 793–9.

Sack, W.H., Seeley, J.R., Him, C. and Clarke, G.N. (1998) Psychometric properties of the Impact of Events Scale in traumatized Cambodian refugee youth. *Personal Individ Diff* **25**, 57–67.

Shannon, M.P., Lonigan, C.J., Finch, A.J. and Taylor, C.M. (1994) Children exposed to disaster: I. Epidemiology of post-traumatic symptoms and symptom profiles. *J Am Acad Child Adolesc Psychiat* **33**, 80–93.

Smith-Fawsi, M.C., Murphy, E., Pham, T., Lin, L., Poole, C. and Mollica, R.F. (1997) The validity of screening for post-traumatic stress disorder and major depression among Vietnamese former political prisoners. *Acta Psychiat Scand* **95**, 87–93.

Stallard, P., Velleman, R. and Baldwin, S. (1999) Psychological screening of children for post-traumatic stress disorder. *J Child Psychol Psychiat* **40**, 1075–82.

Thulesius, H. and Håkansson, A. (1999) Screening for posttraumatic stress disorder symptoms among Bosnian refugees. *J Traum Stress* **12**, 167–74.

Ursano, R.J., Fullerton, C.S. and Kao, T. (1995) Longitudinal assessment of posttraumatic stress disorder and depression following exposure to traumatic death. *J Nerv Mental Dis* **183**, 36–43.

Weathers, F.W., Huska, J.A. and Keane, T.M. (1991) The PTSD Checklist—Civilian Version (PCL-C). Available from F.W. Weathers, National Center for PTSD, Boston Veterans Affairs Medical Center, 150 S. Huntington Avenue, Boston, MA 02130, USA.

Weathers, F.W., Litz, B.T., Herman, D.S., Huska, J.A. and Keane, T.M. (1993) The PTSD Checklist (PCL): reliability, validity, and diagnostic utility. Paper presented at the meeting of the International Society for Traumatic Stress Studies, San Antonio, TX.

Weisaeth, L. (1989) Torture of a Norwegian ship's crew: the torture, stress reactions and psychiatric after-effects. *Acta Psychiat Scand* Suppl. 355, **80**, 63–72.

Wessely, S., Rose, S. and Bisson J.I. (1998) A systematic review of brief psychological interventions ('debriefing') for the treatment of immediate trauma related symptoms and the prevention of posttraumatic stress disorder. *The Cochrane Library*, published on CD-ROM. Oxford: Update Software Inc.

Yule, W. (1997) Anxiety, depression, and post-traumatic stress in childhood. In Sclare, I. (ed.) *Childpsychology Portfolio*. Windsor: NFER-Nelson.

Yule, W. and Udwin, O. (1991) Screening child survivors for posttraumatic stress disorders: experiences from the 'Jupiter' sinking. *Br J Clin Psychol* **30**, 131–8.

13 A new evidence base for making early intervention in emergency services complementary to officers' preferred adjustment and coping strategies

Roderick Ørner

Traditional prescriptions deconstructed

In the search for helpful early interventions after trauma, investigations have tended to focus on individuals and groups who experience adverse reactions and functional impairment (Shalev *et al.*, 2000). This is as true for accidental victims as for high-risk occupational groups, such as the emergency and uniformed services. This historical legacy is not unreasonable considering the aim of early intervention is to offer assistance for acute trauma-related syndromes. However, hindsight also makes us wiser about the biases and blind spots inherent in this particular line of investigation. For instance, it is now recognized that trauma does not invariably result in functional impairments (Lyons, 1991) and can promote positive personal adjustment in the longer term (Tedeschi *et al.*, 1998). Much less is known about the processes that promote post-traumatic coping, post-traumatic competence and post-traumatic mastery than the risk factors associated with adjustment difficulties.

Suitably humbled, psychotraumatology is now discovering that there is a long-established requirement and demonstrated competency within some occupational groups, e.g. emergency and uniformed services, to adjust to recurrent exposures to trauma. They do so in a manner that meets a minimum requirement of maintaining operational readiness. Granted, this is not always possible for everyone (Alexander and Klein, 2001), but officers learn through experience that individual and group actions help mitigate the psychological and somatic sequelae of exposure to trauma. This may go some way towards explaining the fact that occupational satisfaction ratings in these professions are comparable to those reported for other professions not routinely exposed to traumatic stressors (Brown *et al.*, 1996).

An examination of published prescriptions about early intervention reveals that some notional recognition has been given to the organizational and personal imperatives of coping and competence. For instance, Mitchell (1983) claims that the origins of protocol prescriptions for critical incident stress debriefing (CISD) derive from long-established and naturally emergent practices 'in the field'. He argued that special initiatives are required because it is common to experience some level of distress and agitation after critical and traumatic incidents. Clearly, such reactions present a challenge to the officers themselves, their peer groups, their employing organizations and helping professionals to decide how best to confront and come to terms with these reactions.

Given the extensive experience of these organizations and their staff in effecting appropriate adjustments to trauma, it is unclear why Mitchell (1983) advocated introducing mental health workers trained in CISD to promote these ends.

If it is correct that Mitchell's (1983) protocol prescriptions for CISD derive directly from field practice within emergency and uniformed services, it should follow that to call and hold a CISD meeting would be seamlessly integrated as an adjunct to long-established coping and adjustment strategies. Systematic evaluations of CISD suggest otherwise (Carlier, 2001). The seemingly arbitrary introduction of mental health professionals as a standard for early intervention puts paid to that. This recommendation undermines and devalues naturally emergent, sensible and largely informal self and peer group care practices. Such expropriation of coping and competence, by the champions of CISD has caused a shift of emphasis away from naturally occurring adjustment reactions to PTSD psychopathology, presumptions of competence has been replaced by imposed dependence on professional helpers and active mastery has been substituted by pacified consumer discipline.

In fact, there are several profound flaws in the way CISD has been promoted. The most obvious presumption to be challenged is the notion that all responders will wish to attend a group meeting as part of their post-incident adjustment strategy. No evidence base exists that demonstrates all officers want to talk to colleagues about what has happened and listen to their accounts. In the absence of such evidence it is imprudent to prescribe a single early intervention protocol. For similar reasons, the recommendation of mandatory participation in CISD appears wholly perfunctory. A further criticism can be levelled at the implied assumption that administration of protocol driven technical interventions will engender the subtle group processes that occur more or less spontaneously in natural settings. This is not likely since technique is no substitute for process. CISD is further compromised by a failure to differentiate declared objectives from putative aims. These are listed by Mitchell and Everly (1995) as if they are one and the same. For instance, it is a reasonable objective to call a group meeting to share information about a critical event. However, there is no causal link between this objective and the proclaimed aim of effecting a reduction in PTSD symptomatology.

Requests that the evidence base that inspired CISD protocol prescriptions should be brought into the public domain for comment and peer review have been made by Gist and Woodall (1998) and also by Avery *et al*. (1999). But none has been forthcoming. No surprise, therefore, to find an emergent body of opinion which suspects the evidence base for Mitchell's (1983) recommendations is anecdotal, impressionistic and lacking in scientific rigour. Marked discrepancies exist between the prophecies of what CISD and its closely related derivatives can purportedly achieve (Mitchell, 1983; Dyregrov, 1989; Armstrong *et al*., 1991) and demonstrated outcomes documented by systematic research (Rose and Bisson, 1998).

Starting again by coming full circle

For the reasons outlined above it is most unlikely that further methodological refinements of randomized controlled outcome studies will, engender an evidence base for improving standards for CISD. The question therefore arises as to what to do next? Ørner and King (1999) have proposed an entirely different line of enquiry that offers a prospect of resolving the current impasse. They suggest going back to first principles. This involves recognizing that emergency responders have developed competencies for adjusting to trauma. The foremost precondition for sensible practice is to start by systematically investigating how this feat is achieved. Only when this evidence base has been established is it justifiable to propose prescriptive guidelines in respect of early intervention for emergency services staff.

This chapter outlines an emergent evidence base derived from an investigation carried out in accordance with the above suggestions and considers its implications for informed practice in respect of early intervention for emergency services officers.

Subjects and methodology

Examination of standardized self report measures used in earlier studies of coping (Lazarus and Folkman, 1984; Rutter, 1990) revealed these to be insufficiently specific for the purposes of detailing action taken by emergency services officers to specifically mitigate the effects of critical incidents and trauma. To develop an appropriate instrument for this survey a semi-structured pilot interview was carried out with 18 police officers and fire fighters who had recently attended a multiple fatality road traffic accident. All agreed this was one of the worst incidents they had been called to for many years. The emergency responders were asked to give a detailed account of deliberate steps taken during the incident and its aftermath to modulate the distress they felt. Two self-report questionnaires were designed based on their narratives. The first asked respondents to 'think back to a particularly distressing incident at work that affected you more than usually'. Then, keeping this specific event in mind, respondents ticked 65 statements according to the degree to which each described their preferred adjustment strategy in the aftermath of this event. The second questionnaire comprised 19 statements about deliberate steps routinely taken to modulate distress evoked by work-related critical and traumatic events. For all statements a four-point Likert scale was used which for data analysis purposes was reduced to three (often, occasionally and never).

These self-report measures were administered to 217 mostly middle ranking emergency services officers at the start of a series of awareness raising workshops about staff care following critical and traumatic incidents in the workplace. The study period spanned four workshops held during 1999 and 2000. All delegates had line management or supervisory responsibilities and had been nominated by their employing service on the basis of their declared interest in advancing their professional competence in respect of staff support. None refused to participate in the survey and all questionnaires returned were valid for data analysis purposes. The final sample comprised 49 police officers (22.6%), 45 fire fighters (20.7%), 24 ambulance service staff (11.1%), 84 national health service personnel (38.7%) and 15 social services representatives (6.9%). 123 were male (56.7%) and 94 were female (43.3%). The age range was 19–59 years with a mean age of 41.3 years. Time of service with current employer ranged from 1 to 40 years with a mean of 17.7 years.

For data analysis purposes, 118 subjects from police, fire brigade and ambulance services (54.4%) were grouped as front line responders. The remaining 99 (45.6%) from national health and social services were grouped as second line responders. These two groups were comparable for age (Mann-Whitney $U=5096$, $P=0.11$) and length of service (Mann-Whitney $U=10080$, $P=0.12$). Reflecting diverging service specific employment practices, as well as gender career preferences, men were over represented in front line services ($n=108$, 91.5%) as were women in second line services ($n=84$, 84.8%) ($\chi^2=127.89$, df$=1$, $P<0.001$).

Results

Distress evoked by critical incidents

Survey returns confirmed that a career in the emergency services is at some time likely to involve deployment to incidents that evoke high levels of distress. In this sample all subjects could identify one such index event and 158 (72.8%) rated evoked distress as marked or overwhelming. Overall, the intensity of reactions were equally strong within front and second line services ($\chi^2 = 3.29$, df = 1, NS) as it was amongst men and women ($\chi^2 = 2.93$, df = 1, NS).

Early, rather than late identification of distress was the norm for emergency services staff. 132 subjects (60.8%) felt distress during the incident itself and a further 52 (24.0%) did so within 24 hours of finishing their operational involvement. Delayed recognition occurred only for the 16 (7.4%) who first realized the impact of the event between 24 and 48 hours. Another 17 (7.8%) did so after three days or more. This time-related pattern of acknowledging the emotional impact of work related incidents in the emergency services is independent of service groups ($\chi^2 = 2.01$, df = 3, NS) and gender ($\chi^2 = 3.03$, df = 3, NS).

As to the nature of evoked reactions, only 34 (5.7%) confirmed experiencing persistently intrusive sensory impressions as described for DSM-IV diagnoses of Acute Stress Disorder or Post-traumatic Stress Disorder (APA, 1994). Most commonly reported by 161 subjects (74.2%) were enduring feelings of distress perceived as a natural consequence of having witnessed a particularly tragic occurrence. For a further 22 officers (10.1%) distress was attributed to a perceived failure to provide a satisfactory standard of professional service rather than an aspect of the incident itself. This pattern of evoked reactions occurred with comparable regularity in the two service groups ($\chi^2 = 1.79$, df = 2, NS), and was independent of gender ($\chi^2 = 1.29$, df = 3, NS).

In summary, these findings are consistent with previous reports documenting the emotionally evocative nature of some critical incidents to which emergency services staff are called (Alexander and Klein, 2001). A failure to recognize the distinctive status of some such events, against a backdrop of predominantly routine deployments is ill advised. However, emergency services staff give every indication of being aware of these facts and have learned to draw upon adjustment strategies which modulate their reactions. Self-reports or observation of evoked distress does not therefore necessarily constitute a demonstrated need for professionals to provide early intervention. At best, it raises the possibility of extra help and support being welcomed at some stage.

Who is turned to for support after critical and traumatic incidents?

In the first instance, the inclination of 155 subjects (71.4%) was to welcome contact with colleagues when adjusting to a critical incident. Forty-two (19.4%) were indifferent and 20 (10.3%) stated they did not want such contact. This ratio of responses was very similar to that expressed for degrees of welcoming contact with a partner or someone close away from the workplace. Here percentages were respectively 75.6% ($n = 157$), 16.7% ($n = 35$), 7.7% ($n = 16$). Overall, it would appear those who welcomed contact with colleagues reported the same for others with whom they felt close, and vice versa ($\chi^2 = 21.3$, df = 4, $P < 0.001$; see Table 13.1).

It is, however, noteworthy that front and second line service groups differed significantly in ratings given for welcoming contact with colleagues ($\chi^2 = 15.99$, df = 2, $P < 0.001$). This was principally because positive endorsements were given by 84 second line emergency services officers (84.8%), but only 71 (60.7%) in front line services. These findings were associated with contrasting gender preferences ($\chi^2 = 6.84$, df = 2, $P < 0.05$) in so far that in the total sample 76 female subjects (80.9%) welcomed contact with colleagues, whereas only 79 men (64.6%) did so. It would appear therefore that peer support was rated highly within emergency services organizations. This was particularly so in second line services, which predominantly employ female staff. Within front line, male-dominated services there was a higher proportion of officers who did not routinely turn to colleagues for help and support. No statistically significant differences were found for service ($\chi^2 = 0.12$, df = 2, NS) or gender endorsements ($\chi^2 = 0.32$, df = 2, NS) for welcoming contact with someone close away from the workplace.

Table 13.1 Sources of support used by emergency services staff after traumatic events (n = 217)

Sources of support	Contact welcomed	Indifferent to contract	Did not want contact	Service Group	Gender Group
Colleagues	155 (71.4%)	42 (19.4%)	20 (10.3%)	P<0.001*	P<0.05†
Someone close	157 (75.6%)	35 (16.7%)	16 (7.7%)	NS	NS
Welfare department staff	22 (10.1%)	80 (36.9%)	102 (47.0%)	NS	NS
Outside professional helpers	20 (9.2%)	76 (35.0%)	111 (51.2%)	NS	NS

*Higher endorsement rates in second line emergency services group.
†Higher endorsement rates in female emergency services officers group.

Welcome ratings for contact with welfare department staff formed an altogether different pattern. Only 22 (10.1%) welcomed such contact, 80 (36.9%) were indifferent and 102 (47.0%) did not want such contact in the early aftermath of critical events. For contact with outside professionals endorsement levels are even less favourable at 20 (9.2%), 76 (35.9%) and 111 (51.2%). Neither service group nor gender differences for welcoming contact with welfare departments or outside professionals achieve statistical significance. This evidence conveys a clear message for helping professionals not to assume their active involvement in the early aftermath of critical and traumatic events will be welcomed or even be perceived as necessary.

Implications

As revealed in Table 13.1, most emergency service officers actively seek contact with colleagues and others with whom they feel close. However, distinctive service group (front and second line) and gender processes appear to influence ratings given for welcoming contact with colleagues. Health and social services staff appear to function within an organizational culture in which help and support from colleague is given most prominent emphasis. It is of interest to note that these service and gender differences do not seem to generalize to others with whom officers feel close, staff in welfare departments or outside professionals.

Not everyone wants to talk

Early intervention protocols presume emergency services staff wish to talk about what has happened. Over time, this presumption has somehow been elevated to the status of a necessary requirement for post-incident coping and adjustment. The evidence of this survey suggests otherwise. Talking about the event was important for 173 (79.7%) of all respondents. However, this left a substantial proportion of 43 officers (19.8%) who used adjustment strategies that were not primarily contingent on developing a verbal narrative of what had happened. Amongst front line officers the proportion whose preference was not to talk is nearly one in three ($n=34$, 28.8%). In the second line services the proportion was less than one in 10 ($n=10$, 9.2%). The distribution of 'talkers' and 'non-talkers' in the two service groups differed to a statistically significant degree ($\chi^2=12.94$, df=1, $P<0.001$). Gender preferences broke down into similar ratios of talkers and non-talkers. Amongst male and female subjects, respectively, 33 (26.8%) and 10 (10.8%) resorted to adjustment strategies that did not preferentially involve talking about what has happened ($\chi^2 = 8.41$, df = 1, $P < 0.01$).

Implications

This evidence suggests marked service and gender differences exist in respect of the extent to which officers talk about what has happened to their colleagues and those with whom they feel close. It is therefore no longer advisable to insist that talking about what has occurred is necessary for everyone in the aftermath of critical and traumatic incidents. The prescription of relying on structured, talk-based and agenda driven early intervention protocols is brought into further question by other findings. For instance, only 13 subjects (6.0%) endorsed formalized interventions as their preferred means of adjusting to what had happened. 186 (85.7%) preferred an informal and undirected context within which they could use their own adjustment and coping strategies. This preference was shared to a similar extent in both service groups ($\chi^2 = 0.57$, df = 2, NS) and amongst male and female subjects ($\chi^2 = 1.96$, df = 2, NS). Clearly, the emergent principle is that emergency services staff approach post-incident adjustment with an awareness of having a range of adjustment options from which they choose on the basis of circumstances and their subjective preferences of what is appropriate for any given or constantly changing situation.

A time for talking

Survey returns point to an important relationship between time of talking to colleagues and rated helpfulness of doing so. This has major implications for early intervention. Whilst 93 (42.9%) reported not talking to colleagues about their evoked distress during the index event, a similar proportion of 88 (40.6%) actually did and found this to be helpful. Highest helpfulness was derived from talking to colleagues immediately after the event. At this time point, 111 (51.2%) found talking helpful. Thereafter, diminishing returns were reported. 90 (41.5%) found talking helpful during the subsequent 24 hours and this decreased to 82 (37.8%) after more than one day. For those who actually chose to talk, the time-related changes in perceived helpfulness were in the direction of talking becoming neither helpful nor unhelpful, rather than becoming definitely unhelpful. As summarized in Table 12.2, indications are that with the passing of time a greater number of officers choose not to continue to talk about what happened. There is clearly an optimum time for talking to colleagues and results suggest greatest benefits occurred at an early, rather than a later stage post-incident.

Implications

The evidence of this survey suggests that by introducing a delay before considering early intervention emergency services officers will have reached a stage where talking is typically rated as neither helpful nor unhelpful. Good leadership practices encouraging immediate and early peer support is strongly indicated.

Service and gender differences in rated helpfulness of talking

Front line and second line emergency services officers differed markedly in the helpfulness ratings given to talking to colleagues during the event, immediately after incident closure and during the subsequent 24 hours (see Table 12.2). Hospital and social services staff were significantly more likely to give favourable helpfulness ratings for talking during the incident ($\chi^2 = 18.87$, df = 3, $P < 0.001$), during its immediate aftermath ($\chi^2 = 12.01$, df = 3, $P < 0.01$) and the first day after the incident ($\chi^2 = 11.36$, df = 3, $P < 0.05$). Thereafter, service group differences failed to achieve statistical significance ($\chi^2 = 6.27$, df = 3, NS) as the prevailing norm approached that of

Table 13.2 Rated helpfulness of talking (N=217)

	Helpful	Neither helpful or unhelpful	Unhelpful talk	Did not group	Service group	Gender
During an incident						
To colleagues	88(40.6%)	17(7.8%)	19(8.8%)	93(42.9%)	$P<0.001$*	$P<0.05$†
Immediately after incident						
To colleagues	111(51.2%)	20(9.2%)	17(7.8%)	69(31.8%)	$P<0.01$*	NS
To someone close	104(47.9%)	21(9.7%)	10(4.6%)	82(37.6%)	NS	NS
During first day after incident						
To colleagues	90(41.5%)	33(15.2%)	16(7.4%)	78(35.9%)	$P<0.05$*	$P<0.05$†
To someone close	86(39.6%)	37(17.1%)	10(4.6%)	84(38.5%)	NS	NS
After more than one day						
To colleagues	82(37.8%)	36(16.6%)	19(8.7%)	80(36.9%)	NS	$P<0.05$†
To someone close	64(29.5%)	50(23.0%)	13(6.0%)	90(41.5%)	NS	NS

*Highest endorsement rates in second line emergency services group.
†Highest endorsement rates in female emergency services officer group.

not talking. Positive endorsement rates for front and second line services at each of the first three time intervals were, respectively, 36 (30.5%) and 52 (52.5%); 50 (42.4%) and 61 (61.6%); 37 (31.4%) and 53 (53.5%). Gender-related helpfulness ratings followed a similar pattern, but differed in one important respect. Female officers rated talking as significantly more helpful at the time of the incident ($\chi^2=15.27$, df=3, $P<0.01$; 51.1% for female and 32.5% for male officers), during the first day after the incident ($\chi^2=10.74$, df=3, $P<0.05$; 53.2% and 32.5%) and after more than 1 day ($\chi^2=9.29$, df=3, $P<0.05$; 45.7% and 31.7%). Immediately after the incident, however, greater gender consensus prevailed with respect to the helpfulness of talking ($\chi^2=7.41$, df=3, NS; 59.6 and 44.7%).

Implications

These findings reinforce the impression that the optimal time for emergency services staff to talk to colleagues is immediately after a critical or traumatic event, and that this is especially true within second line services. Even under the most difficult circumstances of the career 'worst' incidents of officers who took part in this survey it would appear that they could rely on a sense of self-sufficiency, coping and competence to reduce evoke distress. For instance, 172 (79.3%) confirmed drawing upon the same adjustment strategies used for the index event when trying to modulate distress evoked by other similar incidents. Members of front line and second line emergency services did not differ in respect of the high levels of generalizability of their preferred adjustment strategies ($\chi^2=2.49$, df=1, NS). In this respect gender differences were not significant either ($\chi^2=1.37$, df=1, NS). Also consistent with the impression of competence and autonomy was the finding that 88 (40.6%) preferred to make their own independent decision about whether or not to access early intervention services. Only five (2.3%) would have preferred to be mandated to attend. 44 (20.3%) preferred to decide in consultation with line managers and 48 (22.1%) in consultation with colleagues. In these respects, statistically significant service and gender differences were found. The differentiating factors were that front line responders prefer the most independent decision options whilst second line services staff showed a greater inclination to confer with their peers ($\chi^2=36.19$, df=4, $P<0.001$).

Deliberate actions taken to reduce distress and implications for early intervention

As outlined above, emergency services officers are by no means rendered passively dependent by distress evoked by work-related trauma. Rather, they deliberately draw upon a range of specific, sometimes idiosyncratic adjustment strategies that mitigate the impact of events. Any consideration of early intervention for emergency services staff should therefore be premised by a recognition that these preferred adjustment strategies engender a sense of coping and competence during what may be a time of personal crisis. Early intervention should therefore, at all times, be informed by a resolve to offer help in a manner that recognizes and complements existing personal and organizational resources.

How this can be done is suggested by returns from a questionnaire that listed a range of deliberate coping strategies commonly used by emergency services staff. Each subject ticked a four-point scale to indicate the extent to which each strategy is relied upon to reduce the impact critical and traumatic events have had upon them (0=never, 3=always). When responses were subjected to a five factor principal component analysis the emergent factors could be labelled as follows:

- 'Wait and monitor the nature and course of reactions';
- 'Rest and relaxation';
- 'Re-establish control and routines';
- 'Confront what has happened';
- 'Find release from somatosensory sequelae' (see Table 13.3, column 1).

These five factors account for 41.9% of the total variance of scores observed in the sample surveyed.

Examples of deliberate actions that comprise each of these clusters are listed in Table 13.3, column 2. The levels of endorsement given to each are as in columns 3–5. Comparisons of columns 1 and 2 with column 6, which lists CISD prescriptions for early intervention, reveals striking differences between preferred coping strategies and protocol prescriptions. For instance, whilst CISD prescribes group meetings within days of a critical incident it would appear emergency services officers overwhelmingly prefer to wait and monitor their reactions. Personal and group interests appear to be served by an initial period of waiting. This is sensible to the extent it allows officers to monitor the nature, intensity and course of their reactions. It also allows for simultaneous opportunities to rest and relax after what may have been physically and psychologically exacting experiences. Equally ill advised is the instruction that participation in CISD meetings should be mandatory. Such a prescription runs counter to officers' preferred practices on several counts. It compromises their preferred option to 'wait and see' and, furthermore, cannot be readily reconciled with the stated priority for fostering a sense of personal control and re-establishing routines.

A rare point of convergence between CISD prescriptions and officers' preferred coping strategies is found in a common recognition of the importance of confronting what has happened. For most, but by no means all officers, talking serves this purpose. However, as many as 98 officers (45.6%) acknowledge occasionally deliberately avoiding reminders of what has happened. A further 29 (13.5%) do so often. Such avoidance may be functional to the extent it enhances a sense of subjective control that may be helpful in the longer term. It would appear, therefore, that in the early aftermath of critical and traumatic events control takes precedence over confrontation. This is consistent with Gerson's (2003) suggestion that early intervention should not engender further psychophysiological over arousal at a time when the priority of at least some officers is to rest and relax.

Table 13.3 Deliberate coping strategies used to reduce impact of events (*n*=217)

Guiding principles for coping and competence	Examples for early intervention	Often	Occasionally	Never	CISD prescription
Wait and monitor the nature and course of reactions	Deliberately let time pass	148 (67.9%)	59 (27.4%)	10 (4.7%)	Intervene early (48–72 hours)
Rest and relaxation	Deliberately go somewhere comfortable	139 (64.7%)	58 (27.0%)	18 (8.4%)	Prioritize convening group meeting
	Deliberately relax	140 (65.4%)	62 (29.0%)	12 (5.6%)	
Re-establish control and routines	Deliberately take charge of my life	153 (71.5%)	49 (22.9%)	12 (5.6%)	Mandatory attendance
	Deliberately re-establish routines	146 (67.9%)	49 (22.8%)	20 (9.3%)	
Confront what has happened	Deliberately talk about the event in general terms	170 (78.7%)	45 (20.8%)	1 (0.5%)	Adhere to prescriptive protocol
	Deliberately avoid some reminders	29 (13.5%)	98 (45.6%)	88 (40.9%)	
Find release from somatosensory sequelae	Deliberately use humour	163 (75.5%)	46 (21.3%)	7 (3.2%)	Only talk based
	Deliberately do what releases physical sensations	138 (63.9%)	67 (31.0%)	11 (5.1%)	

Principal component analysis indicates the five clusters in column 1 account for 41.9% of the total variance.

A further element of deliberate coping is to effect relief from somatosensory sequelae of trauma. Officers achieve this by resorting to humour, as well as a various forms of physical activity. Keeping busy, working hard and taking exercise may, for some, be more adaptive than talking. Even for those who rely on talking there appears to be a place for combining this form of confrontation with other non-verbally based coping strategies.

Discussion

This survey confirms previous reports that work related critical incidents and trauma can evoke marked distress reactions in emergency services personnel (Clohessy and Ehlers, 1999; Alexander and Klein, 2001). Not only does this present a personal and occupational challenge, but it also highlights the necessity of making some successful adjustment that will be conducive to maintaining operational readiness and a sense of personal control. Basic competency training for emergency services staff should therefore include awareness raising about the psychological risks of emergency response, especially as it arises in critical and traumatic incidents. Such training can be complemented by recommendations based on the commonly used adjustment and coping strategies that mitigate event-related distress.

When exceptional critical or traumatic events have occurred there may be occasions when specialist help and support should be made available to officers in the emergency services. However, the premises that have so far underpinned prescriptions for early interventions are long overdue for radical review. For emergency services staff, early intervention can now be reconstructed from an empirical evidence base that builds on officers' demonstrated capacity for post-incident coping and competence. Officers called to critical and traumatic events typically recognize their psychological impact during or very shortly after its occurrence. The challenge is therefore immediate and special adjustment strategies are mobilized without delay. On site and back at the operational base officers initially draw on peer support, and later seek help from friends or others with whom they feel close. For eight out of ten responders a core aspect of post-incident adjustment is to talk about and confront what has happened. However, the stated preference is to do so without interference or intrusion from either welfare department staff or outside professionals, such as mental health workers.

The conclusions and recommendations arising from this survey should be qualified by a recognition that the sample is drawn from a single English county, and that the sample has skewed gender distributions in front line and second line services. For these reasons, it has not been possible to establish the extent to which observed differences are related specifically to service and gender variables or interactions between the two. For these reasons, the evidence base should be expanded to encompass all regions of the United Kingdom and other countries. This will help to identify the extent of regional or local variations. Larger numbers will also help clarify the extent to which front line and second line services have developed different adjustment strategies due to the nature of the incidents to which they are called or if gender preferences are the overriding variable. Staff in other public service organizations (e.g. the military, the prison service), should be surveyed to establish appropriate evidence bases for early intervention. The same could be done for volunteer, helpers and accident victims.

All the same the findings of this survey indicate that allowances must be made for important service and gender specific variations. Even when adjustment strategies are incorporated in the organizational cultures and leadership practices of emergency services, not all officers have identical adjustment priorities (Alexander and Walker, 1994). These organizational considerations recommend themselves to the extent they provide flexible scope for each individual to follow his or her own preferred adjustment strategy. The notion that there is a single post-incident adjustment path to be followed under guidance of mental health workers appears ill informed and unhelpful. Reconstructed early intervention therefore has to incorporate recognition that within the emergency services there is no single and universal prescription for adjusting to work-related critical incidents and trauma. In future, early intervention provision for emergency responders should be flexibly planned and delivered in progressive stages. Because no blueprint exists for early intervention the imperative is to enter into consultation and negotiation with possible service users about their needs and preferences. Providers must also be cognisant of the requirement to obtain informed consent. In contrast to past practices, no helpers should claim prescriptive expertise unless a substantiating evidence base exists in support of particular early interventions.

Consistent with the above Avery *et al.* (1998) proposed that the aim of early intervention might usefully be reformulated as 'seeking to effect agreed and operationalized improvement(s) in the quality of the recovery environment'. The platform for achieving this aim within emergency services should, in the first instance be peer support and help from friends away from the workplace.

References

American Psychiatric Association (1994). Diagnostic and statistical manual of mental disorders. Fourth edition (DSM-IV). Washington, D.C. APA.

Alexander, D.A. and Klein, S. (2001) Ambulance personnel and critical incidents. Impact of accident and emergency work on mental health and emotional well-being. *Br J Psychiat* **178**, 76–81.

Alexander, D.A. and Walker, A. (1991) Reactions of police officers to body handling after a major disaster. A before and after comparison. *Br J Psychiat* **159**, 547–55.

Armstrong, K., O'Callahan, W. and Marmar, C. (1991) Debriefing Red Cross disaster personnel: the multiple stressors debriefing model. *J Traum Stress* **4**, 581–93.

Avery, A., King, S. and Ørner, R.J. (1998) First report on psychological debriefing abandoned. The end of an era? *Traum Stress Points* **12**(3), 3–4.

Avery, A., King, A., Bretherton, R. and Ørner R.J. (1999) Deconstructing psychological debriefing and the call for evidence based practice. *Eur Soc Traum Stress Stud Bull* **6**, 7–11.

Brown, J., Cooper, C. and Kilkardy, B. (1996) Occupational stress among senior police officers. *Br J Psychol* **87**, 31–41.

Carlier, I. (2001) What early intervention can achieve. In Ørner, R.J. and Schnyder, U. (eds) *Reconstructing Early Intervention after Trauma*. Oxford: Oxford University Press.

Clohessy, S.W. and Ehlers, A. (1999) PTSD symptoms, response to intrusive memories and coping in ambulance service workers. *Br J Clin Psychol* **38**, 251–65.

Dyregrov, A. (1989) Caring for helpers in disaster situations—psychological debriefing. *Disaster Manag* **2**, 25–30.

Gersons, B.R. (2003) Historical background; social psychology and crisis theory. In Ørner, R.J. and Schnyder, U. (eds) *Reconstructing Early Intervention after Trauma*. Oxford University Press, Oxford.

Gist, R. and Woodall, S.J. (1998) Social Science versus social movements: the origins and natural history of debriefing. *Aust J Disaster Trauma Stud*. Available at: http:/www.massey.ac.nz/~trauma/issues/1998–1/gist1.htm.

Lazarus, R.S. and Folkman, S. (1984) *Stress, Appraisal and Coping*. New York: Springer Publishing Co.

Lyons, J.A. (1991) Strategies for assessing the potential for positive adjustment following trauma. *J Traum Stress* **4**, 93–111.

Mitchell, J.T. (1983) When disaster strikes. The critical incident stress debriefing process. *J Emerg Med Serv* **8**, 36–9.

Mitchell, J.T. and Everly, G.S. (1995) Critical incident stress debriefing (CISD) and the prevention of work related traumatic stress among high risk occupational groups. In G.S. Everly and J.M. Lating (eds) *Psychotraumatology: key papers and core concepts in post traumatic stress*. New York: Plenum Press, pp. 267–280.

Ørner, R.J. and King, S. (1999) *A New Evidence Base for Early Intervention after Trauma*. Paper presented at the 6th European Conference on Traumatic Stress, June 6–9th 1999, Istanbul, Turkey.

Rose, S. and Bisson, J. (1998) Brief early interventions following trauma: a systematic review of the literature. *J Traum Stress* **11**, 697–710.

Rutter, M. (1990) Psychosocial resilience and protective mechanisms. In Rolf, J., Masten, A., Cicchetti, D., Nuechterlein K. and Weintraub, S. (eds) *Risk and Protective Factors in the Development of Psychopathology*. New York: Cambridge University Press, pp. 181–224.

Shalev, A.Y., Yehuda, R. and McFarlane, A.C. (2000) *International Handbook of Human Response to Trauma*. London: Kluwer Academic/Plenum Publishers.

Tedeschi, R.G., Park, C.L. and Calhoun, L.G. (1998) *Posttraumatic Growth: positive changes in the aftermath of crisis*. Mahwah: Lawrence Erlbaum Associates.

Section 4 The evidence base provided by applied early intervention strategies

As explained in other sections of this book, early intervention is not a recent innovation. Its legacy extends into distant times and is characterized by constant change. History reveals its typical position to be on the margins of professional activity and even within the trauma field it has only recently attained status as a mainstream intervention. What is not in doubt, however, is the capacity of early intervention to re-invent itself to accommodate new and changing circumstances. Most transformations have been inspired by pragmatic imperatives of 'having to do' rather than theoretical advances or refinements.

In these respects, early intervention has its own distinct momentum that continues to the present. The process of reconstructing early intervention will therefore not be complete unless account is taken of recent demonstration projects that exemplify informed practice. To this end, Section 4 is a compilation of chapters selected for the guidance offered to those preoccupied with establishing evidence-based service delivery to a wide variety of survivor populations. Suggestions offered about 'how to do' are the personal views of chapter authors and should not be taken to imply they are sanctioned for general use. They are featured in this book on the understanding readers will judge their relative merits and appropriateness for the survivor populations whose needs they seek to address.

The first impression to emerge from Section 4 is the range of survivor populations for whom early intervention is now considered appropriate. In addition to model services for military personnel described by Professor Lars Mehlum of the Norwegian Armed Forces Medical Service, new and innovative schemes are bringing systematic care to populations for whom early intervention has hitherto not been considered a priority. For instance, Drs Josef Ruzek and Matthew Cordova, respectively, of the Veterans Administration Health Care System and Stanford University in Palo Alto, USA, report on the establishment of an early intervention service for patients admitted to hospital for medical care. Screening for a wide variety of medical and psychosocial needs that emerge into prominence in conjunction with hospitalization helps engender a sense of wholistic patient care. By integrating psychosocial perspectives into hospital provision these authors document improved recovery paths for a number of patient groups. A similar scheme has been established and evaluated by Dr Jonathan Bisson for the Accident and Emergency Services Department, University Hospital of Wales in Cardiff, United Kingdom. He too exemplifies the value of screening patients and targeting services at those identified as being in greatest need.

Reconstructed early intervention implies not only flexible service provision informed by survivors' stated preferences, but also some degree of continuity of provision that may extend into the longer term. In keeping with this principle, relatively simple interventions, possibly with a psycho-educational focus, may be strongly indicated once safety and security needs have been addressed. Given their relative simplicity and appropriateness for early stages of post-trauma adjustment, this phase of reconstructed early interventions should be so planned as to anticipate calls to coordinate and deliver information based services targeted at whole populations affected by trauma. Dr Kaz de Jong of Médecins Sans Frontières and Professor Rolf Kleber of the Institute of Psychotrauma at Tilburg and Utrecht Universities, The Netherlands, detail how the provision of services that disseminate of information relevant to trauma survivors comprises a prominent component of early intervention for refugees. This theme is both elaborated and reinforced by Professor Bill Yule of the Institute of Psychiatry, University of London, England, in his chapter titled 'Early intervention strategies with traumatized children, adolescents and families'. He makes a strong case for ensuring information is made available about common reactions to trauma so that these are demystified. Survivors, their relatives and friends will also wish to be advised of other facts pertaining to what has happened. From their points of view immediate and longer-term adjustment will crucially depend upon being able to access information about known casualties, where the injured are, if populations have been displaced into different reception centres, knowing where to go to establish the whereabouts of family members, etc. Group meetings called to share known facts is recommended as one of the means by which awareness raising can be achieved. They also offer an opportunity to carry out informal screening. It is clear, therefore, that information management has emerged as a core element of reconstructed early intervention!

Re-establishing family or social networks and raising awareness can for most survivors, help engender a sense of coping and mastery under difficult circumstances. Establishing services apposite for the early aftermath of trauma typically involves responding to immediate needs, but it is unwise to presume they will necessarily prove to be short-term measures. As reiterated by several authors, reconstructed early intervention involves taking short, intermediate and long-term perspectives on survivors' needs. For the latter two eventualities, brief and focused psychological therapy is indicated subject considerations being given to local culture and conditions.

Several authors make a case for drawing on the evidence base pertaining to cognitive behaviour therapy (CBT) to rationalize its use, and adaptation, for early intervention with trauma survivors. Professor Richard Bryant of University of New South Wales in Sydney, Australia gives a summary of outcome studies for victims of road traffic accidents. A significant body of evidence points to the potential of CBT to exert a marked and positive influence on the course and development of event-related reactions, most especially those identified as symptoms of acute stress disorder and specific phobias. Outcome studies published to date secure a place for CBT and its related approaches in reconstructed early intervention. Bryant also cautions against assuming that these techniques provide a panacea for all accident victims. A decision about which type of therapeutic intervention is most strongly indicated for individual or groups of survivors is therefore unlikely to be a simple matter. This difficulty is repeatedly referred to in Section 4 and a sensible strategy for improving standards of decision-making advocated by several authors is to defer declarations of expert opinion until service users' preferences have been established.

In keeping with the above, Anna Avery and Steven King of the Lincolnshire Joint Emergency Services Initiative based in Lincoln, England describe a radical restructuring of an early intervention service for staff exposed to work-related trauma. In this instance, change was prompted not only by a resolve to link provision to published evidence, but also a recognition that officers draw upon a range of adaptive coping strategies to modulate reactions to extreme events. Personal preferences evolve in conjunction with accumulated experience and consultation with possible service users has therefore become a new imperative of the initiative. Where past recommendations might have included routine group meetings facilitated by healthcare professionals, current practice encourages peer support, good leadership practices plus pre-incident education and training. Their is also the suggestion that the aim of reconstructed early intervention should not primarily be the elimination of symptoms but to effect improvements in the quality of survivors' recovery environment.

Readers wishing to be informed of how to provide reconstructed early intervention for victims of sexual assault can draw upon and extensive evidence base. This is summarized by Drs Heidi Resnick and Ron Acierno, with their colleagues Jane Stafford and Robin Minhinnett at the National Crime Victims Research and Treatment Centre, Charleston, South Carolina, USA. In addition to giving evidence-based rationales for the use of early intervention strategies adapted from CBT these authors draw attention to the scope of using single session interventions to help survivors modulate intense feelings experienced during the very early aftermath of their trauma. In combination with providing personalized support and raising awareness of what is about to happen in unfolding post-trauma situations, such focused approaches hold particular promise. They can help reduce risks of re-traumatization associated with submitting to medical or forensic examinations, assist in preventing feelings engendered by traumatic bereavement from becoming overwhelming, etc. A common element of these focused early interventions is an aspiration to reduce arousal and anxiety at a time that is critically important for the prognosis of trauma reactions. In a separate chapter Dr Chris Freeman of the Rivers Centre in Edinburgh, Scotland, highlights the same principle in his description of the evidence base that informs prescription practices for recently trauma survivors. Psychotropic medication taken in the early aftermath of trauma is helpful to the extent it effects prompt short-term control of emotions. This is associated with positive outcomes in the intermediate or longer term.

With a growing understanding of survivors' needs in the early aftermath of trauma, it has been possible for reconstructed early intervention programmes to concern themselves with pre-incident education and training. This is a significant service evolution that marks a shift from being exclusively preoccupied with the sequelae of trauma to prevention and public health education. Professor Søren Buus-Jensen and Nancy Baron describe three training modules designed in anticipation of meeting trauma survivors' needs at some future date in a variety of contexts. Each module contains elements that may be incorporated in other training programmes established for the purpose of developing appropriate local competencies to deliver reconstructed early intervention. Reflecting their experience of setting up such training schemes these authors strongly advocate regular supervision, monitoring and continuous training to ensure practice remains reconcilable with emergent evidence relevant to the provision of reconstructed early intervention.

14 Cognitive behaviour therapy of acute stress disorder

Richard A. Bryant

An important development in the early intervention of post-traumatic stress disorder (PTSD) occurred when the diagnosis of acute stress disorder (ASD) was introduced in 1994 in the fourth edition of the *Diagnostic and Statistical Manual for Mental Disorders* [DSM-IV; American Psychiatric Association (APA), 1994]. This new diagnosis was important, because its aim was to identify people in the initial month after a trauma that would subsequently develop long-term PTSD. Implicit in this goal was the expectation that successful identification of people at risk of PTSD would receive early intervention to prevent chronic PTSD. This chapter reviews the evidence for the utility of ASD diagnosis as a predictor of subsequent PTSD, critiques the evidence for cognitive behaviour therapy of ASD, and highlights the advantages and disadvantages of early intervention with cognitive behaviour therapy.

Definition of ASD

DSM-IV stipulates that the requisite symptoms to satisfy the criteria for ASD include a fearful response to experiencing or witnessing a threatening event (Criterion A), three dissociative symptoms (Criterion B), one re-experiencing symptom (Criterion C), marked avoidance (Criterion D), marked anxiety or increased arousal (Criterion E), and evidence of significant distress or impairment (Criterion F). The disturbance must last for a minimum of 2 days and a maximum of 4 weeks (Criterion G), after which time a diagnosis of PTSD should be considered. The distinguishing feature of the ASD diagnosis is the requirement that one needs to display at least three of the following dissociative symptoms:

- a subjective sense of numbing or detachment;
- reduced awareness of one's surroundings;
- derealization;
- depersonalization;
- dissociative amnesia (for review, see Bryant and Harvey, 1997).

Rationale of ASD

The ASD diagnosis was driven by the notion that acute dissociative reactions are a crucial mechanism in psychopathological post-traumatic adjustment. This view stems from the early theorizing of Janet (1907), who argued that trauma led to attempts to minimize discomfort by dissociating awareness. Janet proposed that this dissociation resulted in diminished psychological well-being because it drained mental resources that were required for other processes. On the basis of this theory, Janet argued that adaptation to a traumatic event involved integrating the fragmented memories into awareness. Recent adaptations of Janet's (1907) views hold that acutely traumatized individuals will have impaired recovery if their dissociative responses impede access to and resolution of their traumatic experience (van der Kolk and van der Hart, 1989). Specifically, this perspective has stimulated the rationale that the ASD criteria (and, most particularly, the dissociative symptoms) will predict chronic PTSD (Koopman *et al.*, 1995). The ASD diagnosis has been widely criticized for a number of reasons. First, the notion of having a diagnosis to predict another diagnosis is often seen as unnecessary (Marshall *et al.*, 1999). Secondly, some have expressed concern that this diagnosis may potentially pathologize normal and transient responses to trauma (Solomon *et al.*, 1996). Thirdly, at the time of its introduction the ASD possessed very little empirical basis to justify its description (Bryant and Harvey, 1997). Fourthly, the strong emphasis on dissociation was contrary to one view that conceptualized acute dissociation as a protective mechanism that could potentially facilitate adaptation (Horowitz, 1986).

Relationship between ASD and PTSD

There is now an initial body of evidence informing us about the incidence of ASD and the utility of this diagnosis to predict subsequent PTSD. In terms of the incidence of ASD, studies have noted ASD in between 10 and 20% of survivors of motor vehicle accidents (Harvey and Bryant, 1998a), mild brain injury (Harvey and Bryant, 1998b), burns and industrial accidents (Harvey and Bryant, 1999a), and assaults (Brewin *et al.*, 1999). One study found a higher rate (33%) of ASD in a sample of bystanders to a mass shooting (Classen *et al.*, 1998).

The more critical issue is the extent to which ASD predicts subsequent PTSD. The ability to predict PTSD from acute reactions needs to be considered in the context of prospective studies that indicate that the majority of trauma survivors who initially display post-traumatic stress reactions remit over the following 3 months without intervention (Rothbaum *et al.*, 1992; Riggs *et al.*, 1995; Blanchard *et al.*, 1996). In terms of prospective studies of ASD, Harvey and Bryant (1998a) found that 78% of MVA survivors who were initially assessed for ASD were diagnosed with PTSD 6 months post-trauma. Importantly, 60% of those who satisfied all ASD criteria except dissociation (subsyndromal ASD) were also diagnosed with PTSD 6 months post-trauma. When reassessed for PTSD 2 years later (Harvey and Bryant, 1999b), 63% of those who were initially diagnosed with ASD and 70% of those with subsyndromal still had PTSD. In a sample of MVA survivors who had sustained a mild traumatic brain injury, Bryant and Harvey (1998) reported that 82% of those who initially had ASD met criteria for PTSD 6 months post-trauma and 80% still had PTSD 2 years later (Harvey and Bryant, 2000). Brewin *et al.* (1999) found that 83% of assault victims who initially satisfied ASD criteria were subsequently diagnosed with PTSD at 6 months follow-up (although this estimate is very limited by the significant attrition rate at follow-up). Other prospective studies have been conducted that have not indexed the relationship between ASD and subsequent PTSD diagnostic status. By assessing the relationship between acute reactions and arbitrary cut-off scores on general measures of subsequent post-traumatic stress, these studies are not able to infer specific predictive capabilities of ASD in terms of later PTSD. In a prospective study of firestorm survivors that formed the basis for the current ASD criteria, it was observed that three acute dissociative symptoms combined with re-experiencing, avoidance and arousal symptoms best predicted subsequent distress (Spiegel *et al.*, 1996). A later study of survivors of a mass shooting reported that a diagnosis of ASD within 8 days of the trauma was found to be a significant predictor of the level of post-traumatic stress symptoms at 7–10 months post-trauma (Classen *et al.*, 1998).

Overall, these studies provide mixed support for the ASD diagnosis. Although there is strong evidence that the majority of people with ASD will suffer long-term PTSD, there is also strong evidence that many people who did not display acute dissociative reactions will also suffer chronic PTSD. This pattern of findings indicates that provision of early intervention to acutely traumatized individuals should focus on those trauma survivors who display acute symptoms that are predictive of longer-term PTSD.

Assessment of acute stress disorder

Identifying people who are at risk of PTSD is a difficult task because many acutely distressed people will make positive adaptations to what has happened in the ensuing few months. Although DSM-IV states that ASD can be diagnosed after 2 days following the stressor, there is evidence that this time frame may be premature. A study of civilians following bombings during the Gulf War found that many people who displayed distress in the immediate days reported remission in the following week (Solomon *et al.*, 1996). It is possible that attempting to identify people who are at risk of PTSD before 2 weeks have elapsed since the traumatic event may result in identifying an excessive number of people as being at risk of PTSD, but who may adaptively manage their experience in the following weeks and months. Although it is often tempting for practitioners to provide therapeutic interventions as soon as possible after a traumatic event, the available evidence indicates that there is a window of time after a trauma in which many people will resolve their initial distress without receiving formal therapeutic intervention. Not only is prematurely identifying people immediately after a traumatic event unnecessary, it may also have aversive effects because it may communicate to people who are experiencing understandable and transient distress that they are functioning in a maladaptive or pathological manner.

In terms of assessment tools to identify people with ASD, there are three measures currently available. The Stanford Acute Stress Reaction Questionnaire (SASRQ; Cardeña *et al.*, 2000) is a 30-item self-report inventory that has the benefits of rating each symptom on an ordinal scale and encompasses all ASD symptoms. Its major limitation is that there is no data supporting its utility in identifying individuals who meet ASD diagnostic criteria or who subsequently satisfy PTSD criteria. The Acute Stress Disorder Interview ASD (ASDI; Bryant *et al.*, 1998a) is a structured clinical interview that is based on DSM-IV criteria. It possesses reasonable sensitivity (92%) and specificity (93%) relative to independent clinical diagnosis of ASD and has strong test–retest reliability over a period of 1 week ($r = 0.88$). The Acute Stress Disorder Scale (ASDS; Bryant *et al.*, 2000a) is a self-report version of the ASDI, and has been shown to predict 91% of those who subsequently develop PTSD and 93% of those who do not. The major flaw of the ASDS is that one-third of those scoring above the designated cut-off do not develop PTSD.

Treatment of ASD

Treatment of ASD is based on the premise that there is a psychopathological condition that needs to be treated. Accordingly, it is important to refrain from offering active CBT before 2 weeks has elapsed since the precipitating event. This caution is indicated because delaying treatment for several weeks:

- decreases the likelihood of presenting symptoms being transient reactions to the trauma that may abate with time;
- it allows the client additional time to consolidate their resources prior to treatment starting;
- it increases the opportunity for the many practical or contextual problems that can occur with a traumatic event to have settled.

CBT may include prolonged exposure (PE) that may be either imaginal or *in vivo*, cognitive therapy, anxiety management or stress inoculation training (SIT), or a combination of all these components. Theorists propose that successful adaptation to a traumatic experience involves:

- emotionally engaging with and habituating to their traumatic memories;
- organizing their trauma memories in an adaptive manner;
- correcting dysfunctional cognitions about the traumatic experience (Hembree and Foa, 2000).

Accordingly, it is often assumed that therapeutic gains secondary to CBT occur because some or all of these processes are facilitated by the components of CBT. Although there is considerable evidence of the efficacy in reducing chronic PTSD symptoms (see Foa and Meadows, 1996; Bryant, 2000; Foa, 2000), the employment of CBT to prevent PTSD by early treatment of people with ASD is a very recent development.

Prior to the introduction of ASD, a number of studies investigated early intervention with cognitive behaviour therapy with acutely traumatized populations. Kilpatrick and Veronen (1984) provided recent rape victims with either behavioural intervention, repeated assessment, or delayed assessment. Although they reported symptom reduction for all groups at three months follow-up, there were no significant differences between groups. Foa *et al.* (1995) provided recent sexual and nonsexual assault victims with four sessions of either cognitive-behaviour therapy (CBT) or repeated assessments. The CBT program involved trauma education, relaxation training, imaginal exposure, in vivo exposure, and cognitive restructuring. Two months post-trauma, 10% of the CBT group met criteria for PTSD compared to 70% of the repeated assessments group. Although the CBT and control groups had comparable rates of PTSD at the five-month follow-up assessment, the CBT group had less depression and re-experiencing than controls. One problem with these early intervention studies is that their inclusion of all participants who had initial distress resulted in the possibility that a proportion of their sample naturally recovered over time; that is, it is difficult to differentiate the effects of treatment from natural remission in these studies.

In the first study of treatment of ASD, MVA survivors were allocated to either cognitive behaviour therapy (CBT) or supportive counselling within 2 weeks of their MVA (Bryant *et al.*, 1998b). CBT comprised education, prolonged imaginal exposure, cognitive therapy and anxiety management. Supportive counselling involved education, problem-solving and non-directive support. All participants met criteria for ASD, as indexed by the ASDI (Bryant *et al.*, 1998a). Fewer participants in CBT (8%) than supportive counselling (83%) met criteria for PTSD at post-treatment. There were also fewer cases of PTSD in the CBT (17%) than supportive counselling (67%) conditions 6 months post-trauma. At follow-up there were greater statistically and clinically significant reductions in intrusive, avoidance and depressive symptomatology in the CBT than supportive counselling participants. In a subsequent study, Bryant and colleagues investigated the components of CBT that are effective in preventing PTSD (Bryant *et al.*, 1999). Forty-five civilian trauma survivors (either MVA or nonsexual assault) with ASD were given five sessions of either (a) prolonged exposure (PE), (b) a combination of PE and anxiety management (PE+AM), or (c) supportive counselling within 2 weeks of their trauma. Fewer patients allocated to the PE (14%) and PE+AM (20%) conditions, compared to the supportive counselling (56%) condition, met criteria for PTSD at post-treatment. At 6 months follow-up, there were fewer cases of PTSD in the PE (15%) and PE+AM (23%) than SC (67%) conditions. These findings suggested that the combination of imaginal exposure and cognitive therapy might be the critical ingredients in treating ASD. Interestingly, this study found that successful response to treatment was associated with increased use of cognitive strategies that use adaptive reappraisals of the traumatic experience (Bryant *et al.*, 2001a). This finding supports the proposition that CBT is associated with constructive modification of trauma-related cognitions.

Some commentators have argued that the optimal intervention for ASD is hypnosis because this medium may overcome any obstacles associated with dissociative reactions to the trauma (Spiegel and Classen, 1995). The potential utility of hypnosis for treating ASD is indicated by evidence that people with ASD are particularly hypnotizable (Bryant *et al.*, 2001b) and by evidence that hypnosis can enhance the effects of CBT. In a meta-analysis of 18 studies that compared CBT against CBT supplemented by hypnosis, Kirsch *et al.* (1995) found that the average recipient of CBT and hypnosis showed greater clinical gains than 70% of those who received only CBT. In an ongoing study, Bryant and colleagues tested the utility of hypnosis by randomly allocating civilian trauma survivors with ASD ($n=60$) to either cognitive behaviour therapy, cognitive behaviour therapy, plus hypnosis or supportive counselling (Bryant *et al.*, 2000b). This study aimed to enhance the effectiveness of exposure by preceding each imaginal exposure session with a hypnotic induction and suggestions to emotionally engage in the exposure. Both active treatments led to greater reductions in PTSD relative to supportive counselling. The CBT plus hypnosis treatment led to greater reductions in re-experiencing symptoms than CBT at post-treatment, but this difference was not evident at 6 months follow-up. That is, whereas hypnosis did not seem to enhance the benefits of CBT at follow-up, it did lead to faster resolution of those symptoms that were directly targeted in the imaginal exposure.

Overall, the available data suggest that CBT has significant potential for preventing PTSD in a proportion of traumatized people. Prolonged exposure and cognitive therapy appear to be critical ingredients for successful therapy and it seems that hypnosis may play a facilitative role in engaging participants to engage in therapy. It needs to be recognized, however, that these studies have been conducted with survivors of motor vehicle accidents and non-sexual assault. The extent to which these successes are applicable to other traumatized populations awaits further empirical study. It is important that these findings are replicated in different treatment centres and with diverse trauma populations.

Delivering cognitive behaviour therapy

The following steps can be followed in administering CBT to clients with ASD.

Assess suitability for CBT

The client's capacity to engage in therapy and, in particular, in the demanding components of CBT should be carefully assessed. Any indications that the client cannot use therapy constructively at the acute stage or that the client may suffer aversive side effects of early intervention (see below) should be carefully assessed before proceeding.

Education

The next step is to provide a clear outline of the mechanisms that mediate ASD and the rationale for the specific CBT techniques that will be provided. It is important to enhance client participation and motivation by ensuring that the client understands the reasons for the difficult tasks that they will be required to undertake. For example, the client can be informed that the elevated arousal that is inherent and responsible for a range of symptoms, such as insomnia and irritability, in ASD can be reduced by progressive muscle relaxation and controlled breathing. It is critical to emphasize to clients that therapy success depends on their commitment to the programme and their willingness to complete daily homework as directed by the therapist. It is often at this stage that therapists can decide whether a client is ready and motivated to undertake therapy.

If the client displays signs of ambivalence or inadequate motivation, it may be preferable to delay treatment till they are ready to commit themselves fully to the therapy programme.

Anxiety management

It is often best to commence with anxiety management because this provides the client with some initial control over their distress. The prevalence of hyper-arousal symptoms in the acute phase and the role that the play in mediating longer-term PTSD, supports the provision of anxiety management techniques (Shalev *et al.*, 1998; Bryant *et al.*, 2000c). Furthermore, providing clients with strategies to reduce their distress can enhance their motivation to comply with more demanding therapy tasks. In terms of the specific techniques, it common to teach progressive muscle relaxation, isometric muscle relaxation and breathing control (see Bryant and Harvey, 2000). One should be specifically sensitive to clients who report panic sensations. There is evidence that panic is commonly reported by clients with ASD (Bryant and Panasetis, in press). The therapist should teach the client to identify catastrophic interpretations of physical sensations and to learn anxiety management techniques to ensure that panic responses are adequately controlled before proceeding with exposure-based techniques (for a detailed review of managing panic, see Craske and Barlow, 1993).

Cognitive therapy

This approach aims to correct clients' maladaptive interpretation of their trauma and their current environment by teaching them to identify erroneous cognitions and the replace these thoughts with more realistic interpretations (Beck *et al.*, 1979). It is often useful to introduce cognitive therapy prior to exposure because clients can use cognitive therapy techniques more effectively if they have previously learnt this approach before focusing on distressing memories during exposure therapy. The application of cognitive therapy to ASD clients requires an approach that is particularly relevant to acutely traumatized clients. First, many of the beliefs that acutely traumatized clients present with are based on recent and threatening experiences. That is, often their beliefs that the world is dangerous appear to them valid in the context of their recent experience. Clinicians need to be careful that they are not perceived by their clients as invalidating their perceptions of the threat that they have survived. It is easy for clients to interpret cognitive restructuring as a therapists' lack of understanding of the threat that they have recently suffered. Therapists should explain to clients that, whilst the client's reactions are understandable in the wake of their experience, they need to distinguish between realistic and unrealistic perceptions. Considering the brief period of time since the traumatic experience, it is often constructive to focus cognitive therapy in the acute phase on encouraging the client to recognize that the perceptions that they currently hold may change with time. It may be unrealistic to expect a client who has recently been traumatized to modify their trauma-related beliefs within weeks of their trauma. It can be very helpful, however, for the client to learn that the beliefs they do hold in the acute phase may not be permanent and that they can change as time elapses after the trauma. If cognitive therapy in the acute phase can achieve this step, then it opens up considerable opportunity for further cognitive interventions.

Exposure

The therapist should initially clarify the client's suitability for undertaking exposure in the acute phase. It is important to education the client about the rationale of exposure. That is, the client must understand that if they are to habituate their fear, it is essential that they remain in proximity to avoided memories of places until their anxiety subsides. Clients who do not adequately understand this rationale are likely to not comply with the prolonged distress that is associated with this technique. The first step in imaginal exposure is to obtain a narrative from the client because this represents the stimuli that are the focus of exposure. The therapist needs to emphasize that the client is required to 're-live' their experience by narrating their trauma in the first person and present tense, and that they are to engage all of the emotions and sensations that they experienced at the time of the trauma. The client should be informed that the exposure will continue for at least 50 minutes, and they should be told that they will be asked to describe their level of distress regularly throughout the exposure by providing a rating (typically this is on a scale of 0 to 100). If the client completes the narrative in less than 50 minutes, they are asked to repeat the exercise until 50 minutes have expired. The narrative may be audiotaped, which permits the client to listen to it in a structured manner during homework exercises. Once clients have demonstrated that they can perform this task adequately, it is set as daily homework. In session, it is usual for exposure to be followed by cognitive therapy that focuses on the catastrophic interpretations that emerge during exposure.

In later sessions, it is useful to implement *in vivo* exposure, which involves graded exposure to avoided places or situations. The component commences with construction of a hierarchy that typically involves about 10 steps that range from minimally distressing to most distressing. The client is asked to enter these situations and to remain in the situation until the distress rating reduces by at least 50%. Once the client has managed to master one step on the hierarchy, they are then required to proceed to the next step. It is often useful to commence *in vivo* exposure by having a companion accompany the client to often encouragement and to ensure compliance. As therapy progresses, it is usual to reduce the presence of a companion. It is important to recognize that in the acute phase it may be unreasonable to expect the client to reduce avoidance of all situations. For example, a victim of a violent home invasion may be reluctant to return home, while the walls and carpets are still bloodstained. This example points to the need to distinguish between avoidance that is understandable and probably adaptive in the more acute phase, and behaviour that is maladaptively contributing to persistent anxiety and avoidance.

Obstacles to cognitive behaviour therapy

Although most people respond positively to early CBT, there are important contraindications for its use. Bryant *et al.* (1999) reported that 20% of their sample dropped out of treatment and the drop-outs were characterized by more severe ASD than completers. There is increasing evidence that exposure may not be appropriate for all people and this may be especially the case with those who have been recently traumatized. Although early intervention has appeal because it can limit the incidence of PTSD, it needs to be emphasized that it is not a panacea for all survivors of trauma. The demands of therapy and the distress that it can elicit leads to the conclusions that it is useful for the proportion of trauma survivors who can cope with these tasks. It is important to remember that many people who have suffered trauma will adapt more effectively by being offered support and containment of distress, rather than active interventions based on CBT strategies.

Across our treatment studies of ASD, a number of factors have been noted as possible reasons for withholding exposure. Specifically, acutely traumatized people who presents with extreme anxiety, panic attacks, marked dissociation, borderline personality disorder, psychotic illness, significant anger, unresolved prior traumas, severe depression or suicide risk, complex co-morbidity, substance abuse or distressing ongoing stressors may experience deterioration following exposure. These individuals can be offered less demanding interventions, including medication, supportive counselling, anxiety management or possibly cognitive therapy. It is importtant to recognize that early intervention is not imperative and that many people can benefit more effectively when they are offered active treatment after the disruption of the acute post-trauma period has subsided.

Concluding comments

The development of assessment tools that identify acutely traumatized people who are at risk of developing PTSD has paved the way for targeting resources towards those people who need it most. Although the available evidence indicates that early provision of CBT can prevent PTSD in a significant proportion of cases, there are many limitations to our current knowledge of this topic. Future research needs to:

- refine assessment methods to more accurately identify all those who are at risk of developing PTSD and associated psychological disorders;
- increase treatment effectiveness by developing interventions that maximize outcomes and minimizing aversive effects of early interventions;
- expand the early provision of CBT to address the range of co-morbid conditions that can occur after a traumatic event.

Considering the documented difficulties in managing chronic PTSD, there is an important clinical need to continue these initial steps towards developing and evaluating early intervention strategies that reduce psychopathological trauma reactions.

References

American Psychiatric Association (1994) *Diagnostic and Statistical Manual of Mental Disorders*, 4th edn. Washington DC: Author.

Beck, A.T., Rush, A.J., Shaw, B.F. and Emery, G. (1979) *Cognitive Therapy of Depression*. New York: Guilford.

Blanchard, E.B., Hickling, E.J., Barton, K.A., Taylor, A.E., Loos, W.R. and Jones-Alexander, J. (1996) One-year prospective follow-up of motor vehicle accident victims. *Behav Res Ther* **34**, 775–86.

Brewin, C.R., Andrews, B., Rose, S. and Kirk, M. (1999) Acute stress disorder and posttraumatic stress disorder in victims of violent crime. *Am J Psychiat* **156**, 360–66.

Bryant, R.A. (2000) Cognitive behaviour therapy of violence-related posttraumatic stress disorder. *Aggress Violent Behav* **5**, 79–97.

Bryant, R.A. and Harvey, A.G. (1997) Acute stress disorder: a critical review of diagnostic issues. *Clin Psychol Rev* **17**, 757–73.

Bryant, R.A. and Harvey, A.G. (1998) Relationship of acute stress disorder and posttraumatic stress disorder following mild traumatic brain injury. *Am J Psychiat* **155**, 625–9.

Bryant, R.A. and Harvey, A.G. (2000) *Acute Stress Disorder: a handbook of theory, assessment, and treatment*. Washington DC: American Psychological Association.

Bryant, R.A. and Panasetis, P. (in press) Panic symptoms during trauma and acute stress disorder. *Behav Res Ther*.

Bryant, R.A., Harvey, A.G., Dang, S. and Sackville, T. (1998a) Assessing acute stress disorder: Psychometric properties of a structured clinical interview. *Psycholog Assess* **10**, 215–20.

Bryant, R.A., Harvey, A.G., Sackville, T., Dang, S. and Basten, C. (1998b) Treatment of acute stress disorder: a comparison of cognitive-behavioural therapy and supportive counseling. *J Consult Clin Psychol* **66**, 862–6.

Bryant, R.A., Sackville, T., Dang, S.T., Moulds, M. and Guthrie, R. (1999) Treating acute stress disorder: an evaluation of cognitive behaviour therapy and counseling techniques. *Am J Psychiat* **156**, 1780–6.

Bryant, R.A., Moulds, M. and Guthrie, R. (2000a) Acute stress disorder scale: a self-report measure of acute stress disorder. *Psycholog Assess* **12**, 61–8.

Bryant, R.A., Moulds, M., Guthrie, R.M., Nixon, R. and Felmingham, K. (in press) (2000b) *The Additive Benefits of Hypnosis and Cognitive Behaviour Therapy in Treating Acute Stress Disorder*. J Consult Clin Psychol.

Bryant, R.A., Harvey, A.G., Guthrie, R. and Moulds, M. (2000c) A prospective study of acute psychophysiological arousal, acute stress disorder, and posttraumatic stress disorder. *J Abnorm Psychol* **109**, 341–4.

Bryant, R.A., Moulds, M. and Guthrie, R.M. (2001a) Cognitive strategies and the resolution of acute stress disorder. *J Traum Stress* **14**, 213–19.

Bryant, R.A., Moulds, M. and Guthrie, R.M. (2001b) Hypnotizability in acute stress disorder. *Am J Psychiat*. **158**, 600–4.

Cardeña, E., Koopman, C., Classen, C., Waelde, L.C. and Spiegel, D. (2000) Psychometric properties of the Stanford Acute Stress reaction Questionnaire (SASRQ): a valid and reliable measure of acute stress. *J Traum Stress* **13**, 719–34.

Classen, C., Koopman, C., Hales, R. and Spiegel, D. (1998) Acute stress disorder as a predictor of posttraumatic stress symptoms. *Am J Psychiat* **155**, 620–4.

Craske, M.G. and Barlow, D.H. (1993) Panic disorder and agoraphobia. In Barlow, D.H. (ed.) *Clinical Handbook of Psychological Disorders*. New York: Guilford, pp. 1–47.

Foa, E.B. (2000) Psychosocial treatment of posttraumatic stress disorder. *J Clin Psychiat* **61** (Suppl. 5), 43–8.

Foa, E.B. and Meadows, E.A. (1996) Psychosocial treatments for posttraumatic stress disorder: a critical review. *Ann Rev Psychol* **48**, 449–80.

Foa, E.B., Hearst-Ikeda, D. and Perry, K.J. (1995) Evaluation of a brief cognitive-behavioural program for the prevention of chronic PTSD in recent assault victims. *J Consult Clin Psychol* **63**, 948–55.

Harvey, A.G. and Bryant, R.A. (1998a) Relationship of acute stress disorder and posttraumatic stress disorder following motor vehicle accidents. *J Consult Clin Psychol* **66**, 507–12.

Harvey, A.G. and Bryant, R.A. (1998b) Acute stress disorder following mild traumatic brain injury. *J Nerv Ment Dis* **186**, 333–7.

Harvey, A.G. and Bryant, R.A. (1999a) Acute stress disorder across trauma populations. *J Nerv Ment Dis* **187**, 443–6.

Harvey, A.G. and Bryant, R.A. (1999b) Relationship of acute stress disorder and posttraumatic stress disorder: A two-year prospective study. *J Consult Clin Psychol* **67**, 985–8.

Harvey, A.G. and Bryant, R.A. (2000) A two-year prospective evaluation of the relationship between acute stress disorder and posttraumatic stress disorder following mild traumatic brain injury. *Am J Psychiat* **157**, 626–8.

Hembree, E.A. and Foa, E.B. (2000) Posttraumatic stress disorder: psychological factors and psychosocial interventions. *J Clin Psychiat* **61** (Suppl. 7) 33–9.

Horowitz, M.J. (1986) *Stress Response Syndromes*, 2nd edn. New York: Jason Aronson.

Janet, P. (1907) *The Major Symptoms of Hysteria*. New York: Macmillan.

Kilpatrick, D.G. and Veronen, L.J. (1984) Treatment for rape-related problems: crisis intervention is not enough. In Cohen, L.H., Claiborn, W. and Specter, C.A. (eds) *Crisis Intervention*, 2nd edn. New York: Human Services Press, pp. 165–185.

Kirsch, I., Montogomery, G. and Sapirstein, G. (1995) Hypnosis as an adjunct to cognitive-behavioural psychotherapy: a meta-analysis. *J Consult Clin Psychol* **63**, 214–20.

Koopman, C., Classen, C., Cardeña, E. and Spiegel, D. (1995) When disaster strikes, acute stress disorder may follow. *J Traum Stress* **8**, 29–46.

Marshall, R.D., Spitzer, R. and Liebowitz, M.R. (1999) Review and critique of the new DSM-IV diagnosis of acute stress disorder. *Am J Psychiat* **156**, 1677–85.

Riggs, D.S., Rothbaum, B.O. and Foa, E.B. (1995) A prospective examination of symptoms of posttraumatic stress disorder in victims of non-sexual assault. *J Interpers Violence* **10**, 201–13.

Rothbaum, B.O., Foa, E.B., Riggs, D.S., Murdock, T. and Walsh, W. (1992) A prospective examination of post-traumatic stress disorder in rape victims. *J Traum Stress* **5**, 455–75.

Shalev, A.Y., Sahar, T., Freedman, S., Peri, T., Glick, N., Brandes, D., Orr, S.P. and Pitman, R.K. (1998) A prospective study of heart rate responses following trauma and the subsequent development of PTSD. *Arch Gen Psychiat* **55**, 553–9.

Solomon, Z., Laor, N. and McFarlane, A.C. (1996) Acute posttraumatic reactions in soldiers and civilians. In van der Kolk, B.A., McFarlane, A.C. and Weisaeth, L. (eds) *Traumatic Stress: the effects of overwhelming experience on mind, body, and society*. New York: Guilford, pp. 102–14.

Spiegel, D. and Classen, C. (1995) Acute stress disorder. In Gabbard, G.O. (ed.) *Treatments of Psychiatric Disorders,* Vol. 2. Washington, DC: American Psychiatric Press, pp. 1521–35.

Spiegel, D., Koopman, C., Cardeña, E. and Classen, C. (1996) Dissociative symptoms in the diagnosis of acute stress disorder. In Michelson, L.K. and Ray, W.J. (eds) *Handbook of Dissociation: empirical, theoretical, and clinical perspectives*. New York: Plenum, pp. 367–80.

van der Kolk, B.A. and van der Hart, O. (1989) Pierre Janet and the breakdown of adaptation in psychological trauma. *Am J Psychiat* **146**, 1530–40.

15 Drugs and physical treatment after trauma

Chris Freeman

Introduction

There is now a large and impressive evidence base for the treatment of PTSD using either drugs or psychological treatments. There is also an emerging evidence base for the treatment of Acute Stress Disorder with brief psychological treatments and a consensus that one-off individual debriefing post-trauma does no good and may do harm. Drug treatments have a long history in the management of Acute Stress Reactions after trauma and are still widely used. Self-medication with alcohol is undoubtedly the major intervention practised in the western world.

Why then has virtually no attention been paid to the evaluation of drug treatments, acutely post-trauma? Why have researchers felt the need to carry out over 11 randomized controlled trials of one-off psychological debriefing, sufficient to produce two editions of a Cochrane Review, along with considerable debate and acrimony in the traumatic stress world, but hardly examined drug treatment at all? It seems bizarre and perverse that the traumatic stress field should have got so worked up, in recent years, about a semi-structured talking treatment given in a single session of between 30 and 90 minutes long, and its power to prevent or induce PTSD, whilst completely ignoring interventions such as 2 weeks of high dose benzodiazepines, the early prescription of antidepressants and the use of major tranquillizers. There may be a number of reasons for this:

- Perhaps the traumatic stress field is just perverse.
- The field has been dominated by psychological therapists not psychopharmacologists.
- Drug interventions are usually given by non-specialists in the emergency room or by GPs.
- Such interventions are probably not regarded as treatments, but just as symptom relief, in the same way that painkillers are given acutely for pain or antacids for dyspepsia.
- There have not been high profile promoters of acute drug treatment in the same way there have been for psychological debriefing, EMDR and cognitive therapy.
- Post-trauma sufferers may be resistant to taking drugs for a reaction they regard as normal and understandable.

The pharmacotherapeutic guidelines published by the International Society for Traumatic Stress Studies ISTSS (Friedman and Keane, 2000) are, of course, guidelines for the treatment of PTSD, not Acute Stress Reaction or Acute Stress Disorder, but they do highlight how little evidence was available up until that point, and it is striking that Bryant and Harvey's excellent book on Acute Stress Disorder has absolutely nothing on drug treatments and drugs are not even mentioned in the index (Bryant and Harvey, 1999).

It is tempting, therefore, to conclude that this should be a 1-line chapter as follows: 'There is no evidence base for the use of drugs, acutely after trauma, either for prophylaxis or for treatment and they should not be used'. I would be quite content with this if it weren't for the fact that drugs do continue to be used often in idiosyncratic or unusual ways.

What questions need to be answered?

There are a number of important questions and as yet there are answers to none of them. They involve the purpose, timing and type of drugs that might be used:

- Do drugs have any role in preventing the development of Acute Stress Disorder or PTSD?
- If so, which drugs should be given, in what dosage, and how soon after the trauma?
- Should drugs be offered to everyone or only to high-risk individuals, and how would high risk be defined?
- Is drug treatment useful for targeting specific symptoms such as hyperarousal or sleep disturbance and, if so, does treatment of these symptoms simply relieve stress in the short term or does it prevent future development of other psychological disorders?
- Do drugs do harm? Does reducing arousal impair cognitive and/or emotional processing, and make longer-term psychological reactions more likely?
- Are there drug treatments for Acute Stress Disorder and, if so, do the same drugs that successfully treat PTSD, treat ASD also?
- Given that PTSD can be diagnosed within 1 month of a trauma and becomes chronic after 3 months, how quickly should drug treatment be offered?
- Given that there is now an impressive evidence base for selective serotonin reuptake inhibitors (SSRI's) in the treatment of PTSD, would a reasonable health intervention be to offer SSRI's to all who meet criteria for PTSD as soon as they do so?

It would be nice to have an answer to even one of these questions, but presently we have answers to none of them. What follows is a review of what little is known from both clinical practice and a small number of clinical trials.

What might a rationale for drug treatment be?

A full discussion of the neuroendocrine and physiological responses to trauma is beyond the scope of this chapter. In brief, acute stress results in an increase of both catecholamines and cortisol, and the greater the severity of the stressor, the higher the level of these two hormones.

Catecholamines promote greater blood glucose going to muscles and vital organs, allowing the fight or flight response. In contrast, cortisol helps shut down and acts as an anti-stress hormone. The time response of these two hormones is different with a catecholamine response starting within seconds, and a cortisol response over the minutes and the first few hours. The main centres in the brain mediating the stress response and trauma memories, the hypothalamus, hippocampus and amygdala are all rich in glucocorticoid receptors.

McFarlane et al. (1997) looked at blood samples 1–2 hours after trauma and measured the cortisol response to a motor vehicle accident. Six months later the subjects were rated for PTSD. Those who had developed PTSD had a blunted cortisol response, suggesting that there may be abnormalities in the HPA axis and cortisol response in those who go on to develop PTSD, and that this is detectable very early. Similarly, Resnick et al. (1995) demonstrated that women who had been raped or assaulted before had lower cortisol levels immediately after a subsequent rape. Shalev has shown that resting heart rate in the emergency room of recently traumatized individuals predicts PTSD in subsequent months (Shalev et al., 1998).

Interesting though such findings are, it is far too early to recommend that we should be using drugs in the acute phase post-trauma to correct them. Though it is tempting to think that damping down arousal in those who are hyperaroused may be indicated.

What then can we learn from history and from clinical practice?

Much of clinical practice in this area is simply not documented. The best records are from military psychiatry, where there is a long history of frontline psychiatrists.

World War I

One of the most well recorded treatment centres was Craiglockhart War Hospital, Edinburgh were Dr W. H. R. Rivers treated Sigfried Sassoon. Rivers was transferred to Craiglockhart in January 1916. He promoted a humane regime stressing that successful treatment of war neuroses required a close relationship between physician and patient, and furthermore, that this patient must have a true understanding of his condition and must have the ability to confront it courageously (Anon., 1993). He commented that the usual advice given to patients up till then had been that they should put their war experiences out of their minds and try not to think of them, but because their experiences would come flooding back at night, it was far better that the patient should be encouraged to face up to his memories by talking about their painful experiences (Rivers, 1917).

Sassoon (1936) gave vivid descriptions of these nightmares in *Sherston's Progress*:

> One became conscious that the place was full of men whose slumbers were morbid and terrifying—men muttering uneasily or suddenly crying out in their sleep. Around me was that underworld of dreams haunted by submerged memories of warfare ... each man was back in his doomed sector of a horror-stricken Front Line, where the panic and stampede of some ghastly experience was re-enacted among the vivid faces of the dead.

When I reviewed the notes from Craiglockhart, it was clear that as well as the psychological treatments promoted by Rivers, sedative medication was often recorded. Drugs such as bromide and laudanum were frequently prescribed. In other hospitals hypnosis and suggestion were widely used, often with service men held at bases in France and hypnotized there (Myers, 1916). Bennett-Tombleson (1916) claimed to have cured all 60 of the cases of war neuroses he saw between 5 and 60 days with hypnosis.

The urgent need to do something led to the introduction of unusual and controversial treatments such as electric shocks. Garton (1917), and Adrian and Yealland (1917) practised galvanism or faradization. Yealland reported effective cure in 95% of 250 cases. This technique was not electro-convulsive therapy (ECT), but involved applying an increasingly powerful electric current to disabled parts of the soldier's body until they spoke, screamed or recovered function. In France, the technique was called Torpillage and was also practised in Germany. The aim of the treatment was literally to provoke the soldier into some sort of functional response, whether he was malingering or suffering from hysterical conversion. A wide variety of other physical treatments were employed such as massage, sinusoidal electric baths, and the slow administration of chloroform to induce a state of hypnosis or suggestibility.

World War II

Grinker and Spiegel devote a whole chapter to narcosynthesis giving detailed guidelines and case histories (Grinker and Spiegel, 1945). Pentothal (2.5 or 5%) was slowly injected until the appropriate stage of narcosis was reached. The purpose was to induce an abreaction of facts, thoughts and feelings about both traumatic and early experiences. They stress this process was rarely punitive in itself, but was the beginning of the process of giving insight with subsequent interviews required to work through the material. They used narcosynthesis both in the US and in theatres of war abroad.

Sargent and Slater (1942) used pentothal somewhat differently, to induce what they called 'hypnoanalysis' or 'narcoanalysis'. The purpose here was not abreaction, but the use of hypnosis and strong suggestion to overcome the symptoms, rather than uncovering and working through them.

Narcosis or continuous sleep treatment was used by both the American Eighth Army and by UK psychiatrists (Sargent and Slater, 1942; Hastings *et al.*, 1944) who both reported favourable results and high rates of return to active service. Grinker and Spiegel (1945) were disappointed with their results. Both in the North African campaign and in the US, most soldiers were treated within a month of removal from the combat zone. Length of sleep varied for 27–110 hours. They abandoned the technique and recommended its place in war treatments be checked (Kubic, 1943).

Ergotamine was recommended because of its properties of inhibiting sympathetic activity and Heath and Powdermaker (1944) reported successful results in 20 cases. Again, when tested by Grinker and Spiegel (1945), 13 of 16 soldiers developed toxic reactions, and only two showed benefit with reduction in tremor and they recommended it should not be used.

Sedatives were widely used for agitated patients and for sleep disturbance and a wide range of barbiturates were available (barbital, nembutal and amytal) (Macy 1944).

Kubic (1943) recommended rapid wakening in the early morning to avoid a period of light sleeping before awakening when nightmares could be troublesome. Grinker and Spiegel (1945), concerned about barbiturate dependence, substituted placebo tablets to good effect.

One might think that the dramatic coercive treatments used in World War I had dropped into misuse by World War II, but new drugs and physical treatments had replaced them. Sargent (Sargent and Slater, 1940; Sargent and Craske, 1941; Sargent, 1967) reported the use of new drugs, insulin coma therapy, ECT and even leucotomy, though much of these treatments must have been for established PTSD not for acute reactions.

Vietnam

It is clear from Camp's description (1993) that as well as vigorous use of the PIE System (proximity, immediacy and expectancy) as part of forward psychiatry, drugs were also used. 'In November, 1971, Corporal A, a 20-year-old infantryman, who had been assigned to Vietnam for five months, was transported by helicopter to an Army Evacuation Hospital along with other combat casualties. Upon his arrival he was observed to be mute, grunting incomprehensibly, and posturing. He was quite disorganized and could not communicate with his examiners. He was easily startled by noise and walked with a slow, shuffling gait. When he sat in a chair, he rocked with his eyes closed and occasionally mumbled 'Mamma'. The results of his physical investigations were otherwise normal'.

Corporal A was given a shower and was put to sleep 'with Chlorpromazine. When he woke up, eighteen hours later he seemed alert, coherent and rational ... ' Corporal A described in a group session, that day, how six of his friends had been killed and mutilated in front of him. He was given a further dose of chlorpromazine that night, a fresh uniform and returned to his unit the following day with a diagnosis of combat exhaustion. No follow-up is reported. We are left to wonder if he went back into the front line sedated by a major tranquillizer.

It seems then that there is little that we can learn from a historical perspective, except perhaps that Psychiatry's track record in treating acute stress reactions with drugs and physical treatments is no better than its track record in other areas where 'heroic' physical treatments were used.

In a review article in 1993, Friedman *et al.* produced a set of recommendations for psychotropic drugs in recently evacuated military casualties. They recommended withholding all medication for at least 48 hours and then using drugs such as clonidine, propranolol, lorazepam and antidepressants depending on symptom pattern.

What then is the current situation with drugs that are available?

Benzodiazepines

This group of drugs were widely used for treatment of acute stress and may still be in many countries in Europe. In the UK benzodiazepine prescribing has markedly decreased, partly because of increasing use of antidepressants, but mainly because of increasing awareness of the addictive and dependence producing properties of these drugs. The idea benzodiazepines may actually do harm in acute situations, particularly when someone is grieving, has also gained acceptance. This is reflected in the British National Formulary (BMA of the Royal Pharmaceutical Society, 2000) and the Committee on Safety of Medicines (1988) both of which advise against using benzodiazepines after bereavement and suggest that such compounds may inhibit the grieving process.

This advice appears to emanate from clinical opinion and anecdote, rather than a secure evidence base, but Warner *et al.* (2001) recently conducted a randomized controlled trial to examine this. They randomly allocated 30 recently bereaved subjects to either diazepam or placebo. Dosage of diazepam was up to 2 mg three times daily. Doses were low because subjects were given a bottle of 20×2 mg diazepam to take as they wished up to three times daily over the next 6 weeks. The authors concluded that diazepam had a neutral effect on the grieving process. Diazepam certainly did not lessen distress, but a conclusion that it was neutral requires some caution. Those subjects taking placebo reported better sleep quality, less difficulty getting off to sleep and fewer bad dreams. The sample size was small and only a big difference between groups could have been detected. The doses of diazepam were low and no subjects appeared to develop tolerance in dependence.

Parkes (1964) reported that benzodiazepines were prescribed to between 25 and 50% of people recently bereaved of a spouse in the 1960s, whereas rates had fallen dramatically to 10–15% by the early 1990s (Warner and King, 1997). The latter authors certainly questioned the hypothesis that benzodiazepines inhibit the grieving process and wonder if some people are being deprived of effective control of their acute distress. Woods and Winger (1995) have described the rational prescribing of longer acting benzodiazepines, such as diazepam and chlordiazepoxide, in low doses for short periods and suggest that this may be regaining acceptance.

Two studies of recently traumatized subjects gave different results. Mellman *et al.* (1998) showed in a pilot study that specifically targeting sleep disturbance with a benzodiazepine hypnotic markedly reduced subsequent PTSD symptoms. In contrast, Gelpin *et al.* (1996) found that the use of clonazepam and alprazolam in the days after traumatized subjects presented at an emergency room showed no preventative action on the later development of PTSD. A similar result was found by Braun *et al.* (1990) who found that the core symptoms of PTSD were not improved by alprazolam.

The self-appointed international consensus group on depression and anxiety (Ballenger *et al.*, 2000) say that four consecutive nights of sleep disturbance is an appropriate threshold for providing symptomatic relief, but that the benzodiazepines should not be used to treat acute sleep disturbance. In preference, non-benzodiazepine hypnotics should be prescribed, but they don't say which.

Beta blockers

We have recently reviewed the efficacy of beta blockers such as propranalol across the whole range of anxiety disorders (SIGN, 2001). Beta blockers have an established place in the treatment of anxiety, certainly in the UK and are often used in preference to benzodiazepines. To our surprise, there is little or no evidence for their efficacy, and no evidence at all for their efficacy in the treatment of PTSD. There are no randomized controlled trials of propranalol for anxiety disorders.

There is one study on a small group of children (Fanularo 1988). Eleven children who had been physically or sexually abused or both, and who presented in an agitated hyper-aroused state were treated with propranalol. There was a 6-week placebo running followed by 6 weeks of active drug and then 6 weeks of placebo again. The children did show fewer PTSD type symptoms during the 6 weeks on active drug; however, it is difficult to interpret this as a treatment for acute stress disorder. Pitman (2002) has recently described a study of propranalol used acutely shortly after trauma. It did seem to have some acute effect, but no effect on preventing PTSD.

The alpha-2 agonist clonidine has been shown to be effective in some open studies for treatment of PTSD, but not in the treatment of Acute Stress Disorder (Friedman and Keane, 2000).

Antidepressants

There is now clear evidence for efficacy of the selective serotonin reuptake inhibitors (SSRI's) in the treatment of established PTSD. The strongest evidence is for sertraline and paroxetine, although the first trial showing clear evidence was with fluoxetine. The database for both sertraline and paroxetine is large and impressive (Freeman, 2001) with over 1100 patients in the paroxetine studies. These show that paroxetine works in both men and women, for all the main symptom clusters of PTSD, irrespective of trauma type and irrespective of time since trauma.

This latter fact may seem a useful guide for the use of SSRI's in Acute Stress Disorder. However, neither the sertraline nor paroxetine trials included subjects with very recent trauma. The average time from duration of trauma to treatment was 7 years and the range was extremely wide (1–50 years).

We know that depressive symptoms can begin early after trauma and Shalev *et al.* (1996) postulates that it is depressive symptomatology on top of normal intrusiveness and re-experiencing that drives the patient towards PTSD. Therefore, there might be a cogent rationale for treating such individuals early, either with an effective brief psychological treatment (Interpersonal Therapy or Cognitive-Behavioural Therapy) or for with an SSRI. There is an urgent need for a randomized controlled trial of the use of SSRI's in Acute Stress Disorder and/or acute PTSD.

The older antidepressants, tricyclics and monoamine oxidase inhibitors have a much weaker evidence base in the treatment of PTSD, and are no longer recommended as first line drug treatment. They are still widely used in general practice because of their sedative and sleep-inducing properties.

As early as 1986 Blake reported three patients with acute PTSD treated with tricyclic antidepressants with a favourable response. He recommended tricyclics because of their anti-anxiety and antidepressant properties.

Robert *et al.* (1999) reported a pilot study of children with burns and acute stress disorder treated with imipramine. This is one of the few randomized controlled trials. Twenty-five children aged 2–19 years were randomly allocated to either imipramine or chloral hydrate for 7 days. Burns were severe (mean total burn surface 45%) and, although one patient was 19 and therefore not a child, the mean age was 8 (SD + 6). Ten out of 12 (83%) low dose imipramine patients were positive responders compared with five of 13 (35%) chloral hydrate patients. The authors are cautious in their conclusions and there is no longer-term follow-up.

So, in contrast to drug treatment of established PTSD where SSRI's are the clear first choice, for acute PTSD there is slightly more evidence for tricyclics.

Antipsychotics

Despite the anecdotes quoted above there is very little evidence for antipsychotics. Stanovic *et al.* (2001) in an uncontrolled trial treated 10 recent burn victims with risperidone in low dosage (0.5–2 mg at bed time). The average dose was 1 mg. All 10 patients had acute stress symptoms of nightmares, flashbacks, hyperarousal and disturbed sleep. All 10 patients reported clear reduction of symptoms 1–2 days after starting risperidone. None reported side effects.

Recommendations and conclusions

Given such a dismal and disappointing literature, what can be concluded? Birmes and Schmitt (2001) published a French language review of biological therapies for acute trauma reactions recommending the use of psychotropic drugs to reduce or abate the acute symptoms, and facilitate response to psychotherapy, but I don't think the evidence supports their conclusions:

- Military psychiatry has a poor record, and all the drug and physical treatments that have been used should no longer be used.
- There is no evidence to support the use of major tranquillizers in Acute Stress Disorder/acute PTSD except one uncontrolled study of risperidone.
- There is no evidence to support the use of benzodiazepines in the treatment of Acute Stress Disorders/ acute PTSD.
- Small studies on propranalol and on imipramine are insufficient to make firm recommendations but the only positive randomized controlled trial is with imipramine.
- Although there are no trials, clinical expediency means that targeting specific symptoms if they are very disturbing or troublesome, such as marked agitation, marked arousal or severe sleep disturbance, may be necessary.
- Given the effectiveness of SSRI's over a very wide range of traumas and a wide time frame since trauma, it may just be justifiable to use them in acute PTSD (1–3 months after trauma), but a trial in this area is urgently needed.
- Physical and drug-related treatments, such as abreaction, and electrical treatments have no place in post-trauma treatment.

References

Adrian, E.D. and Yealland L.R. (1917) The treatment of some common war neuroses. *Lancet* **i**, 867–72.
Anon (1993) W. H. R. Rivers and the anthropology of psychiatry. *Soc Sci Med* **36**, 1.
Ballenger, J.C. *et al.* (2000) Consensus statement on Post-Traumatic Stress Disorder from the International Consensus Group on Depression and Anxiety. *J Clin Psychiat* **61** (Suppl. 5): 60–6.
Bennett-Tombleson, J. (1916) A series of military cases treated by hypnotic suggestion. *Lancet* **ii**, 707–9.
Birmes, P. and Schmitt, L. (2001) Biological therapies of acute traumatic psychological reactions. *Rev Francoph Stress Trauma* **2**, 143–7.
Blake, D.J. (1986) Treatments of Acute Post-Traumatic Stress Disorder with tricyclic antidepressants. *Sthn Med J* **79**, 201–4.
Braun, P., Greenberg, D., Dashber, G. and Lever, B. (1990) Core symptoms of PTSD unimproved by Alprazolam. *J Clin Psychol* **516**, 236–8.
British Medical Association of Royal Pharmaceutical Society of Great Britain (2000) *British National Formulary*. London: BMJ Books Pharmaceutical Press.
Bryant, R.A. and Harvey, A.G. (1999) *Acute Stress Disorder*. Washington DC: American Psychological Press.

Camp, N.M. (1993) The Vietnam War and the Ethics of Combat Psychiatry. *Am J Psychiat* **150**, 1000–10.

Committee on Safety of Medicines. (1988) *Current Problems No 21*. Quoted in British Medical Formulary 42 September 2001 Royal Pharmaceutical Society of Great Britain, London.

Fanularo, R., Kinscherff, R. and Fenton, T. (1988) Propranalol Treatment for Childhood Post-Traumatic Stress Disorder, Acute Type. *American Journal of Diseases of Children*, **142**, 1244–1247.

Freeman, C.P.L. (2001) *Drug Treatment for PTSD*. Presentation at ECNP, Munich.

Friedman, M.J. and Keane, T. (2000) Pharmacotherapy. In Foa., E., Keane, T. and Friedman, M.J. (eds) *Effective Treatments for PTSD*. New York: Guildford Press.

Friedman, M.J., Southwick, S.M. and Charney, D.S. (1993) Pharmacotherapy for recently evacuated military casualties. *Military Med* **158**, 493–7.

Garton, W. (1917) Shellshock and its treatment by cerebrospinal galvanism. *J Roy Army Med Corps* **28**, 600–4.

Gelpin, E., Bonne, O., Peri, T., Brandes, D. and Shalev, A. (1996) Treatment of recent trauma survivors with benzodiazepines. A prospective study, *J Clin Psychiat* **57**, 390–4.

Grinker, R. and Spiegel, J.P. (1945) *Men Under Stress*. Philadelphia: Blakiston.

Hastings, D.W., Wright, D.G. and Gleueck R.C. (1944) *Psychiatric Experiences of the Eighth Air Force, First Year of Combat (July 4 1942–July 4, 1943)*. New York,

Heath, R.G. and Powdermaker, F. (1944) The use of ergotamine tartrate as a remedy for 'battle reaction'. *J Am Med Ass* **125**, 111.

Kubie, L.S. (1943) Manual of emergency treatment of war neurosis. *War Medicine* **4**, 582.

Macy, J. (1944) Sodium amytal narcosis in treatment of occupational fatigue in combat air crews, *War Med* **5**, 368.

MacFarlane, A.C., Atchison M. and Yehuda R. (1997) The acute stress response following vehicle accidents and its relation to PTSD. *Annl NY Acad Sci* **821**, 437.

Mellman, T.A., Byers, P.M. and Augenstein, J.S. (1998) Pilot evaluation of hypnotic medication during acute traumatic stress response. *J Traum Stress* **11**, 563–9.

Myers, C. (1916) Contributions to the study of shell shock. *Lancet* **iii**, 608–13.

Parkes, C.M. (1964) Effects of bereavement on physical and mental health. A study of medical records of widows. *Br Med* **2**, 274–9.

Pitman, R., Sanders, K., Zusman, R., Randall, M., Healey, A.R., Cheema, F., Lasko, N., Cahill, L. and Orr, S.P. (2002) Pilot study of secondary prevention of posttraumatic stress disorder with propranolol. *Biological Psychiatry* **51**, 189–92.

Resnick, H.S., Yehuda, R. and Pitman, R.K. and Shalev, A. (1995) Defective previous trauma on acute plasma cortisol level following rape. *Am J Psychiat* **152**, 1675–7.

Rivers, W.H.R. (1917) Freud's psychology and the unconscious. *Lancet* **I**, 912.

Robert, R., Blakeney, P.E., Villarreal, C., Rosenberg, L. and Meyer, W.J. (1999) Imipramine treatment in pediatric burn patients with symptoms of acute stress disorder: a pilot study. *J Am Acad Child Adolesc Psychiat* **38**, 873–8.

Sargent, W. (1967) *The Unquiet Mind. The Autobiography of a Physician in Psychological Medicine*. London: Heinemann.

Sargent, W. and Craske, N. (1941) Modified insulin therapy in war neuroses. *Lancet* **ii**, 212–14.

Sargent, W. and Slater, E. (1940) Acute War Neuroses. *Lancet* **ii**, 1–2.

Sargent, W. and Slater, E. (1942) Physical treatment of acute war neuroses. *Br Med J* **2**, 574.

Sassoon. S. (1936) *Sherstons Progress*. London: Faber and Faber.

Shalev, A.Y., Peri, T., Kanneti, L. and Scheiber, S. (1996) Predictors of PTSD in recent trauma survivors: a prospective study. *Am J Psychiat* **153**, 219–25.

Shalev, A.Y., Sahar, T., Freedman, S. and Peri, T. and Yehuda, R. (1998) A prospective study of heart rate responses following trauma and the subsequent development of PTSD. *Arch Gen Psychiat* **55**, 553–9.

SIGN (2001) *Scottish Intercollegiate Guidelines Network. Consensus Conference Primary Care Guidelines on the Treatment of Specific Anxiety Disorders*. Stirling: SIGN.

Stanovic, J.K., Kelly, J.A. and Van Deuse, C.A. (2001) The effectiveness of risperidone on acute stress symptoms in adult burn patients: a preliminary retrospective pilot study. *J Burn Care Rehab* **22**, 210–13.

Warner, J., Metcalfe, C. and King, M. (2001) Evaluating the use of benzodiazepines following recent bereavement. *Br J Psychiat* **178**, 36–41.

Warner, J. P. and King, M.B. (1997) The use of benzodiazepines after bereavement. *Bereav Care*, **16**, 14–15.

Woods, J.H. and Winger, G. (1995) Current benzodiazepine issues. *Psychopharmacol* **118**, 107–15.

16 Early intervention strategies with traumatized children, adolescents, and families

William Yule

A high proportion of children and adolescents have been shown to develop serious stress reactions and other psychopathology after a wide variety of group and individual traumatic experiences (Bolton *et al.*, 2000; Yule *et al.*, 2000). This chapter will address the question of how mental health and other professionals can, through early intervention, best respond to the specific needs of these young victim groups so as both to reduce levels of distress and prevent later, more serious disorders.

The immediate distress associated with exposure to traumatic events is a powerful motivator to act. Early intervention strategies may serve a variety of needs simultaneously. These include the need for people to provide assistance and to show concern, the need of survivors to talk about and understand what has happened and to gain control, and the need of those not directly affected to overcome feelings of helplessness, guilt at having survived and to experience and master vicariously the traumatic encounter. As far as children are concerned there is also the need to reunite the children with their parents or other family members. Thus, there is also an imperative to do something and, in this increasingly litigious society, to be seen to be doing something. Over a very short period, survivors of disasters have come to expect that some form of counselling will be offered for them.

Given that treatment of chronic disorders can be lengthy and expensive, and in a world where health care resources are scarce, brief preventive interventions are attractive. The question remains as to what forms such interventions should take and their effectiveness in reducing both immediate and long-term psychopathology.

The nature of traumatic experience for children and adolescents

Children are exposed to a diverse range of traumatizing experiences. They may survive a bizarre, life-threatening accident, such as electrocution or near drowning; they may be survivors of road traffic accidents, either as pedestrians or passengers; they may be the victims of deliberate attacks, either physical or sexual; they may survive a natural disaster or a mass transportation disaster. Most of these, apart from secretive, chronic abuse, will be sudden, one-off events in the course of normal experiences. Some, like war, will be repeated over long periods. Clearly, the nature of the events and the contexts in which they occur will, in part, determine how the children respond, when they are psychologically available to benefit from help and what form that help should take.

Very young children will probably require different forms of intervention from older, more mature and more verbal children.

Where a disaster affects a whole community it makes sense to think of initial interventions that target the whole community and aim to mobilize its resources. As far as children are concerned, in most communities, the school is a major focus of their world and so it often makes sense to think of delivering services through schools. Teachers, after all, can monitor how well and how quickly children are recovering from any ill effects.

Where children are physically hurt in an incident or accident, the current received wisdom is that no psychological intervention can reasonably get under way until the child's physical needs have been met. Put this way, it seems obvious and it highlights the need to consider carefully the timing of any intervention.

It is sometimes easier to consider the issues involved in planning services for children and adolescents by examining the needs evoked in a radically different situation to that which faces people dealing with small-scale traumas within the context of readily available child and adolescent mental health services.

Large-scale interventions

Ten years on from the genocide in Rwanda there have been many other wars and massive natural disasters. Hundreds of thousand of children have been made homeless and had to flee their birthplaces, following tragedies like the earthquakes in Turkey, Greece, Taiwan, El Salvador and India or the floods in Mozambique and Bangladesh. Equally notable for their impact on children and adolescents are the political upheavals in Kosovo, and the fighting in Afghanistan, Chechnya, Sri Lanka or Algeria. One is confronted with the question of what can be done to alleviate suffering on such a large scale?

Obviously, the first need is to ensure the safety of the children and to meet their physical needs. Of these, food, shelter, clean water and sanitation are paramount, whilst making sure they are in contact with their families is also important. Then there is the need to provide some form of schooling both to continue to improve the skills of the children, and to provide a much needed predictability and routine to their unsettled lives. When these basic requirements are met, then one can help to bring relief to their psychological distress.

Meeting the psychological needs of the children should be built in to all emergency and rebuilding initiatives. Staff involved in setting up tent cities, be they civilian or military, can be advised about the importance of play and education for the children who will live in the camps. The imperative of finding ways to reunite children with their families, as they get lost in the vast impersonal rows of canvas should also be explained. Those providing education should have appropriate preparation and support in order that they can provide some emotional first aid to children in their care.

There is fairly widespread agreement that part of any early crisis intervention should involve a psycho-educational component (Cohen *et al.*, 2000). Within the international relief and UN agencies this is often referred to as a psychosocial response. Parents, teachers and children themselves are provided with simplified and accessible information on how the disaster, war or other incidents may affect them. This is part of a process of raising awareness so that what are, to them, unpleasant, distressing reactions are duly recognized and understood, not as indications they are going mad, but as 'normal reactions to an abnormal event'.

Of course, the question must be put as to whether even this well-intentioned, apparently benign act may have unintended consequences? Even if it is widely reported that survivors greatly appreciate all forms of help, we all too often forget there are wide individual differences in how people respond to apparently similar situations. For instance, in a study of adult survivors of the

Herald of Free Enterprise, all of whom had been sent the then-current version of a leaflet about 'Coping with a Personal Crisis', the vast majority recalled receiving the leaflet at follow-up and reported finding it helpful. However, a sizeable minority of around 15% said the leaflet had been definitely unhelpful. I know of no similar evaluation of children's responses to receiving explanatory leaflets about reactions to trauma. However, there is every reason to assume, as with other public health and total population interventions there will invariably be a minority who are damaged by interventions that are helpful to the vast majority.

In other words, in planning for early interventions following any emergency one has to think carefully about the nature of the emergency, the ages of the children involved, whether they were at or away from home, how and when to reunite them with their parents, whether their basic needs for safety and shelter have been met, whether they require any physical medical interventions, and how soon initial psychological help should be offered. Strangely, many professionals offering help to adult survivors of trauma have inexplicably overlooked this last point. To many of us who have experience of working in the field it seems self-evident that in the first few days after any major life-threatening incident the survivors are in no state to benefit from most psychological interventions. They report that they are in shock. They are numb, may be dissociating and/or are highly aroused. All the same it is important that emergency response teams somehow establish contact with survivors and make them aware that help will be on hand, at an appropriate time, to deal with their emotional reactions. Even so, at this early stage, one should not under-estimate the value of a sympathetic hug, a cup of (sweet) tea (at least in the UK), and help with contacting loved ones. As has been repeatedly stated, 'Interventions offered by "professionals" should not interfere with or undermine the natural coping responses of a community affected by disaster. Nor should it be assumed that help will not be needed in the future even if it is not appropriate immediately' (Canterbury and Yule, 1999).

Crisis intervention

While the overall aim of crisis intervention is to prevent later problems emerging, it also serves other purposes (Cohen *et al.*, 2000). Getting children together in groups gives group leaders an opportunity to screen for immediate distress and problems (Yule and Udwin, 1991). This is effectively a form of triage that allows help to be targeted at those most in need. One aim of early intervention with children and adolescents must therefore be to identify healthy coping strategies that are already being used, to reinforce their use and to inform other group members about their value. As noted earlier, this is also an opportunity to educate the children about stress reactions and elementary first aid to deal with them.

We have argued elsewhere (Yule and Gold, 1993) that preparation for the eventuality or possibility of disaster or critical incidents is preferable to panic. This is especially apposite for children and adolescents who, because they spend most of their childhood years in school will find that many of the disasters that happen to them occur in relation to school. Therefore, it is far better for schools to be properly prepared to respond to such crises, rather than try to reinvent the wheel when it occurs. As we put it, it is good to be 'wise before the event'.

Good guidance is available as to how to respond to the needs of children after a crisis. The best articulated approach is that of psychological debriefing adapted by Dyregrov (1991) from the original guidelines issued for critical incident stress debriefing (CISD).

Critical incident stress debriefing

Psychological debriefing was originally developed to assist emergency personnel adjust to their emotional reactions to events encountered in the course of their rescue work. It makes use of group support techniques within a predominantly male culture where expressing and sharing feelings is not the norm. Dyregrov (1991) adapted it for use with groups of children, again making use of group dynamics to assist recovery.

Within a few days of an incident, the survivors are brought together in a group with an outside leader. During the introductory phase, the leader sets the rules for the meeting emphasizing that they are there to share feelings and help each other, and that what goes on in the meeting is private. The information should not be used to tease other children. No one *has* to talk, although all are encouraged to do so. They then go on to clarify the facts of what actually happened in the incident. This offers an early opportunity to dispel incorrect rumours. Participants are asked about what they thought when they realized something was wrong, and this leads naturally into discussions of how they felt and of their current emotional reactions. In this way, children share the various reactions they have experienced and usually learn that others have similar feelings, too. The leader labels their responses as normal (understandable) reactions to an abnormal situation. Many children are relieved to learn, not only that there is an explanation for how they feel, but also that they are not the only ones experiencing what may be to them rather strange reactions and that they are not going mad. The leader summarizes the information arising in the group and educates the children into what simple steps they can take to control some of their reactions. They are also told of other help available should their distress persist.

There is some evidence that this structured crisis intervention is helpful in preventing later distress in adults (Dyregrov, 1988, 1997; Duckworth, 1986; Robinson and Mitchell, 1993; Canterbury and Yule, 1999). However, recent criticisms (see Rose *et al.*, this volume) have been raised about the lack of proper randomized control trials to establish the distinctive contributions that psychological debriefing (PD) can make. Some studies that have not used the PD model, but have instead been based on providing individualized crisis interventions, have not only failed to find evidence in favour of such support when provided for adults, but even claim that some participants are made worse by this form of early intervention (Wessely *et al.*, 1997; Rose and Bisson, 1998). Indeed, a 3-year follow up of 30 road traffic accident (RTA) survivors given a 1 hour 'debriefing' by a researcher within 24–48 hours of the accident found members of this group to have more problems than the 31 survivors not given the intervention (Mayou *et al.*, 2000). Thus, both the nature of the crisis intervention and its timing are crucial issues that require further careful study.

Fortunately, the situation with children is a little more optimistic. Yule and Udwin (1991) describe their use of psychological debriefing with girls who survived the sinking of a passenger ship in Greek waters. Self-report data 5 months after the incident suggest that this early intervention had reduced levels of stress and particularly those event-related reactions manifested as intrusive thoughts (Yule, 1992). Stallard and Law (1993) showed that debriefing greatly reduced the distress of seven girls who survived a school bus crash. However, we still do not know when best to offer this form of early intervention to survivors of disasters, nor indeed whether all survivors will benefit.

Pynoos and Nader (1988) describe a different form of psychological first aid for groups of children following crises. Professionals asked to provide early intervention for children and adolescents subjected to trauma should consult the references cited above. These contain suggestions for sensible ways to offer and deliver help so that the difficult events that have happened can be talked about and steps be taken to gain some mastery over the strong emotional reactions that may have been evoked.

What this amounts to is that many inspired attempts have been made to try to respond to the perceived needs of children following emergencies. There has been a great lack of theory driven interventions and very few attempts to systematically evaluate early interventions that have been implemented. In part, this reflects the relatively low number of professionals who work with children within a clinical research structure. Also important is the lack of appropriate measuring and evaluation instruments that can serve both as screening tools and outcome measures. Thus, there are still very few empirical studies of early intervention for children and adolescents the results of which can be used to provide a foundation for evidence based practice.

Working in the real world

Having had experience of working in a number of emergency situations, six of us (Atle Dyregrov, Rolf Gjestad, Leila Gupta, Patrick Smith, Sean Perrin and I) met in Norway during the summer of 1998 to discuss which recommendations could be offered to those responding to future major incidents and disasters. From our brain storming session, we developed a manual for *Children and Disaster: teaching recovery techniques* (Smith *et al.*, 1999). We wanted to develop flexible materials that could address common early distressing reactions experienced by children so as to help them on the road to recovery. The intervention should be capable of being delivered by sensitive people who get on well with children, but who probably would have little or no child mental health experience. Our strong recommendation is that they make arrangements for there to be two group leaders for each group of 10 children. The early intervention might consist of three half-day modules for all children, followed by a fourth meeting for those who have been bereaved. An essential element in the package of recommendations is a one-session meeting for parents to explain the intervention and give suggestions on how to help their children in the early aftermath of a traumatic incident.

The philosophy behind the manual is that, wherever possible, the advice should be based on good empirical evidence. However, we recognize that children cannot wait while all the evidence is collated. Therefore, some of the suggestions are drawn from our own clinical experience and that of others. Because of this, we see it as vital that whoever uses the manual must evaluate its effects. To that end, we supply an up to date version of our core battery of screening and outcome measures and insist that those who use the package, under licence from the Foundation for Children and War, which owns the copyright, send their outcome data to us so that we can adapt the package in the light of new evidence.

We had intended evaluating the package ourselves before releasing it for more general usage. However, the spate of natural disasters and wars at the end of the twentieth century and the demand for some concerted action to address needs prompted us to licence its early use by some colleagues. By mid-2001, initial impressions and results are being fed back to us as requested. There is considerable enthusiasm for the package of measure and many positive comments from the workers who have used it, most recently in Turkey. However, in spite of our qualified optimism, a concern is that when chaos reigns, anything available for use may seems better than nothing at all. The spectre of possible harm arising from inappropriate applications still hangs over the enterprise. For these reasons, it was exciting to get some preliminary results from a study carried out in Athens, Greece. Here, mental health professionals, who were largely unfamiliar with cognitive behavioural techniques, implemented the manual. They found the suggestions and exercises brought immediate relief to children in their groups, and this was confirmed in self-report questionnaire data from the children themselves (I. Giannopolou, 2000, personal communication).

The three main sessions concentrate on helping children deal with the troubling symptoms of intrusion, arousal and avoidance. Children are taken through various warm-up exercises, and helped to adopt a problem-solving and group-sharing approach to these difficulties. With regard to intrusion, they are taught about how traumatic reminders can be upsetting. They practice various imagery techniques to demonstrate to themselves that they can gain some control over the intrusive images that may have been troublesome. They are also introduced to distraction techniques, dual attention techniques (similar to some of the EMDR techniques) and how to manage frightening, repetitive dreams.

To reduce arousal, they are first helped to identify their reactions and are then taught the skills that enable them to relax at will. They are also encouraged to make use of their own techniques to induce relaxation and, where possible, bolster these by breathing exercise and muscle relaxation. They are helped to schedule their activities, to look at better sleep hygiene, and to develop and practice self-statements that enhance a sense of coping.

With respect to avoidance, the exercises introduce the children and adolescents to the concept of graded exposure, giving short practice in imaginal exposure followed by self-reinforcement. They are encouraged to draw, write and talk about the incidents, and above all to look to the future rather than the past.

In other words, this is a psychosocial educational programme. It is designed to be delivered by people with a minimum of experience, but with supervision from someone with more mental health expertise. Under the auspices of the Foundation for Children and War, we intend developing and refining the package, since there is clearly a great demand for effective, low-cost early interventions that can be used with large numbers of children following a broad range of catastrophes.

Conclusions

Children suffer from many man made and natural emergencies. Their suffering can be serious and long lasting. Early intervention offers a promise of preventing initial distress becoming chronic disorder. However, evidence is not yet available to demonstrate that the types early crisis intervention currently practised does in fact achieve this aim. Indeed, it has to be conceded that, since all types of intervention with children of necessity involve re-exposure to the frightening events, it is possible that badly handled or badly timed, such interventions might make things worse.

Clinical experience suggests that most children rate early intervention positively, and most professionals who have participated in this form of help and support for children believe they do more good than harm. However, this is no substitute for harder evidence of efficacy. Initial group meetings usually require a few hours, and are usually linked to the later provision of small group or individual therapy. Recent experience with the use of a manualized early intervention for children affected by earthquakes and war shows considerable promise for delivering some alleviation of the cardinal traumatic stress symptoms experienced by children.

What is now needed is better planning of responses to emergencies that incorporate appropriate screening measures administered both before and after early interventions. More thought needs to be given to the timing of these interventions, as well as to the training requirements of the professionals who are to lead the groups. Thought should also be given to the type of early intervention offered to individuals who, in relative isolation, survive traumas. After all, PD is primarily a group intervention that relies on unfolding group processes to exert its influence (Dyregrov, 1997) and altogether different techniques may need to be applied to help individual survivors (Bisson *et al.*, 2000).

References

Bisson, J.I., McFarlane, A.C. and Rose, S. (2000) Psychological debriefing. In Foa, E.B., Keane, T.M. and Friedman, M.J. (eds) *Effective Treatments for PTSD*. New York: Guilford Press, pp. 39–59.

Bolton, D., O'Ryan, D., Udwin, O., Boyle, S. and Yule, W. (2000) The long-term psychological effects of a disaster experienced in adolescence: II. General psychopathology. *J Child Psychol Psychiat* **41**, 513–23.

Canterbury, R. and Yule, W. (1999) Debriefing and crisis intervention. In Yule, W. (eds) *Post Traumatic Stress Disorder: concepts and therapy*. Chichester: Wiley, pp. 221–38.

Cohen, J.A., Berliner, L. and March, J.S. (2000) Treatment of children and adolescents. In Foa, E.B., Keane, T.M. and Friedman, M.J. (eds) *Effective Treatments for PTSD*. New York: Guilford Press, pp. 106–38.

Duckworth, D. (1986) Psychological problems arising from disaster work. *Stress Med* **2**, 315–23.

Dyregrov, A. (1988) *Critical Incident Stress Debriefings*. Unpublished manuscript, Research Center for Occupational Health and Safety, University of Bergen, Norway.

Dyregrov, A (1991) *Grief in Children: a handbook for adults*. London: Jessica Kingsley Publishers.

Dyregrov, A. (1997) The process in critical incident stress debriefings. *J Traum Stress*, **10**, 589–605.

Mayou, R., Ehlers, A. and Hobbs, M. (2000) Psychological debriefing for road traffic accident victims. *Br J Psychiat* **176**, 589–93.

Pynoos, R.S. and Nader, K. (1988) Psychological first aid and treatment approach for children exposed to community violence: research implications. *J Traum Stress,* **1**, 243–67.

Robinson, R.C. and Mitchell, J.T. (1993) Evaluation of psychological debriefings. *J Traum Stress*, **6**, 367–82.

Rose, S. and Bisson, J. (1998) Brief early psychological intervention following trauma: a systematic review of the evidence. *J Traum Stress*, **11**, 697–710.

Smith, P., Dyregrov, A., Yule, W., Gupta, L., Perrin, S. and Gjestad, R. (1999) *Children and Disaster: teaching recovery techniques*. Bergen: Norway: Foundation for Children and War. (cf: www.childrenandwar.org)

Stallard, P. and Law, F. (1993) Screening and psychological debriefing of adolescent survivors of life-threatening events. *Br J Psychiat* **163**, 660–5.

Wessely, S., Rose, S. and Bisson, J. (1997) *A Systematic Review of Brief Psychological Interventions (Debriefing) for the Treatment of Immediate Trauma-related Symptoms and the Prevention of Posttraumatic Stress Disorder (Protocol)*, The Cochrane Library (CD-ROM). Oxford: Update Software Inc.

Yule, W. (1992) Post traumatic stress disorder in child survivors of shipping disasters: the sinking of the 'Jupiter'. *Psychother Psychosom* **57**, 200–5.

Yule, W., Bolton, D., Udwin, O., Boyle, S., O'Ryan, D. and Nurrish, J. (2000) The long-term psychological effects of a disaster experienced in adolescence: I. The incidence and course of post traumatic stress disorder. *J Child Psychol Psychiat* **41**, 503–11.

Yule, W. and Gold, A. (1993) *Wise before the event: Coping with Crises in Schools*. London: Calouste Gulbenkian Foundation.

Yule, W. and Udwin, O. (1991) Screening child survivors for post-traumatic stress disorders: Experiences from the 'Jupiter' sinking. *British Journal of Clinical Psychology*, **30**, 131–138.

17 Early psychosocial interventions for war-affected populations

Kaz de Jong and Rolf Kleber

Introduction

Médecins Sans Frontières (MSF) is an independent, humanitarian organization working with international and national volunteer staff in 87 countries worldwide. In its 29 years of existence, MSF has developed specialist knowledge in providing health support to populations in emergency and crisis settings.

MSF has been involved in mental health interventions since 1990. The decision to intervene in the early stage of an emergency is largely based on operational observations and compassion of field workers. The usefulness of intervening in early stages of a crisis has been documented in a number of settings (Brom and Kleber, 1989). However, the relative novelty of psychosocial care programmes in large emergencies (often in non-western settings) requires an ongoing search for valid cross-cultural appraisal techniques, appropriate frameworks for intervention and programme evaluation. This chapter aims to add to the knowledge base that informs provision of early psychosocial intervention programmes in emergencies involving refugees and war-affected populations, and seeks to foster discussion about this form of help. In particular, we draw attention to key principles that inform MSF service provision. A description is also offered that outlines a general framework and activities incorporated in MSF psychosocial programmes for refugees and displaced people after man-made disasters. The chapter is concluded with lessons learned to date.

Focus on the psychosocial effects of violence

In its role as a provider of relief in emergencies MSF seeks to prioritize interventions focusing on the psychosocial needs that arise in the course of a crisis. The operational definition of psychosocial needs and problems adopted by the organization refers to those problems and needs that have a psychological (referring to emotions, behaviour, cognition and individual coping resources) and/or a social (mainly referring to the support mechanisms necessary for a collective coping process) origin.

Basic principles of an intervention

Cultural sensitivity

Respect for cultural differences is a prerequisite when planning early intervention for refugees and societies affected by war. Programmes of help and support should aim to create a common and shared approach, while avoiding the enforcement of Western methods and values upon other culture and populations.

To ensure appropriate cultural input from the onset MSF trains locally-based personnel to provide psychosocial support to people in their own communities. Implementation is facilitated by expatriate staff who assist and guide national staff in the planning and delivery of services that are tailored to specific cultures or needs. Although the local culture is respected the general ethical principles that underpin the work of MSF are paramount. For instance, whilst in some early intervention programmes it is culturally desirable to involve traditional healers, it is also important to have some oversight over their activities so as not to endanger the physical and mental integrity of those who make use of available services. Finding a balance between specific cultural values and general ethical principles is a crucial consideration, and it is rarely a routine or simple aspect of care planning and implementation.

A programme by local people for local people

MSF has come to appreciate that local capacity building is a prerequisite for early intervention to be viable and sustainable. By adopting the principle of implementing 'programmes by local people for local people' an attitude of self-control and self-help is engendered. Expatriate staff seek to support and facilitate processes that promote self-repair and healing. In order to build and consolidate a local professional capacity, as well as to guarantee quality standards set for the developing services, the national staff are trained and coached on the job by MSF expatriate staff or nationals with appropriate training and experience, if these are available. Only in exceptional cases is therapeutic assistance and treatment provided by expatriate workers.

Overcoming helplessness

Poor and difficult conditions of living and the loss of a life perspective that incorporates a sense of purpose carried into the future often lead to profound feelings of helplessness. Adaptation to and coping with extreme stresses are facilitated by fostering conditions in which a person can be helped to feel more in control during and after an event (Kleber and Brom, 1992). Basic assumptions of trust, certainty and control are shattered, and in need of repair (Janoff-Bulman, 1992). Whether subjective or factual, a sense of mastery is essential. MSF psychosocial programmes, therefore specifically concentrate on enhancement of control that counteracts patterns of learned helplessness (Peterson and Seligman, 1983). In the experience of this organization, the most effective way of achieving this is to train national staff and foster community-focused approaches.

Coping with extreme stress

War is not a singular traumatic event, but a sequence of extremely disruptive events to which are added prolonged hardships. The concept of post-traumatic stress disorder (PTSD) is frequently used in connection with traumatic events (APA, 1994), but may, in fact, be rather less useful for service planners than has often been assumed. An analysis of human responses to extreme and catastrophic experiences reveal these to be much more diverse and varied than what is included in symptom criteria that comprise PTSD.

A first consideration is that not all mental distress after traumatic events can be described in terms of PTSD. In other words, it is not necessarily the only expression of extreme distress manifest after traumatic events. This is recognized by implication within the classification system offered by DSM-IV (Shalev and Yehuda, 1998). For instance, co-morbidities, such as depression, substance abuse, dissociative disturbances, etc., have been found to be much more prominent in trauma patients than was originally assumed (Kleber, 1997). A further, and in our opinion more important consideration, is that although many people confronted with war experience some negative responses, such as nightmares, fears, shock reactions and despair, approximately 60–90% do not go on to develop diagnosable mental disorders (Kleber and Brom, 1992). An exclusive emphasis on PTSD overlooks the normal and healthy ways in which many victims adapt to extreme stress. As explained by cognitive theories, the general psychological and physical processes that follow in the wake of trauma can be useful in helping to integrate traumatic experiences and should, in principle, not be regarded as pathological responses (Creamer, 1995).

A framework for early intervention

Cognitive processing models (Horowitz, 1986; Creamer, 1995) describe the integration of traumatic experiences as occurring through oscillations between intrusions involving some form of re-experiencing of critical events and avoidance of distressing reminders. It is assumed this is part of a process of adjustment that helps realize adaptations to what has happened.

These processes do not occur in isolation (Lazarus, 1981). Many factors shape the coping process in a positive way so as to engender protection from adverse effects of trauma, whilst others may increase the risk of negative outcome. The interaction between such factors determines, together with the traumatic situation itself, the eventual outcomes of coping processes (Kleber and Brom, 1992). Many humanitarian crises are characterized by omnipresent risks, whilst protective mechanisms such as social support may be largely absent. Under such circumstances coping is likely to be more difficult and the number of people at risk of developing severe traumatic stress-related complaints, psychosocial problems, or even chronic mental disorders is higher than under less disruptive or non-violent conditions.

It is for these reasons that MSF's psychosocial programmes do not specifically set out to address psychopathology (see Fig. 17.1). Rather they seek to provide support at an early stage of a humanitarian crisis with the explicit aim of helping put in place help and support that will strengthen the coping resources available to survivor populations. One of the aims is to foster

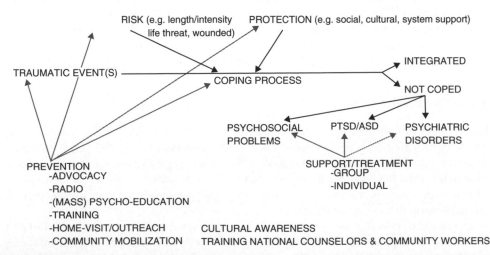

Figure 17.1 Overview of adaptation processes after traumatic experiences and the focus of MSF psychosocial programme activities.

greater resilience. The aim is not necessarily to heal or to cure. Curative approaches (e.g. counselling, brief therapy) are indicated under some circumstances, especially if there is a recognized need to prevent or help minimize the development of further psychopathology. If patients require treatment for severe mental disorders, referrals can be made to specialist services. However, in war situations, where confrontations and violence is persistent and ongoing, such idealistic aims cannot always be realized.

In line with the framework for early intervention described above MSF psychosocial programme activities are characterized by three themes:

- cultural awareness;
- prevention;
- support or treatment.

MSF psychosocial programme activities

Cultural awareness while capacity building

Psychosocial or primary mental health care services are poorly developed in many countries affected by major traumatic disruptions. Where such services exist they are frequently insufficiently equipped or resourced to deal with the increased demands for support and help that arise in the early aftermath of an emergency. Such was the situation that arose when MSF became involved in Bosnia-Herzegovina in 1994. What follows is an example of how help and support can be offered.

In Sarajevo and other parts of the country staff were recruited to new counselling centres from health services (nurses, medical doctors, psychologists, psychiatrists), social services departments (social workers) and educational organizations that had been fully operational before the war. Relevant authorities were engaged in selection of staff so as to avoid further depleting scarce resources and expertise available in the community provision.

After recruitment a training course was organized based on the principle of 'learning by doing'. The preferred strategy was to enrol national mental health experts as trainers. However, as proves to be the case in many countries, the availability of local personnel was limited. MSF was therefore forced to largely depend on expatriate staff to run these courses. The training in Bosnia-Herzegovina lasted 3 months (de Jong *et al.*, 2001) and set out to increase knowledge about traumatic stress reactions, as well as to foster skills and applied strategies for supporting and treating traumatized people. The course consisted of various topics: the concepts of stress and trauma, the psychosocial consequences of violence and the evidence base provided by social psychiatry. Skills training focused on counselling (listening, interviewing, confronting and structuring) with particular reference to the needs of internally displaced, women and children. Introductory training in group and family therapy was also provided.

During the training sessions that were based on the principles of brief trauma-focused therapy (Brom *et al.*, 1989), opportunities were offered for the participants to talk about and try to work through their own traumatic experiences. This part of the training was perceived by trainees to be particularly important because of the beneficial effects it had upon their own psychological condition. Also the experience of being put in the position of a client or service user added to the learning process.

The training programme provided the setting for an encounter between two cultures. West European knowledge was mixed with, translated or adapted so that it could be incorporated into the prevailing culture and language. This was largely achieved by time set aside during training for participants and trainers to exchange views, and make joint decisions about culturally acceptable intervention techniques, appropriate monitoring of clients and use of rituals that enjoyed a high level of local acceptance. Culturally appropriate psycho-education tools (brochures and posters) and methods of dissemination (mass media, groups) were also developed.

This training provided participants with sufficient knowledge and skills to start to address the psychosocial problems of their clients (de Jong *et al.*, 2001). However, the training provided by MSF in Bosnia-Herzegovina was regarded as a means to an end rather than an end in itself. All too often, agencies involved in implementing early psychosocial interventions regard formal training and developing local competencies as their main objective. In the Bosnia-Herzegovina programme our experience was that by far the most important learning processes for counsellors started when they implemented the planned services. This involved exposure to experiences of working with clients presenting with real life problems and difficulties. Through training on the job, supervision and supplementary follow-up workshops on special topics, such as sexual violence and orphan caregivers support, the programme established opportunities for continuous learning. For expatriate staff this ongoing training process helped promote a deeper understanding of local norms and attitudes, as well as the nature of local, culture specific healing systems and practices.

This notion of ongoing mutual exchanges of experience and learning is now incorporated in all MSF psychosocial programmes. The level and duration of training depend on the extent of existing knowledge and expertise amongst local staff, the needs of target population and the phase a crisis may have reached. For instance, in other emergency settings, such as Macedonia (de Jong *et al.*, 1999), Sierra Leone (de Jong *et al.*, 2000), Tajikistan and Lebanon, crash courses were held of varying length ranging from several days to two months.

Prevention

Advocacy to reduce risk factors

Through direct contact with traumatized populations, as well as observations and experiences of expatriates it was possible for staff in Bosnia-Herzegovina to speak out publicly about the abuse suffered by their clients. Such reporting of human rights violations serves to support international efforts to bring perpetrators to justice and to record a history of events. It also allows for the objective recognition of collective trauma. However, advocacy should not be confused with counselling since the specific information obtained through this form of service provision must be kept confidential and should therefore not be used for advocacy.

Advocacy is not restricted to human rights abuses only. In the Sierra Leone emergency programme, staff contributed more directly to the reduction of human suffering through advocacy for basic resources required for making food, clean water and shelter. In Sri Lanka it was possible to prevent further traumatization through advocacy for rights of minority groups.

Mass psycho-education in support of the normal coping process

The process of adjusting to major trauma is invariably difficult. It is, however, what most people do and have to do after such events. They suffer from various symptoms, feel ill or may be extremely distressed. In Bosnia-Herzegovina psycho-education was used to explain the origins of symptoms being experienced, the normality of these reactions, self-help measures that might reduce their impact, how to help others and where to go when additional support was needed.

To increase the effect of psycho-education, several means of disseminating the essential messages were used. Through a weekly, live phone-in radio programme, awareness was raised in the general public. The stigma of weakness, the acknowledgement of suffering and the shame that so often surrounds traumatized people became a collective experience. Greater closeness with those who needed support and help was established through a tailor-made approach for neighbourhoods and vulnerable groups. Counsellors raised awareness and educated people in factories, homes for the elderly, orphanages, community centres, etc. Their presence stimulated self-help mechanisms and modelled a caring attitude in the community.

Lastly, primary health care workers and staff in the emergency health services received special training in how to give psycho-education to their patients and identify those experiencing major violence-related problems.

Increasing protective factors through community mobilization

Restoring social networks and stimulating social support (Eitinger, 1964; Maddison and Walker, 1967) can facilitate coping with and adjusting to trauma. The extent of social support correlates negatively with symptoms of illness (Sarason and Sarason, 1985) and even with mortality (Berkman and Syme, 1979).

During emergencies disruptions occur in protective mechanisms usually provided by families, the community, familiar environments and rituals. The sense of a previously existing social cohesion may be lost. However, the resilience of people even under the horrendous conditions caused by war should not be overlooked. The personal strengths and social resources of a local population must be recognized, and developed further in psychosocial programmes.

In Bosnia-Herzegovina outreach activities were organized to identify and support those who had withdrawn from social life or had isolated themselves. Activities included monitoring the status of vulnerable individuals and groups, such as refugees, women, children and the elderly. Whenever possible, the individuals concerned were linked to care-givers in their environment. Self-help initiatives for groups or individuals within the community were given direct support. Counsellors established strong links with local organizations that sought to foster new levels of social activities for orphans, the resumption of local arts and crafts, and community theatre groups. This public mobilization was structured through the establishment of regular meetings with local authorities, organizations and non-governmental organizations (NGOs).

In other MSF, early intervention programmes implemented in Indonesia and Sierra Leone cultural repair and restoration of community systems were facilitated through involvement of individuals recognized to hold particularly important cultural positions. For instance, traditional healers and religious leaders acted as advisors or implementing partners in the programmes.

A guiding principle of these low profile inputs is to foster a measure of community mobilization without being seen to take local control. The natural protective and healing capacities available within communities are stimulated and learned helplessness is minimized. Furthermore, the focus on communities, rather than specific target populations, prevents the marginalization and stigmatization of survivors of violence.

Support or treatment

Clients identified as being in need of special support either presented themselves directly to the established counselling centres in Bosnia-Herzegovina or were referred there by local health workers. After having their need assessed by means of interview and questionnaires clients received assistance through a local counsellor. They sought to apply the specific interventions and counselling techniques learned and developed during the training programme described above. To a large extent, those who sought help were given the opportunity to discuss their problems and advice was given as to what might be helpful under prevailing circumstances. To support self help mechanisms they also received psycho-education as well as instruction in various skills that promote problem solving or improve conflict management.

To help traumatized survivors of violence the Bosnia-Herzegovina programme, as well as other MSF psychosocial projects, draw extensively on principles derived from brief trauma focused therapy (Brom *et al.*, 1989; Foa *et al.*, 1995). Its core components comprise the following.

First, the process of regaining control is stimulated through providing psycho-education. Existing, positive coping mechanisms are reinforced and new self-help techniques are taught. A second important component of this assistance is to focus on confrontation with traumatic experiences and related losses. Counsellors listen to the story told by their clients and structure their content. Depending on the client and the narrative recited, attempts are made to link event to experienced emotions (Pennebaker, 1997). A last element of the psychosocial care is the restoration of bonds between survivors and the communities to which they belong. In this way, families or community systems become involved in healing processes. Clients are also asked to re-engage with their communities by taking up social activities. Advice is given on how to deal with daily problems and where to go for specific social support. These elements were an integral part of the psychosocial project in Bosnia-Herzegovina (de Jong *et al.*, 2001).

When implementing this part of MSF programmes group interventions are, whenever appropriate, preferred because of the secondary benefits that derive directly from sharing and providing mutual support (Walker, 1981). Despite this preference individual support is also made available. Treatment provision for traumatized people is usually time limited to approximately 10–15 sessions (Marmar *et al.*, 1993). By keeping the period of treatment short, it is possible for staff to help a greater number of traumatized clients. Offering long-term treatment would have reduced the overall number of beneficiaries. Moreover, it has been found that brief therapy focusing specifically on trauma-related reactions, including PTSD can make a clinically significant impact (Marmar *et al.*, 1993). Prescription of psychotropic drugs was kept to a minimum and was only undertaken by professional medical staff. Psychiatric cases or those requiring more intensive, specialist services were referred on as appropriate.

National and expatriate mental health professionals supervised counselling support provided for clients. In the Bosnia-Herzegovina project individual case supervision was provided on request. Arrangements were in place for weekly sessions in which the counsellors discussed case management of difficult clients in small groups. During these group discussions facilitators would include elements of counsellors' own emotions. This proved an opportunity to vent frustrations felt in conjunction with their work.

Daily confrontations with the stories of their clients and the exposure to intense human misery placed our staff at risk of secondary traumatization. A 'Helping the Helpers' service was therefore organized through a national expert, who provided individual counselling support to our staff. This level of provision is now mandatory in all MSF psychosocial programmes. Where there are no national experts available to provide help expatriates provide this early intervention service for staff.

Programme evaluation and audit

The systematic monitoring of programme activities and the benefits accruing for clients receiving assistance are important elements of MSF early psychosocial interventions. For instance, as part of its provision in Bosnia-Herzegovina, MSF and Utrecht University in The Netherlands developed a comprehensive monitoring system (Mooren *et al.*, 2001).

Perspectives

Mental health and psychosocial problems have until recently been largely neglected in international humanitarian assistance. It is therefore regrettable that the boom in provision of such programmes has often resulted in exaggerated expectations on the part of the beneficiaries, over-optimistic claims made about their likely impact, and subsequent criticisms of poorly formulated or ill advised service delivery (Summerfield, 1999).

The years ahead are therefore going to be particularly important for the development of programmes of early psychosocial intervention. Acquired knowledge and accumulated experience needs to be expanded and shared. There are also fundamental issues that need to be addressed through systematic research. In particular, these include cross-cultural assessments of psychosocial problems and needs, cross-cultural validation of PTSD and other stress-related concepts, cross-cultural assessments of the relevance of assistance to be offered, appropriate early intervention programmes and programme evaluation. Operational issues, such as the basic principles that should inform planning and delivery of early intervention, setting programme objectives and deciding on what constitutes appropriate programme activities, warrant more detailed discussion. In this respect, a promising initiative is the formulation of draft guidelines for psychosocial programmes (Aarts *et al.*, 2000).

The chief lessons learned over the past 10 years are that fine tuning interventions to the cultural settings and specific community contexts in which they are to be provided is vital for their acceptance and uptake of services. Knowledge about processes and practicalities of bridging cross-cultural differences and how to adapt services to local needs are limited, and rarely applied with due consideration. To overcome this problem it is strongly recommended that both NGOs and expatriates adopt a more listening attitude, and a more modest disposition in which helping takes precedence over healing. MSF has found that over time the content and methodology of our training and support has undergone marked changes. Our initial interventions in non-western settings, such as Lebanon, Sierra Leone, Indonesia, Colombia and Tajikistan, taught us to balance our western MSF perspectives with the explanatory models and language used by beneficiaries. It is our experience that national staff are well able to act as cross-cultural translators and negotiators when given the opportunity to do so.

Furthermore, MSF has found that training of national staff cannot be achieved by single 'one-off' training programmes. Regular and systematized coaching on the job and case supervision should complement formal training. These are regarded as essential to ensuring that learning becomes a continuous process for all involved. It also goes some way towards guaranteeing the quality of services provided. This support should be available and accessible every day. To implement early intervention programmes for refugees and populations affected by war usually requires a longer-term commitment to local involvement, and consistency in provision.

Another important finding relates to the balance between psychological and social aspects of assistance. Too much emphasis on clinical services may have resulted in stigmatization and in under-used services. If local populations are not informed of what services are setting out to do in their communities their expectations may be unrealistic. Conversely, an exaggerated emphasis on the social and awareness components of psychosocial programmes can result in ever increasing demands for more in-depth support, counselling and therapy that are not available. It is our experience that the balance between the 'psycho' and 'social' needs and provision is subject to cultural variations, and fluctuate according to contextual factors.

In spite of the dearth of information regarding psychosocial programmes, the experience of MSF strongly supports the notion that early psychosocial programmes are commendable. During emergencies, the shattered emotional worlds, the broken trust and the eroded belief in the benevolence of human beings need to be addressed. Early support of coping and adaptation processes plus the prompt provision of practical help, and the immediate facilitation and restoration of a sense of community carries the implicit and crucial message that someone cares.

Acknowledgements

I would like to thank Nathan Ford, V. Puratic, S. Kulnovic, Y. Ruvic and Health Net International for their contributions to this article.

References

Aarts, P.G.H., Graaf, P., Jong, K. de., Kleber, R.J. and Put, W., van der. (2000) *Guidelines for Programmes. Psychosocial and Mental Health Care. Assistance in (Post) Disaster and Conflict Areas*, draft. Institute for Care and Welfare (NIZW), Utrecht, The Netherlands.

American Psychiatric Association (1994) *Diagnostic and Statistical Manual of Mental Health Disorders*, 4th edn (DSM-IV). Washington DC: APA.

Berkman, L.F. and Syme, S.L. (1979) Social networks, lost resistance and mortality: a nine-year follow-up study of Alameda county residents. *Am J Epidemiol* **109**, 186–204.

Brom, D. and Kleber, R.J. (1989) Prevention of posttraumatic stress disorders. *J Traum Stress* **2**, 335–51.

Brom, D., Kleber, R.J. and Defares, P.B. (1989) Brief psychotherapy for post-traumatic stress disorder. *J Consult Clin Psychol* **57**, 607–12.

Creamer, M. (1995) A cognitive processing formulation of posttrauma reactions. In Kleber, R.J., Figley, Ch.R. and Gersons, B.P.R. (eds) *Beyond Trauma: societal and cultural dimensions*, pp. 55–74. New York: Plenum.

Eitinger, L. (1964) *Concentration Camp Survivors in Norway and Israel*. Oslo: University Forlaget.

Foa, E.B., Hearst-Ikeda, D. and Perry, K.J. (1995) Evaluation of a brief cognitive behavioural program for the prevention of chronic PTSD in recent assault victims. *J Consult Clin Psychol* **63**, 948–55.

Horowitz, M.J. (1986) *Stress Response Syndromes*, 2nd edn. San Francisco: Jossey-Bass.

Janoff-Bulman. R. (1992) *Shattered Assumptions: toward a new psychology of trauma*. New York: Free Press.

Jong, K., de., Ford, N. and Kleber, R.J. (1999) Mental health care for refugees from Kosovo: the experience of Mèdecins Sans Frontières. *Lancet*, **353**, 1616–17.

Jong, K., de., Mulhern, M., Ford, N., van der Kam, S. and Kleber, R.J. (2000) The trauma of war in Sierra Leone. *Lancet*, **355**, 2067–8.

Jong, K., de., Kleber, R.J. and Puratic, V. (2001) *Mental Health Programs in War-stricken Areas: the MSF counselling centers in Bosnia-Herzegovina*. (submitted)

Kleber, R.J. (1997) Psychobiology and clinical management of posttraumatic stress disorder. In den Boer, J.A. (ed.) *Clinical Management of Anxiety: theory and practical applications*. New York: Marcel Dekker Inc., pp. 295–319.

Kleber, R.J. and Brom, D. (1992) *Coping with Trauma: theory, prevention and treatment*. Amsterdam: Swets and Zeitlinger International.

Lazarus, R.S. (1981) The stress and coping paradigm. In Eisdorfer, C., Cohen, D., Kleinman, A. and Maxim, P. (eds) *Models for Clinical Psychopathology*, pp. 177–214. New York: Spectrum.

Maddison, D.C. and Walker, W.L. (1967) Factors affecting the outcome of conjugal bereavement. *Br J Psychiat* **113**, 1057–67.

Marmar, C.R., Foy, D., Kagan, B. and Pynoos, R.S. (1993) An integrated approach for treating post-traumatic stress. *Am Psychiat Press Rev Psychiat* **12**, 239–72.

Mooren, G.T.M., Jong, de K.T., Kleber, R.J., Kulenovic, S. and Ruvic, J. (2003) The efficacy of a mental health program in Bosnia-Hercegovina: Impact on coping and general health. *Journal of Clinical Psychology* **59**(1), 1–13.

Pennebaker, J.W. (1997) *Opening up: the healing powers of expressing emotions*. New York: Guildford Press.

Peterson, C. and Seligman, M.E.P. (1983) Learned helplessness and victimization. *J Soc Iss* **39**, 103–16.

Sarason, I.G. and Sarason, B.R. (1985) *Social Support: theory, research and applications*. Dordrecht: Martinus Nijhoff Publishers.

Shalev, A.Y. and Yehuda, R. (1998) Longitudinal development of traumatic stress disorders. In Yehuda, R. (ed.) *Psychological Trauma*. Washington DC: American Psychiatric Press, pp. 31–66.

Summerfield, D. (1999) A critique of seven assumptions behind psychological trauma programs in war-affected areas. *Soc Sci Med* **48**, 1449–62.

Walker, J.I. (1981) Group therapy with Vietnam Veterans. *Int J Gp Psychother* **31**, 379–89.

18 Early intervention strategies applied following rape

Heidi Resnick, Ron Acierno, Jane Stafford, and Robin Minhinnett

Introduction

In this chapter we provide a brief review of the literature related to development and implementation of early intervention strategies following completed rape of women by men. Most, if not all, of the principles in this chapter may be applicable to sexual assault more broadly defined including, but not limited to attempted sexual assault, contact sexual molestation, sexual assault of girls, boys and men, same-gender sexual assault and sexual harassment. However, the large majority of controlled studies of sexual assault have been conducted with women raped by men. Thus, it is on this body of literature that we focus. For information regarding prevalence, impact of and treatment approaches related to other types of sexual assault (e.g. molestation, attempted rape) and/or assaults affecting other groups (e.g. boys and men) we recommend the following data-based papers and reviews (Goyer and Eddleman, 1984; Friedrich *et al.*, 1988; Garnets *et al.*, 1990; Beitchman *et al.*, 1992; Fitzgerald, 1993; Kendall-Tackett *et al.*, 1993; Koss, 1993; Polusny and Folette, 1995; Heflin and Deblinger, 1996; Scarce, 1997; Schneider *et al.*, 1997; Wolfe and Birt, 1997; Hodge and Canter, 1998; Holmes and Slap, 1998; McLeer *et al.*, 1998).

Prevalence of rape

Approximately 12,100,000 (12.7%) adult women in the USA aged 18 years or older have, at some point in their lives, been victims of completed rape. Rape is defined as an event that occurred without the woman's consent, involved the use of force or threat of force, and involved sexual penetration of the victim's vagina, mouth or rectum (Resnick *et al.*, 1993). Moreover, it is estimated that in the USA more than 683,000 adult women are raped each year. Children and adolescents experience even greater levels of rape (Kilpatrick *et al.*, 1992). About half of all rape victims reported they feared being seriously injured or killed during the assault, and approximately 30% actually did sustain physical injury (Kilpatrick *et al.*, 1992). Recent data on rates of sexual assault in Latin American, Africa and Asia indicate rates ranging from less than 1 to 8%. However, these rates are thought to be underestimates due to methodological or other factors (Garcia-Moreno, 2000). The World Health Organization (WHO) has developed a database on violence against women in an attempt to collect information on this topic from all over the world (Garcia-Moreno, 2000). In 2001, WHO's Violence and Injury Prevention Department published the first World Report on Violence and Health. It contains information on the prevalence of sexual assault in various countries and can be accessed on the WHO's website: http://www.who.int/violence_injury_prevention.

Emergency health care and community care programmes for recent rape victims who report the crime to police

Health care

The crime of rape is unique in that all rape victims in the USA who report the crime to police within approximately 72 hours post-assault will, whenever possible, be seen for an evidentiary medical examination. During this examination a specific evidentiary protocol is followed, prophylactic treatment for sexually transmitted diseases is administered; and treatment of any injuries is provided (Young *et al.*, 1992). Data from the National Women's Study indicated that only 20% of adult rape victims reported the crime to police and that the majority who reported the crime also stated they received acute medical care (71.4%). A small proportion of women who did not report the assault to police (15.1%) also reported seeking medical care within days or weeks after a rape (Resnick *et al.*, 2000a).

Women who reported the crime to police were more likely to report fear of death or injury during the assault, and/or did, in fact, incur actual injury. Both of these factors are known to increase the risk of subsequently developing post-traumatic stress disorder (PTSD). Thus, for the subgroup of victims who report the crime to police and who are at high risk for PTSD the infrastructure exists in which to provide an early intervention within hours after rape. Such an intervention is currently being implemented in a hospital-based medical programme that provides post-rape medical care in a southeastern state in the USA (Resnick *et al.*, 1999). It is described in more detail in the last section of this chapter.

Community care

Rape crisis advocacy centres are established across the USA. As noted by Kilpatrick *et al.* (1992) over 2000 such agencies have been active over the past 20 years. Other countries, such as Israel (Edlis, 1993), Malaysia and Thailand (Garcia-Moreno, 2000), are adopting similar programmes, which are often hospital-based. However, little or no evaluation of these programmes has taken place. In addition, the resources available in many countries are extremely limited (i.e. private rooms for medical interviews), making it difficult to implement appropriate treatment (Garcia-Moreno, 2000).

A critical mandate of rape crisis centres in the USA is to provide advocates to meet with victims who are seen for post-rape medical care. In most agencies, advocates include staff and trained volunteers. They are available 24 hours a day to provide hospital accompaniment for those rape victims who are brought to a hospital by police or who present directly for medical care. During this accompaniment advocates provide non-judgmental support to the rape victim and information about what to expect during medical and forensic procedures is shared. In many programmes, advocates may sit in with victims during their medical exam subject to the woman's permission having been given. These agencies also offer follow-up referrals and services related to mental health, social service and criminal justice system needs.

Risk factors for PTSD

Rape-related PTSD is prevalent and frequently enduring among victims. For example, Rothbaum *et al.* (1992) found that 94% of rape victims met symptom criteria for PTSD at approximately 2 weeks post-rape and about 50% continued to meet criteria 3 months later. In an epidemiological study, Kilpatrick *et al.* (1987) showed that PTSD was present 17 years after assault in 16.5%

of cases. Kilpatrick *et al.* (1989) found that three factors significantly predicted PTSD within a community sample of women:

- experience of completed rape;
- reported injury during a crime of any type;
- fear of serious injury or death during the crime.

Kilpatrick and colleagues (1989) also found that rape was a significant predictor of PTSD even after controlling for injury and threat characteristics. A majority (78%) of women reporting all three history characteristics met criteria for PTSD.

Other factors that may increase risk for PTSD, or other negative mental or physical health outcomes include prior history of sexual or physical assault (Ellis *et al.*, 1982; Kramer and Green, 1991; Resnick *et al.*, 1995; Follette *et al.*, 1996; Kilpatrick *et al.*, 1998). Such a history may thus be an important factor to assess and control for in evaluation of treatment efficacy for early intervention approaches that are designed to prevent or reduce negative consequences of rape. The importance of prior history was illustrated in a rape prevention program conducted by Hanson and Gidycz (1993). They found that a rape prevention program that was effective for women without prior history of rape had no impact for women with a prior history.

Initial distress and panic symptoms as a risk factor for PTSD

In addition to prior history of traumatic events and crime characteristics noted above, a major predictor of rape-related PTSD is initial level of distress (Kilpatrick *et al.*, 1985a; Girelli *et al.*, 1986; Rothbaum *et al.*, 1992). Results of several studies indicate that acute physiological arousal and self-reported panic symptoms are significantly associated with later PTSD. Data from two studies indicated that those who later developed PTSD had higher resting heart rates measured at the hospital shortly following physical assaults or accidents (Shalev *et al.*, 1998; Bryant *et al.* 2000). Retrospective self-report of panic attacks occurring during rape or other civilian trauma were found to be significantly associated with later PTSD (Resnick *et al.*, 1994) and Acute Stress Disorder symptoms (Bryant and Panasetis, 2001). Resnick *et al.* (1994) found that 90% of rape victims assessed within 72 hours post-rape reported four or more panic symptoms occurring during the rape while Bryant and Panasetis (2001) found that 53% of recent accident or assault victims reported panic attacks during the traumatic event. Consistent with these findings, factor analytic data from the DSM-IV PTSD field trial study indicated that the largest factor characterizing initial reactions to stressor events was comprised of panic attack symptoms including dizziness, shortness of breath and choking sensations (Kilpatrick *et al.*, 1998b). As suggested by Bryant and Panasetis (2001), these findings indicate that early post-trauma treatment to address distorted beliefs about physiological arousal might be a useful component of intervention strategies to prevent PTSD. Given the fact that many components of the forensic rape examination (e.g. pelvic exam) may evoke strong rape-related cues, it is possible these procedures may increase victims' acute post-rape anxiety symptoms . This, in turn, may increase risk for more chronic distress. We have hypothesized elsewhere (Resnick *et al.*, 1999) that reducing anxiety and distress at the time of the post-rape medical exam might help facilitate long-term recovery.

Acute stress disorder

The fourth edition of the *Diagnostic and Statistical Manual of Mental Disorders* (DSM-IV, American Psychiatric Association, 1994) includes the formal diagnosis of Acute Stress Disorder (ASD). The ASD diagnosis allows for classification of early distress requiring the presence of at least three dissociative symptoms, and at least one symptom of re-experiencing, avoidance and arousal symptoms within 1 month post-trauma. Harvey and Bryant (1999) have noted that a potential limitation of the ASD diagnosis as currently specified is that individuals who have arousal symptoms of PTSD, including increased heart rate, may fail to meet ASD criteria due to the requirement of displaying at least three symptoms of dissociation. This may be particularly problematic given findings noted above regarding associations between acute panic symptoms and longer-term PTSD. Harvey and Bryant (1999) suggest the need to re-evaluate ASD criteria based on empirical findings related to early symptom patterns that are most predictive of PTSD.

The data indicating the predictive utility of early distress for the diagnosis of PTSD suggest that it may be important to control for this factor when evaluating the efficacy of early interventions (Kilpatrick and Calhoun, 1988). For example, Rothbaum et al. (1992) found that, while approximately 95% of women met symptom criteria for PTSD 2 weeks following a rape, this percentage dropped to roughly 45% by 3 months post-rape. This pattern of symptom prevalence over time has been found in a variety of populations (e.g. Calhoun et al., 1982; Kilpatrick and Veronen, 1984; McFarlane, 1988). Thus, an intervention implemented within the first few months following a sexual assault may appear to be quite effective when the reduction in symptoms may in fact be due to a natural process of recovery. The findings reviewed above, indicating that intensity of initial distress or early patterns of symptoms within 1 month post-rape are predictive of PTSD, point to the importance of treatment evaluation studies controlling for the likelihood of naturalistic recovery.

Co-morbidity of PTSD and other mental health outcomes

Rates of major depression, suicidal ideation and suicide attempts are increased among those with histories of rape (Frank et al., 1979; Atkeson et al., 1982; Frank and Stewart, 1984; Kilpatrick et al., 1985b, 1992; Steketee and Foa, 1987; Resick, 1993; Boudreaux et al., 1998). In addition to PTSD and depression, panic disorder or panic attacks have been observed to occur among a substantial subgroup of victims (Kessler et al., 1995; Falsetti and Resnick, 1997)

Many investigators have found high co-morbidity between assault-related PTSD and substance abuse disorders (e.g. Breslau et al., 1991; Brady et al., 1994; Kessler et al., 1995). Moreover, prospective data from the National Women's Study (Kilpatrick et al., 1997) demonstrated that rape and physical assault may lead to illicit drug and alcohol abuse in women who previously reported no history of such problems.

Another behavioural problem for many rape victims is sexual dysfunction (Becker et al., 1982, 1986; Letourneau et al., 1996). These researchers note that, these problems with sexual functioning are consistent with learning theory models of post-trauma distress that posit ongoing anxiety and avoidance cues associated with the original traumatic event.

Post-traumatic sequelae of sexual assault, including PTSD, depression, drug and alcohol use, panic and sexual dysfunction are clearly relevant areas that could be targeted in early intervention for many victims of rape. Additional data indicate that rape victims display poorer social adjustment, as well following assault (Resick, 1993). Thus, it is recommended that assessment and early interventions following rape focus on these relevant multiple indicators of problems in functioning, in addition to PTSD.

Concerns about negative health outcomes should also be addressed. Problems may include direct injuries or health risks (e.g. sexually transmitted diseases STD's). Rape victims should be counselled about medical care, and options for testing and prevention of unwanted pregnancy and sexually transmitted diseases (Resnick et al., 2000a).

Early intervention studies conducted with victims of rape

Only four controlled studies of early intervention in rape victims have been conducted to date. Kilpatrick and Veronen (1983) compared a 4–6-hour cognitive-behavioural coping skills intervention with control conditions comprised of repeated and delayed assessment for 49 recent rape victims. The intervention included recounting of the rape incident to a supportive counsellor, education about common trauma reactions, a normalization of cognitive aspects of guilt and blame typically reported by rape victims, and coping skills training. The latter included helping victims to resume activities that may have been avoided, since the assault and to face stresses such as dealing with police, etc. Specific skills included instruction in deep breathing and muscle relaxation. No additional benefit of this form of early intervention was noted at 3 months post-rape assessment. However, this investigation suffered from several limitations including non-randomization to treatment condition. The study was also conducted prior to the existence of the PTSD diagnosis or data being available regarding the predictive utility of patterns of initial distress. Thus, the investigators were unable to evaluate treatment effects controlling for indicators of risk for long term PTSD.

More recently, Foa et al. (1995) conducted a preliminary evaluation of a brief intervention aimed at arresting development of PTSD symptoms. Ten recently assaulted female victims diagnosed with PTSD received four weekly sessions of a brief preventive cognitive behavioural program and were compared to matched participants who underwent monthly assessments in the absence of treatment. Treatment included psycho-education, anxiety management training, imaginal and in-vivo exposure, and cognitive restructuring techniques and related homework assignments. As described in Foa et al. (1995), treatment sessions were 2 hours long and began with an initial session focused on education about typical reactions to assault and development of a list of currently avoided situations. The subsequent session included teaching the participants deep muscle relaxation and breathing control techniques. In addition, clients were taught to rate their distress in order to monitor progress in dealing with exposure to avoided situations and assault related memories. After a rationale for the treatment had been explained participants engaged in imaginal exposure during each of the subsequent 3 sessions. Imaginal exposure consisted of clients relating the specific details of the trauma in the present tense and with eyes closed. This was followed by evaluation and discussion of any distorted beliefs about safety and competence that these exercises may have identified. Sessions were audiotaped so that victims could listen to the tapes several times as homework on their own between sessions. Other homework included engaging in situations that had been identified from the list of avoided behaviours or situations.

Half of the participants in each early intervention group, which included 10 members, were rape victims. Blind assessments of participants receiving the brief intervention were conducted within the first 3 weeks of the assault, immediately following the 4-week treatment and 5.5 months post-assault. Participants in the assessment control condition were assessed five times during the 12 weeks period and then again at the 5.5 months post-assault point. Results were moderately positive, with significantly fewer subjects in the treatment group (10%) retaining their PTSD diagnosis immediately following treatment than the assessment control group (70%). No significant diagnostic differences were noted at the 5.5 months assessment point in terms of meeting PTSD criteria. Of course, this is not altogether unexpected, given some reduction in symptoms over time that has been noted by Rothbaum et al. (1992). Results of continuous measures of subjective intensity of PTSD and depressive symptoms were also positive. Overall, PTSD symptom severity was reduced in both groups, but significant between group differences were evident only at the second assessment point. Participants receiving the brief intervention also demonstrated significantly lower Beck Depression Inventory scores at the third assessment point when compared to control participants. Overall, this brief intervention was effective in arresting PTSD symptoms in the short-term, but did not differ significantly from the assessment control condition at 5.5 months post-assault.

As pointed out by the investigators, several methodological weaknesses of this preliminary study should be considered. For instance, participants were not randomly assigned to conditions and originated from different time cohorts. Non-specific therapist effects (i.e. time with therapist) were not controlled and the failure to find significant differences at the follow-up point may be attributable to limited statistical power associated with the small size of the groups studied

A subsequent study by Foa *et al.* (2000a) of 93 recent civilian trauma victims, 61% of whom had experienced sexual assault, compared the brief intervention described above, with either assessment control or supportive counselling groups. Results indicated no differences between the groups on PTSD diagnosis at post-treatment or 6 months follow-up. Those in the brief intervention group were higher on a measure of 'good end state functioning' at post-treatment based on a combination of scores reflecting lower PTSD, depression and anxiety symptoms. However, there were no differences between the groups at a 6 months assessment. So, findings of this study failed to replicate those of Foa *et al.* (1995) with regard to reduced PTSD diagnoses at post-treatment.

Resnick and colleagues Acierno, Holmes and Kilpatrick (Resnick *et al.*, 1999) are currently conducting a fourth early intervention study with victims of rape. We are evaluating the impact of a brief (one session) treatment administered to rape victims within 72 hours post-assault at a southeastern medical centre. Thus, this intervention is delivered at an earlier point in time post-trauma than the studies reviewed thus far. The intervention is delivered via a 17-minute videotape shown *prior* to the rape exam. The treatment strategies include modelling of exam procedures, psycho-education about physiological, cognitive and behavioural reactions to rape, and instructions in the use of *in vivo* exposure to rape-related cues. Rationales for the development of the treatment approach included the previously cited findings indicating that initial levels of post-rape anxiety are predictive of longer-term functioning (Kilpatrick *et al.*, 1985a; Girelli *et al.*, 1986; Rothbaum *et al.*, 1992). One major component of the intervention is a segment aimed at reducing anxiety at the time of the medical examination via modelling of medical procedures that will take place. In turn, this might lead to a reduction in acute distress, and subsequently lower rates of PTSD and other psychopathology in the weeks and months following rape. Thus, we hypothesized that it would be important to help prepare women for the potential stress of coping with the medical exam.

A major component of the psycho-educational information provided in the treatment is focused on describing the normal physiological reactions that may occur during rape or other trauma. Thus, physiological reactions of panic attacks are described as actually functional responses to a potentially life or death situation that are automatic in such a situation. Information about the physiological processes that take place during the stress response is similar to that provided by Barlow and Craske (1988) for treatment of panic disorder. Similar to the treatment for those with chronic PTSD and co-morbid panic attacks developed by Falsetti and Resnick (2000) described below, subsequent panic attacks or physiological arousal to reminders of assault are described as part of the normal course of recovery following traumatic events such as rape. Specific responses, including increased heart rate, changes in breathing pattern, etc., are outlined and victims are told that these reactions may reoccur in response to reminders of the assault, but that they are not dangerous and that they will decrease over time with repeated exposure to realistically non-dangerous reminders. Women are instructed that they may be experiencing these physiological sensations as they wait for their medical exam to take place, along with the information that such reactions are normal and predicted to decrease over time.

Previous research has shown that cognitive behavioural approaches that included instructions for exposure had been successfully used to reduce panic frequency at follow-up in an emergency room population with panic disorder (Swinson *et al.*, 1992). Importantly, Swinson *et al.* (1992) found that psycho-education alone, in the absence of instructions for exposure was less effective. Thus, the intervention we developed includes not just education about common physical and emotional reactions to rape. It also includes information about exposure exercises that can be used by victims to get over feared activities or situations (e.g. darkness, being outdoors) that may have been paired with the rape. As with the section of the videotape that includes modelling of medical exam procedures, a model also demonstrates using repeated exposure and coping with physiological arousal symptoms in response to typical rape related cues such as sleeping with lights switched off during the night.

Finally, based on data indicating high rates of other co-morbid mental and physical health problems among rape victims, the intervention addressed symptoms of depression, and other mental and physical health concerns of rape victims in addition to PTSD. Thus, education about depression and modelling of activities and social interaction was included, as was a section addressing use of alcohol or other drugs to avoid emotional distress.

As in most cities in the USA, all rape victims in our area who report the assault to police within 72 hours are seen at the local medical centre for post-rape medical examinations. Since this is typical of other programmes throughout the USA, findings from the ongoing study may provide support for implementation of similar preventive strategies elsewhere. A very important rationale for evaluating an intervention at this very early stage is that it may be the only opportunity at which to provide treatment for some women because many women may not seek traditional mental health or other follow-up services. Preliminary results of our ongoing study have been reported in Resnick *et al.* (1999). All eligible participants presenting to the medical centre were randomly assigned to either the brief cognitive behavioural intervention delivered via videotape prior to the medical exam, or to standard medical treatment and rape crisis advocacy support. Pre- and post-medical exam measures of anxiety are administered during the hospital visit. In addition, women are re-interviewed at 6 weeks and 6 months post-rape to determine mental health status at those time points. In addition to measures of PTSD, depression, and drug and alcohol use women were asked to answer a set of true or false questions that related to information contained in the videotape. Video content questions included items such as; 'Rape is experienced as a life or death type of situation by most women', 'Depression or sadness after rape is a common reaction' and 'Physical reactions, such as your heart beating faster, or breathing in and out very quickly are dangerous and are not part of the body's normal stress reaction.'

Preliminary data from a sample of 46 women (13 video and 33 non-video) indicated that, after controlling for reported levels of pre-examination distress, women who watched the video based intervention were significantly less distressed following the rape examination than women who received standard treatment. In addition, level of distress following the medical examination was significantly positively associated with measures of PTSD and depressive symptom intensity at six weeks post-rape (Resnick *et al.*, 1999). More recent findings with a larger sample of 124 women (63 video and 61 non-video) who have now completed the 6-week follow-up assessment indicated a trend for a lower rate of PTSD based on the PTSD Symptom Scale Self-Report (Foa *et al.*, 1993) among those in the video group (37 *v.* 49%; Fisher's Exact $P=0.11$; Resnick *et al.*, 2000b).

Our preliminary data also indicated that education about physiological arousal sensations that comprise panic attacks might be an important component of the intervention that is related to reduction in the rate of PTSD. Specifically, women who were in the video condition were significantly more likely to correctly identify as false the statement above that proposes that physiological arousal symptoms are dangerous (68% *v.* 39%; x^2 $(1,116)=8.71$, $P<0.005$). Understanding that physiological arousal symptoms are not in themselves dangerous was in turn significantly related to PTSD at 6 weeks post-rape. Those who correctly answered the item were significantly less likely to meet criteria for PTSD than those who were incorrect (30% v. 55%; x^2 (1,116)=6.18, $P<0.05$).

These preliminary data provide some initial support for the efficacy of providing an intervention at the acute post-rape medical exam that may reduce anxiety in the medical setting and that may be related to reduction of PTSD, and other long-term mental health problems among rape victims. The evaluation of the efficacy of the treatment is continuing for the next 4 years. Additional questions being addressed include identification of specific components of the intervention that may be most effective.

In general, findings related to early intervention with rape victims have yielded mixed results. Further research needs to be conducted to evaluate which components of treatment strategies such as imaginal or *in vivo* exposure, psycho-education and cognitive restructuring are effective. In addition, optimal timing of specific intervention strategies post-trauma needs to be assessed. For example, there may be differences in efficacy of imaginal exposure as a function of recency of trauma and number of treatment sessions employed. It may also be important to control for history of prior traumatic events or other patient history characteristics when evaluating effects of treatment. Efficacious treatments will also need to be replicated and their usefulness will need to be evaluated in effectiveness studies across a range of settings.

Specific techniques that may be adapted for use in early interventions with rape victims

The various techniques that have been used in early interventions with rape victims have been outlined above. While it is beyond the scope of this chapter to provide step-by-step instructions in the delivery of these techniques, there are several resources available that do provide in-depth coverage of the rationale, supporting evidence for and application of empirically-supported cognitive behavioural techniques (Foa *et al.*, 2000b). Similar to the strategies described above (Foa *et al.*, 1995), these effective techniques could be further evaluated for their utility in briefer format early interventions with recent victims of rape or other traumatic events. These resources also provide guidelines to comprehensive assessment.

In their book entitled *Treating the Trauma of Rape*, Foa and Rothbaum (1998) provide detailed session-by-session information regarding assessment and cognitive behavioural treatment of PTSD following sexual assault. Treatment strategies described include *in vivo* and imaginal exposure, cognitive restructuring, thought stopping, guided self-dialogue, relaxation training (deep muscle, cue-controlled and differential relaxation), role-play and covert modelling.

Resick and Schnicke (1993) developed and described a 12-session treatment called cognitive processing therapy (CPT) for rape victims with PTSD and depression. CPT is based on a cognitive processing theory of reactions to traumatic events, and involves exposure to the traumatic memory through writing assignments, psycho-education regarding the connection between events, thoughts and feelings, and training in challenging thinking patterns.

Other treatments are under evaluation for treatment of PTSD and other co-morbid disorders. Data indicate that victims of crime commonly experience panic attack symptoms as well as PTSD (Falsetti and Resnick, 1997). Based on the observation that some individuals with PTSD experienced panic levels of anxiety during standard exposure-based treatment, Resnick and Newton (1992) proposed that treatment with interoceptive exposure (Barlow and Craske, 1988) prior to imaginal exposure to trauma-related memories (as in prolonged therapeutic exposure for PTSD) might be beneficial. Interoceptive exposure exercises developed by Barlow and Craske include teaching clients to practice exercises that elicit physiological symptoms similar to those experienced during panic attacks. Exercises such as hyperventilation, step-ups, etc., are practiced repeatedly until anxiety decreases in response to the physiological arousal symptoms produced by the exercises. Resnick and Newton hypothesized that for individuals who experience panic reactions during traditional flooding therapy, initial exposure to somatic cues might reduce anxiety to more manageable levels prior to exposure to memories of the trauma.

Falsetti et al. (1995) proposed that panic sensations may have initially occurred as a response to exposure to traumatic events. Thus, exposure to trauma-related memories could trigger these intense levels of physiological arousal and panic. Based on this theory and data indicating a high prevalence of co-morbid panic attacks among PTSD patients, Falsetti and Resnick (2000) developed a 12-session treatment package called Multiple Channel Exposure Therapy (M-CET) for the treatment of individuals with civilian trauma-related PTSD and co-morbid panic attacks. M-CET was adapted from cognitive processing therapy (Resick and Schnicke, 1993), stress inoculation training (Kilpatrick et al., 1982) and mastery of anxiety and panic (Barlow and Craske, 1988). Thus, this treatment includes exercises in interoceptive exposure (exposure to physiological symptoms of arousal derived from Barlow and Craske, 1988), as well as cognitive/imaginal exposure to the memory of the traumatic event, plus behavioural exposure to avoided cues or situations. Preliminary data indicate this approach may be effective for the treatment of those with PTSD and panic attacks (Falsetti and Resnick, 2000).

Recognition of the problem of co-morbid PTSD, and substance abuse among rape and other trauma victims has also led to the development of treatments designed to address these problems (Dansky et al., 1994; Najavits et al., 1996).

Summary

This chapter contains descriptions of early intervention strategies for use with victims of rape. Data indicate that behavioural approaches appear to show some promise of reducing distress fairly soon after intervention or at longer-term follow-up.

For instance, preliminary data from our own ongoing research indicates that an intervention approach designed to reduce initial distress, PTSD and other mental health outcomes may be administered within hours post-trauma. The intervention is associated with reduced initial anxiety symptoms and lower prevalence of PTSD at 6 weeks post-rape.

Further research is needed to evaluate the efficacy of this approach, as well as other early intervention strategies that adapt empirically supported treatment for use in the acute aftermath of rape or other traumatic events. For a subset of individuals with specific mental health problems brief early interventions may be sufficient, whereas others may benefit from more intensive treatment strategies in the weeks or months following rape.

Acknowledgements

We wish to acknowledge the work of investigators on the ongoing research to develop and evaluate an early intervention for PTSD and other psychopathology following rape. Co-investigators include Melisa Holmes and Dean G. Kilpatrick at the Medical University of South Carolina, Charleston, SC.

This research was supported by the National Institute on Drug Abuse and NIH Inter-agency Consortium on Violence Against Women and Violence in the Family, grant no. R01 DA11158 entitled 'Prevention of Post Rape Psychopathology in Women'; Medical University of South Carolina Healthy South Carolina Grant-in-Aid Initiative entitled 'Multidisciplinary Treatment of Acute and Long Term Health Effects of Rape Victimization: Development of A Model Program'; NIH sponsored Medical University of South Carolina General Clinical Research Center Supported Study, 5M01 RR01070; and Centers for Disease Control and Prevention Grant No. U49/CCU415877–0, entitled 'National Violence Against Women Prevention Research Center'.

References

American Psychiatric Association (1994) *Diagnostic and Statistical Manual of Mental Disorders*, 4th edn. Washington DC: Author.

Atkeson, B.M., Calhoun, K.S., Resick, P.A. and Ellis, E.M. (1982) Victims of rape: repeated assessment of depressive symptoms. *J Consult Clin Psychol* **50**, 96–102.

Barlow, D.H. and Craske, M.G. (1988) The phenomenology of panic. In Rachman, S. and Maser, J.D. (eds) *Panic Psychological Perspectives*. Hilldale: Lawrence Erlbaum Associates, pp. 11–35.

Becker, J.V., Skinner, L.J., Abel, G.G. and Treacy, E.C. (1982) Incidence and types of sexual dysfunctions in rape and incest victims. *J Sex Marit Ther* **8**, 65–74.

Becker, J.V., Skinner, L.J., Abel, G.G. and Cichon J. (1986) Level of postassault sexual functioning in rape and incest victims. *Arch Sex Behav* **15**, 37–49.

Beitchman, J.H., Zucker, K.J., Hood, J.E., DaCosta, G.A., Akman, D. and Cassavia, E. (1992) A review of the long-term effects of child sexual abuse. *Child Abuse Neglect* **16**, 101–18.

Boudreaux, E., Kilpatrick, D.G., Resnick, H.S., Best, C.L. and Saunders, B.E. (1998) Criminal victimization, post-traumatic stress disorder and comorbid psychopathology among a community sample of women. *J Traum Stress* **11**, 665–78.

Brady, K.T., Kileen, T., Saladin, M.E., Dansky, B. and Becker, S. (1994) Comorbid substance abuse and post-raumatic stress disorder. *Am J Addict* **3**, 160–4.

Breslau, N., Davis, G.C., Andreski, P. and Petersen, E. (1991) Traumatic events and post-traumatic stress disorder in an urban population of young adults. *Arch Gen Psychiat* **48**, 216–22.

Bryant, R.A. and Panasetis, P. (2001) Panic symptoms during trauma and acute stress disorder. *Behav Res Ther* **39**, 961–6.

Bryant, R.A., Harvey, A.G., Guthrie, R. and Moulds, M. (2000) A prospective study of acute psychophysiological arousal, acute stress disorder and post-traumatic stress disorder. *J Abnorm Psychol* **109**, 341–4.

Calhoun, K.S., Atkeson, B.M. and Resick, P.A. (1982) A longitudinal examination of fear reactions in victims of rape. *J Counsel Psychol* **29**, 655–1.

Dansky, B.D., Brady, K.T. and Roberts, J.T. (1994) Post-traumatic stress disorder and substance abuse: empirical findings and clinical issues. *Substance Abuse* **15**, 247–57.

Edlis, N. (1993) Rape crisis: development of a center in an Israeli hospital. *Soc Work Hlth Care* **18**, 169–78.

Ellis, E.M., Atkeson, B.M. and Calhoun, K.S. (1982) An examination of differences between multiple and single incident victims of sexual assault. *J Abnorm Psychol* **91**, 221–4.

Falsetti, S.A. and Resnick, H.S. (1997) Trauma, post-raumatic stress disorder and panic attacks: frequency, severity and implications for treatment. *J Traum Stress* **10**, 683–9.

Falsetti, S.A. and Resnick, H.S. (2000) Treatment of PTSD using cognitive and cognitive behavioural therapies. *J Cognit Psychother* **14**, 261–85.

Falsetti, S.A., Resnick, H.S., Lydiard, R.B. and Kilpatrick, D.G. (1995) The relationship of stress to panic disorder: cause or effect? In Mazure, C.M. (ed.) *Does Stress Cause Psychiatric Illness*. Washington, DC: American Psychiatric Press, pp. 111–48.

Fitzgerald, L.F. (1993) Sexual harassment: violence against women in the workplace. *Am Psycholog* **48**, 1070–6.

Foa, E.B. and Rothbaum, B.O. (1998) *Treating the Trauma of Rape: cognitive-behavioural therapy for PTSD*. New York: Guilford Press.

Foa, E.B., Riggs, D.S., Dancu, C.V. and Rothbaum, B.O. (1993) Reliability and validity of a brief instrument for assessing post-traumatic stress disorder. *J Traum Stress* **6**, 459–73.

Foa, E.B., Hearst-Ikeda, D. and Perry, K.K. (1995) Evaluation of a brief cognitive-behavioural program for the prevention of chronic PTSD in recent assault victims. *J Consult Clin Psychol* **63**, 948–55.

Foa, E.B., Zoellner, L., Feeny, N.C., Meadows, E. and Jaycox, L. (November 16–19 2000a) *Evaluation of a Brief Cognitive-behavioural Program for the Prevention of Chronic Ptsd in Recent Assault Victims*. Paper presented at the 34th Annual Convention of the Association for the Advancement of Behaviour Therapy, New Orleans, LA.

Foa, E.B., Keane, T.M. and Friedman, M.J. (2000b) *Effective Treatments for PTSD*. New York: Guilford Press.

Follette, V.M., Polusny, M.A., Bechtle, A.E. and Naugle, A.E. (1996) Cumulative trauma: the impact of child sexual abuse, adult sexual assault and spouse abuse. *J Traum Stress* **9**, 25–35.

Frank, E. and Stewart, B.D. (1984) Depressive symptoms in rape victims: a revisit. *J Affective Disord* **7**, 77–85.

Frank, E., Turner, S.M. and Duffy, B. (1979) Depressive symptoms in rape victims. *J Affect Disord* **1**, 269–77.

Friedrich, W.N., Beilke, R.L. and Urquiza, A.J. (1988) Behaviour problems in young sexually abused boys: a comparison study. *J Interpers Viol* **3**, 1–28.

Garcia-Moreno, C. (2000) Violence against women; international perspectives. *Am J Prevent Med* **19**, 330–3.

Garnets, L., Herek, G.M. and Levy, B. (1990) Violence and victimization of lesbians and gay men: mental health consequences. *J Interpers Viol* **5**, 366–83.

Girelli, S.A., Resick, P.A., Marhoefer-Dvorak, S. and Hutter, C.K. (1986) Subjective distress and violence during rape: their effects on long-term fear. *Viol Victims* **1**, 35–45.

Goyer, P.F. and Eddleman, H.C. (1984) Same-sex rape of nonincarcerated men. *Am J Psychiat* **141**, 576–9.

Hanson, K.A. and Gidycz, C.A. (1993) Evaluation of a sexual assault prevention program. *J Consult Clin Psychol* **61**, 1046–52.

Harvey, A.G. and Bryant, A.B. (1999) The relationship between acute stress disorder and post-traumatic stress disorder: a 2-year prospective evaluation. *J Consult Clin Psychol* **67**, 985–8.

Heflin, A.H. and Deblinger, E. (1996) Treatment of an adolescent survivor of child sexual abuse. In Reinecke, M., Dattilio, F., *et al.* (eds) *Cognitive Therapy with Children and Adolescents: a casebook for clinical practice*. New York: Guilford Press, pp. 199–226.

Hodge, S. and Canter, D. (1998) Victims and perpetrators of male sexual assault. *J Interpers Viol* **13**, 235–61.

Holmes, W.C. and Slap, G.B. (1998) Sexual abuse of boys: definition, prevalence, correlates, sequelae and management. *JAMA* **280**, 1855–62.

Kendall-Tackett, K.A., Williams, L.M. and Finkelhor, D. (1993) Impact of sexual abuse on children: a review and synthesis of recent empirical studies. *Psycholog Bull* **113**, 164–80.

Kessler, R.C., Sonnega, A., Bromet, E., Hughes, M. and Nelson, C.B. (1995) Post-traumatic stress disorder in the National Comorbidity Survey. *Arch Gen Psychiat* **52**, 1048–60.

Kilpatrick, D.G. and Calhoun, K.S. (1988) Early behavioural treatment for rape trauma: Efficacy or artifact? *Behav Ther* **19**, 421–7.

Kilpatrick, D.G. and Veronen, L.J. (1983) Treatment for rape-related problems: crisis intervention is not enough. In Cohen, L., Claiborn, W. and Specter, G. (eds) *Crisis Intervention*, Community Clinical Psychology series, 2nd edn, pp. 165–85, New York: Human Services Press.

Kilpatrick, D.G., Veronen, L.J. and Resick, P.A. (1982) Psychological sequelae to rape: assessment and treatment strategies. In Doleys, D.M., Meredith, R.L. and Ciminero, A.R. (eds) *Behavioural Medicine: assessment and treatment strategies*. New York: Plenum Publishing Corporation, pp. 473–97.

Kilpatrick, D.G., Veronen, L.J. and Best, C.L. (1985a) Factors predicting psychological distress among rape victims. In Figley, C.R. (ed.) *Trauma and Its Wake*. New York: Brunner/Mazel, pp.113–41.

Kilpatrick, D.G., Best, C.L., Veronen, L.J., Amick, A.E., Villeponteaux, L.A. and Ruff, G.A. (1985b) Mental health correlates of criminal victimization: a random community survey. *J Consult Clin Psychol* **53**, 866–73.

Kilpatrick, D.G., Saunders, B.E., Veronen, L.J., Best, C.L. and Von, J.M. (1987) Criminal victimization: lifetime prevalence, reporting to police and psychological impact. *Crime Delinq* **33**, 479–89.

Kilpatrick, D.G., Saunders, B.E., Amick-McMullan, A., Best, C.L., Veronen, L.J. and Resnick, H.S. (1989) Victim and crime factors associated with the development of crime-related post-traumatic stress disorder. *Behav Ther* **20**, 199–214.

Kilpatrick, D.G., Edmunds, C.N. and Seymour, A.K. (1992) *Rape in America: a report to the nation*. Arlington: National Victim Center and Medical University of South Carolina.

Kilpatrick, D.G., Acierno, R., Resnick, H.S., Saunders, B.E. and Best, C.L. (1997) A 2-year longitudinal analysis of the relationships between violent assault and substance use in women. *J Consult Clin Psychol* **65**, 834–47.

Kilpatrick, D.G., Resnick, H.S., Saunders, B.E. and Best, C.L. (1998a) Rape, other violence against women and post-traumatic stress disorder: critical issues in assessing the adversity-stress-psychopathology relationship. In Dohrenwend, B.P. (ed.) *Adversity, Stress and Psychopathology*, pp. 161–76. New York: Oxford University Press.

Kilpatrick, D. G., Resnick, H. S., Freedy, J. R., Pelcovitz, D., Resick, P., Roth, S. and van der Kolk, B. (1996b) Post-raumatic stress disorder field trial: evaluation of the PTSD construct: Criteria A through E. In Widiger, T.A., Frances, A.J., Tincas, H.A., Ross, R., First, M.B., Davis, W. and Kline, M. (eds) *DSM-IV Sourcebook*, Vol. 4. Washington DC: American Psychiatric Association, pp. 803–844

Koss, M.P. (1993) Detecting the scope of rape: a review of prevalence research methods. *J Interpers Viol* **8**, 198–222.

Kramer, T.L. and Green, B.L. (1991) Post-traumatic stress disorder as an early response to sexual assault. *J Interpers Viol* **6**, 160–73.

Letourneau, E.J., Resnick, H.S., Kilpartrick, D.G., Saunders, B.E. and Best, C.L. (1996) Comorbidity of sexual problems and post-raumatic stress disorder in female crime victims. *Behav Ther* **27**, 321–36.

McFarlane, A.C. (1988) The longitudinal course of post-raumatic morbidity: the range of outcomes and their predictors. *J Nerv Ment Dis* **176**, 30–9.

McLeer, S.V., Dixon, J.F., Henry, D., Ruggiero, K.J., Escovitz, K., Niedda, T. and Scholle, R. (1998) Psychopathology in non-clinically referred sexually abused children. *J Am Acad Child Adolesc Psychiat* **37**, 1326–33.

Najavits, L.M., Weiss, R.D. and Liese, B.S. (1996) Group cognitive-behavioural therapy for women with PTSD and substance use disorder. *J Subst Abuse Treat* **13**, 13–22.

Polusny, M.A. and Follette, V.M. (1995) Long-term correlates of child sexual abuse: theory and review of the empirical literature. *Appl Prevent Psychol* **4**, 143–66.

Resick, P.A. (1993) The psychological impact of rape. *J Interpers Viol* **8**, 223–55.

Resick, P.A. and Schnicke, M.K. (1993) *Cognitive Processing Therapy for Rape Victims: a treatment manual*. Newbury Park: Sage Publications.

Resnick, H.S. and Newton, T. (1992) Assessment and treatment of post-raumatic stress disorder in adult survivors of sexual assault. In Foy, D.W. (ed.) *Treating PTSD*. New York: Guilford Press, pp. 99–126.

Resnick, H.S., Kilpatrick, D.G., Dansky, B.S., Saunders, B.E. and Best, C.L. (1993) Prevalence of civilian trauma and PTSD in a representative sample of women. *J Consult Clin Psychol* **61**, 985–91.

Resnick, H.S., Falsetti, S.A., Kilpatrick, D.G. and Foy, D.W. (November 5–9 1994) *Associations Between Panic Attacks during Rape Assaults and Follow-up Ptsd or Panic Attack Outcomes*. Paper presented at the 10th Annual Meeting of the International Society for Traumatic Stress Studies, Chicago, IL.

Resnick, H.S., Yehuda, R., Pitman, R.K. and Foy, D.W. (1995) Effects of previous trauma on acute plasma cortisol level following rape. *Am J Psychiat* **152**, 1675–7.

Resnick, H., Acierno, R., Holmes, M., Kilpatrick, D. and Jager, N. (1999) Prevention of post rape psychopathology: Preliminary evaluation of an acute rape treatment. *J Anx Disord* **13**, 359–70.

Resnick, H.S., Holmes, M.M., Kilpatrick, D.G., Clum, G., Acierno, R., Best, C.L. and Saunders, B.E. (2000a) Predictors of post-rape medical care in a national sample of women. *Am J Prevent Med* **19**, 214–19.

Resnick, H., Acierno, R. and Kilpatrick, D. (November 15–19 2000b) *Acute Psychological Distress and PTSD Following Rape*. Paper presented at the 16th Annual Meeting of the International Society for Traumatic Stress Studies, San Antonio, TX.

Rothbaum, B.O., Foa, E.B., Riggs, D.S., Murdock, T. and Walsh, W. (1992) A prospective evaluation of post-traumatic stress disorder in rape victims. *J Traum Stress* **5**, 455–75.

Scarce, M. (1997) Same-sex rape of male college students. *J Am Coll Hlth* **45**, 171–3.

Schneider, K.T., Swan, S. and Fitzgerald, L.F. (1997) Job-related and psychological effects of sexual harassment in the workplace: empirical evidence from two organizations. *J Appl Psychol* **82**, 401–15.

Shalev, A.Y., Sahar, T., Freedman, S., Peri, T., Glick, N., Brandes, D., Orr, S.P. and Pitman, R.K. (1998) A prospective study of heart rate responses following trauma and the subsequent development of PTSD. *Arch Gen Psychiat* **55**, 553–9.

Steketee, G. and Foa, E B. (1987) Rape victims: post-traumatic stress responses and their treatment: a review of the literature. *J Anx Disord* **1**, 69–86.

Swinson, R.P., Soulios, C., Cox, B.J. and Kuch, K. (1992) Brief treatment of emergency room patients with panic attacks. *Am J Psychiat* **149**, 944–6.

Wolfe, V.V. and Birt, J. (1997) Child sexual abuse. In Mash, E.J. and Terdal, L.G. (eds) *Behavioural Assessment of Childhood Disorders*, 3rd edn. New York: Guilford Press, pp. 569–623.

Young, W.W., Bracken, A.C., Goddard, M.A., Matheson, S. and the New Hampshire Sexual Assault Medical Examination Protocol Project Committee. (1992) Sexual assault: review of a national model protocol for forensic and medical evaluations. *Obstet Gynecol* **80**, 878–83.

19 A brief early intervention service for accident and assault victims

Jonathan I. Bisson

Psychological sequelae to accidents and assaults are common. Breslau *et al.* (1991) interviewed 1007 American adults aged between 21 and 30. Almost 40% had been exposed to a major traumatic event of which accidents and assaults were the most common. Kessler *et al.* (1995) in their large epidemiological survey in the USA found lifetime prevalence of PTSD following serious accident to be 20.7% in men and 23.6% in women. For physical attack the rates were 12.4% in men and 30.8% in women, and for rape 65% in men and 45.9% in women. In Breslau *et al.*'s (1991) study 11.6% of those who had suffered a sudden injury or serious accident and 22.6% of those physically assaulted developed PTSD compared to 80% of women who reported rape. The presence of high levels of psychological morbidity following accidents and assaults has major implications for hospital trauma services including orthopaedic surgery, general surgery, accident and emergency medicine, ophthalmology and maxillo-facial surgery in addition to primary care and mental health services.

Many attempts have been made in recent years to identify effective means of preventing the development of PTSD and other psychiatric disorders in individuals involved in traumatic events. Much attention has been paid to one-off interventions such as psychological debriefing (PD) (Mitchell, 1983; Dyregrov, 1989). Unfortunately, despite its good face validity, psychological debriefing has not lived up to the expectation of many that it would be able to prevent PTSD and other conditions. The latest Cochrane systematic review, which is featured in this book (Rose *et al.*, chapter 3) shows that there are now 11 randomized controlled trials (RCT) that have considered one-off interventions following trauma. Over half of these have dealt specifically with individuals following accidents and assaults. No convincing evidence has been found that one-off interventions reduce psychological symptoms and it seems inappropriate to recommend such provision. Unfortunately, there have been no RCTs of group PD, but the majority of accidents and assaults occur to individuals or a small number of people and, therefore, early group interventions are unlikely to represent a pragmatic intervention approach.

The absence of evidence for the effectiveness of one-off interventions has led to interest in multiple session early interventions. The first reported RCT was by Brom *et al.* (1993) who studied 151 motor vehicle accident victims in the Netherlands. Individuals were randomly allocated to a three to five session intervention that stressed the importance of practical help and information, support, reality testing, confrontation with the experience, early recognition of disorders and referral to psychotherapeutic treatment. The intervention occurred between 1 and 3 months following the accident. The subjects in the intervention group were reported to have appreciated the intervention, but there were no statistically significant differences in outcome between the two groups. Ten per cent of both groups were suffering from PTSD at follow-up 6 months later.

Bryant *et al.* (1998) considered 24 individuals who satisfied the criteria for a diagnosis of acute stress disorder, a common precursor of PTSD, within 2 weeks of a road traffic accident or industrial accident. They found that five 90-minute sessions of cognitive behavioural therapy (CBT) was more effective than five 90-minute sessions of supportive counselling (SC) in reducing psychological distress and preventing the development of PTSD. One (8%) of the CBT group satisfied PTSD criteria immediately post-intervention compared to 10 (83%) of the SC group ($P<0.001$). Two (17%) of the CBT group satisfied PTSD criteria at 6 months compared to eight (67%) of the SC group ($P<0.05$). Bryant *et al.* (1999) subsequently studied 66 survivors of road accidents or non-sexual assault with acute stress disorder. This time individuals were randomly allocated to one of three intervention groups: prolonged exposure, prolonged exposure plus anxiety management and supportive counselling. Immediately post-treatment, 14% of the prolonged exposure group, 20% of the prolonged exposure plus anxiety management group and 56% of the supportive counselling group satisfied the criteria for a diagnosis of PTSD. The differences were maintained at 6 months follow-up (15 *v.* 23 *v.* 67%; see also Bryant, Chapter 14 in this book).

Andre *et al.* (1997) compared one to six sessions of cognitive behavioural therapy with standard care in 132 French bus drivers who had been attacked. At 6 months follow-up there was a small, but significantly greater reduction in anxiety and intrusive symptoms in the treatment group, but no statistically significant differences in depression and avoidance measures. These studies suggest that early brief cognitive behavioural therapy may help individuals experiencing acute psychological distress following a traumatic event.

The apparent promise of more complex early interventions particularly if focused on those individuals with psychological symptoms led us to develop a four-session early intervention, which included elements of exposure therapy and cognitive restructuring. This was used in a randomized controlled trial of 152 individuals presenting to the Emergency Unit in Cardiff following physical injury as a result of accidents or assaults. The intervention was found to significantly reduce symptoms of PTSD using the Impact of Event Scale as the main outcome measure at 13 months after the trauma (Bisson *et al.*, 2000). The intervention was delivered by a relatively inexperienced research psychologist suggesting that it can be implemented by trained and supervised individuals who are not mental health professionals. Adequate training, supervision and audit are vital to achieve the level of competency that is necessary for the successful delivery of any intervention.

The Cardiff & Vale NHS Trust Traumatic Stress Initiative

A close partnership has been developed in Cardiff between the Traumatic Stress Service and the Emergency Planning Unit. This has led to the development of a team of 10 counsellors trained and supervised in the provision of a brief focused cognitive behavioural intervention by a psychiatrist and psychologist. The aim of the initiative is to provide a pre-planned psychosocial response should a disaster occur locally. In order to develop their skills the counsellors are involved in the psychosocial aftercare of individuals presenting to the local Emergency Unit as a result of road traffic accidents, assaults and industrial accidents.

Overview of the service

Following presentation to the local Emergency Unit individuals are screened for the presence of psychological distress. If present the individual is then approached and offered assessment for the brief intervention. If the individual's primary difficulty appears to be symptoms of acute PTSD the intervention is delivered and follow-up occurs. If the individual is not symptomatic or their symptoms are significantly improving they are advised of how to contact us should the need arise. If they appear to be experiencing psychological difficulties that are not predominantly PTSD based, they are directed to the appropriate service for further assessment/management. At follow-up immediately post-intervention and 3 months later, individuals are reassessed, which may result in further management.

Screening

Various studies have considered screening for psychological symptoms in an attempt to predict the development of psychological sequelae. Bisson *et al.* (1997) showed that junior dental house officers with no formal psychiatric training were as good at predicting those individuals who developed traumatic stress difficulties as screening with a standard questionnaire. Several studies have found that early psychological distress is a good predictor of later difficulty. Depressive (e.g. Freedman *et al.*, 1999), intrusive (e.g. Brewin *et al.*, 1998) and dissociative (e.g. Harvey and Bryant, 1998) symptoms have all been shown to have predictive value.

If those individuals dealing with accident victims in the front line such as Emergency Unit personnel are aware of early psychological responses this can help improve rate of detection. We also advocate the use of a standard questionnaire such as the Trauma distress scale developed by Brewin *et al.* (1998). This is easy to administer, acceptable to patients who complete it and has been associated with a high predictive value. Other factors could also help us to identify individuals at higher risk. Family history of psychiatric disorder (Breslau *et al.*, 1991; Davidson *et al.*, 1991), reduced social support (Davidson *et al.*, 1991), and pre-trauma anxiety or depression (McFarlane, 1988; Breslau *et al.*, 1991; Resnick *et al.*, 1992) and reduced cortisol levels (Yehuda *et al.*, 1998) have been shown to be predictive of the development of traumatic stress difficulties. It is also important to remember the other disorders that commonly occur following traumatization, such as substance misuse, depression and other anxiety disorders.

Information

In addition to an adequate screening protocol there needs to be an adequate information policy. Ideally, there should be written information regarding typical symptoms that may be experienced following involvement in a traumatic event. Information should emphasize the normality of experiencing a psychological response following a traumatic event and promote resiliency factors, but should not over-normalize symptoms that may develop. It should contain descriptions of the types of emotions, feelings and symptoms that may develop along with guidance of when and how to obtain help and suggestions regarding successful coping. It is helpful to provide contact phone numbers for potential sources of help. For example, charitable organizations, such as victim support, are very useful to some individuals as is the primary care system (general practitioner).

Assessment

Before offering a brief early intervention it is important to perform a standardized assessment that should confirm the nature of an individual's difficulties and their needs. Standard features of an appropriate assessment include a full history, mental state examination, risk assessment and preparation for the intervention. It is vital to ensure that the individual is aware of the nature of the intervention and willing and motivated to engage in this.

Intervention

The intervention used in Cardiff was designed as a four sessions intervention for a randomized controlled trial as discussed above. It will be described in this way, but in clinical practice it is important to exercise some flexibility in its delivery. In some individuals it will be appropriate to deliver the intervention over a longer period, perhaps six or eight sessions. However, it is strongly recommended that the individual is contracted to a certain number of sessions, which may be extended following reassessment of the situation. We initially offer four weekly sessions of 1 hour duration to individuals with persisting traumatic stress symptoms or for those whose reactions are not significantly reducing one month following a traumatic event. Traumatic stress symptoms are the main indication for the intervention. There are no absolute contraindications, but some individuals feel overwhelmed by their symptoms and may be re-traumatized by exposure work. It is then important to focus on the development of appropriate coping strategies before commencing exposure work and aim to reduce levels of arousal. Usually, this is done through cognitive-behavioural techniques, but may involve pharmacotherapy.

Session One

The accident or assault and psychological symptoms are discussed in some detail. Participants are educated regarding the stress response to a traumatic event, reassured that a significant proportion of people experience similar symptoms following physical injury and receive an explanation of the rationale behind the intervention. There should be a degree of normalization, but it should be remembered that the individuals are receiving the intervention because of their high risk of going on to develop more significant symptoms and, therefore, over-normalization should be avoided. The individual is then encouraged to describe the traumatic incident in detail, in the first person present tense, including thoughts, feelings, sights, smells, noises, emotions and physical reactions. This technique mirrors a standard approach used in exposure therapy for the treatment of established PTSD (e.g. Foa *et al.*, 1992). We have found that it is helpful for the therapist to record the sequence of events on paper. On completion the individual is asked to read the account aloud in session and rate their level of distress to it using a 0–10 subjective units of distress scale (SUDS). At the end of the session, the participant is asked to read it at least once a day as homework. Ideally, this should take at least half-an-hour and may involve reading it several times. It is important that time is allowed for the individual to habituate to the reading task, rather than it merely serving as a re-traumatizing experience.

Session Two

The session starts with a review of functioning over the past week with a 0–10 SUDS rating. The difficulties and achievements are considered along with discussion of homework compliance, and any issues around this. The participant is asked to read the text aloud in session and it is audio-recorded. At this time it is important for the therapist to note down areas where distorted thinking is recognized or issues associated with avoidance. These are discussed with the individual. Specific areas to consider are any distorted cognitions or issues around blame, shame, guilt, criticism and revenge. It is useful to challenge these using traditional cognitive therapy methods such as scenarios using different people/events, Socratic questioning, role reversal and percentages of responsibility. Avoidance issues are confronted and habituation discussed. The session ends with a discussion of skills learnt during the session for example the identification and challenging of irrational beliefs. Homework involves listening to the audiotape recording for at least half an hour every day.

Session Three

The week is again reviewed and achievements/difficulties discussed along with homework compliance. The audiotape is listened to during the session and distress again rated. Discussion then focuses on areas where habituation is not taking place and a number of approaches are suggested to overcome any avoidance including Image Habituation Training (Vaughan and Tarrier, 1992), where an individual is asked to keep the most traumatic images in their minds as vividly as possible for more prolonged periods, say half a minute or as long as possible. This should facilitate habituation and avoid the subtle avoidance that can occur in standard exposure therapy where an individual may ignore some of the most traumatic images. The focus then moves to the avoidance of real life cues. For example, with road traffic accident victims avoidance of car travel is very common. Daily activities such as driving are reviewed and compared to before the accident. Difficulties associated with avoidance are discussed and a graded *in vivo* exposure programme devised if the participant is avoiding real life situations. This involves creating a hierarchy of avoided situations, rationale explanation, discussion of starting points, ways of tackling tasks and coping strategies such as support from others and breathing techniques. Cognitive distortions are again discussed, and the session ends with a recap of the session and the setting of homework in the form of ongoing exposure to the audiotape, graded exposure tasks and/or a cognitive diary as indicated.

Session Four

The week is again reviewed and rated. The tape is listened to and rated during the session. Any specific areas of concern are discussed. The participant is then given a written summary of approximately one or two sides of A4 paper that outlines successes, areas for attention, potential problem areas, and how to cope with these and any other relevant details. They are reassessed and their scores on the assessment battery of tests are reviewed and discussed. This and the therapy is discussed in some detail. Participants are asked to consider the therapy as having equipped them with some new skills that may be beneficial to them in the future. They are encouraged to continue with their exposure work and challenging of cognitive distortions. In the majority of cases the individual is discharged with a follow-up contact arranged for 3 months later. In some instances, the individual's ongoing symptoms will be such that further immediate intervention is required.

Further intervention

Individuals who continue to experience difficulties are reassessed by an experienced member of the Traumatic Stress Service. Whenever their primary difficulty appears to be PTSD or subsyndromal PTSD they are offered another evidence-based intervention for PTSD. This may involve more focused cognitive work particularly where engagement in exposure work has proved difficult. Alternatively antidepressant medication or Eye Movement Desensitization and Reprocessing (Shepherd *et al.*, 2000) are used.

Evaluation

In order to monitor the individual's progress and the effectiveness of the service and the intervention individuals are asked to complete standard measures on entry to the service, post-intervention and at follow-up. At present these include the Davidson Trauma Scale, Clinician Administered PTSD Scale, Beck Depression Inventory and Beck Anxiety Inventory. The service and intervention are viewed as representing good practice with the evidence available at present. The development of the service has provided several important learning experiences. It has encouraged us to move away from considering a single blanket intervention as appropriate for everyone with traumatic stress symptoms following a traumatic event. Indeed, some individuals may become more symptomatic as a result of psychological intervention. It is therefore vital that adequate assessment and monitoring occurs. It is hoped that our approach will evolve and improve as a result of ongoing monitoring and evaluation, and through incorporating the results of future research in this area.

References

Andre, C., Lelord, F., Legeron, P., Reigner, A. and Delattre, A. (1997) Effectiveness of early intervention on 132 bus driver victims of aggression: a controlled study. *Encephale* **23**, 65–71.

Bisson, J.I., Shepherd, J.P. and Dhutia, M. (1997) Psychological sequelae of facial trauma. *J Trauma Injury Infect Crit Care* **43**, 496–500.

Bisson, J.I., Shepherd, J.P., Joy, D. and Probert, R. (2000) Randomised controlled trial of a brief psychological intervention following acute physical injury, Abstracts of papers for 23rd European Conference on Psychosomatic Research. *J Psychosom Res* **48**, 224.

Breslau, N., Davis, G.C., Andreski, M.A. and Peterson, E. (1991) Traumatic events and post-traumatic stress disorder in an urban population of young adults. *Arch Gen Psychiat* **48**, 216–22.

Brewin, C.R., Andrews, B., Rose, S. and Kirk, M. (1998) Acute stress disorder and post-traumatic stress disorder in victims of violent crime. *Am J Psychiat* **156**, 360–6.

Brom, D., Kleber, R.J. and Hofman M.C. (1993) Victims of traffic accidents: Incidence and prevention of post-traumatic stress disorder. *J Clin Psychol* **49**, 131–40.

Bryant, R.A., Harvey, A.G., Dang, S.T., Sackville, T. and Basten, C. (1998) Treatment of acute stress disorder: a comparison of cognitive-behavioral therapy and supportive counselling. *J Consult Clin Psychol* **66**, 862–6.

Bryant, R.A., Sackville, T., Dang, S.T., Moulds, M. and Guthrie, R. (1999) Treating acute stress disorder: an evaluation of cognitive behavior therapy and supportive counselling techniques. *Am J Psychiat* **156**, 1780–6.

Davidson, J.R., Hughes, D., Blazer, D.G. and George, L.K. (1991) Post-traumatic stress disorder in the community. *Psycholog Med* **21**, 713–21.

Dyregrov, A. (1989) Caring for helpers in disaster situations: psychological debriefing. *Disast Manag* **2**, 25–30.

Foa, E.B., Rothbaum, B.O., Riggs, D.S. and Murdock, J. (1992) Treatment of posttraumatic stress disorder in rape victims: a comparison between cognitive-behavioural procedures and counselling. *J Consult Clin Psychol* **59**, 715–23.

Freedman, S.A., Brandes, D., Peri, T. and Shalev, A. (1999) Predictors of chronic post-traumatic stress disorder. *Br J Psychiat* **174**, 353–9.

Harvey, A.G. and Bryant, R.A. (1998) The relationship between acute stress disorder and post-traumatic stress disorder: a prospective evaluation of motor vehicle accident survivors. *J Consult Clin Psychol* **66**, 507–12.

Kessler, R.C., Sonnega, A., Bromet, E., Hughes, M. and Nelson, C.B. (1995) Post-traumatic stress disorder in the national comorbidity survey. *Arch Gen Psychiat* **52**, 1048–60.

McFarlane, A.C. (1988) The longitudinal course of post-traumatic morbidity: the range of outcomes and their predictors. *J Nerv Ment Dis* **176**, 30–9.

Mitchell, J.T. (1983) When disaster strikes … the critical incident debriefing process. *J Emerg Med Serv* **8**, 36–9.

Resnick, H.S., Kilpatrick, D.G., Best, C.L. and Kramer, T.L. (1992) Vulnerability-stress factors in development of post-traumatic stress disorder. *J Nerv Ment Dis* **180**, 424–30.

Shepherd, J., Stein, K. and Milne, R. (2000) Eye movement desensitisation and reprocessing in the treatment of post-traumatic stress disorder: a review of an emerging therapy. *Psycholog Med* **30**, 863–71.

Vaughan, K. and Tarrier, N. (1992) The use of image habituation training with post-traumatic stress disorders. *Br J Psychiat* **161**, 658–64.

Yehuda, R., McFarlane, A.C. and Shalev, A.Y. (1998) Predicting the development of posttraumatic stress disorder from the acute response to a traumatic event. *Biolog Psychiat* **44**, 1305–13.

20 The Lincolnshire Joint Emergency Services Initiative: an early intervention protocol for emergency services staff

Anna Avery and Stephen King

Establishment of the original service

The First European Conference on Traumatic Stress held in Lincoln, England in 1988 highlighted the impact disasters can have on rescue personnel, as well as primary victims. A major achievement of this scientific meeting was to foster an appreciation that both these groups, as well as those described by Figley (1995) as being at risk for secondary 'vicarious reasons', should be studied and understood as part of the endeavours of modern psychotraumatology.

At the conference delegates were advised of the Critical Incident Stress Debriefing model promoted by Mitchell (1983) for use with staff groups and individuals recently exposed to trauma and critical incidents. It had been claimed that this early intervention (conducted within 24–72 hours of the traumatic event) would, amongst other achievements, effectively prevent the subsequent development of trauma related symptomatology. After the conference a report of the proceedings of the First European Conference was sent to senior officers within emergency services in Lincolnshire, England. It proposed to establish a new local and dedicated early intervention service for staff at risk following exposure to critical and traumatic events in the course of their work. This proposal found unanimous support from the Police, Ambulance and Fire Brigade in Lincolnshire, as well as the local National Health Service and Social Services departments. The Lincolnshire Joint Emergency Services Initiative for Staff at Risk Following Critical Incidents (LJESI) was formally constituted by a working group that met in December 1988, and has remained operational ever since. Each participating emergency service has nominated senior and middle ranking officers who provide a formal link to the LJESI, either as members of a county wide support group (the responder team) or serve on the Steering Group of the Initiative (its management team). Some individuals are active in both groups. No one is paid for their involvement with the LJESI, but it is understood that time spent in providing early support services for staff can be claimed back as 'time owing'. It has been estimated the Initiative requires a resource investment by each participating emergency service of approximately 10 working days per year. With the initiative in place it is possible to provide staff training, incident and post-incident advice to front line incident controllers and managers plus post-incident staff support meetings free of charge to the participating emergency services. Time has also proven the Initiative to be a crucial resource for conducting research into aspects of staff welfare within emergency services.

The working group that founded the LJESI in 1988 decided to give first priority to promoting awareness of what was then known about critical incident stress reactions amongst staff in the emergency services. Initially, this was achieved by holding a series of 2-day workshops, which used didactic teaching, group work and self-disclosure. Their aim was to foster a professional climate that is accepting of the notion that particular work-related events can have significant psychological ramifications for emergency responders. The workshops also gave consideration to the then diagnostic criteria for Post-traumatic Stress Disorder (DSM-III; American Psychiatric Association, 1980) and what were believed, at that time, to be the core elements of good staff support practices following major incidents. Half a day was dedicated to presentations made by senior officers whose emergency services had been called out to recent well-publicized disasters such as the Kings Cross Fire, the Hungerford Massacre, the Clapham Rail Disaster, etc. So it came to be that the main focus and activity of the Initiative is to implement an educational and training strategy for staff. Only some 3 years later did the LJESI establish its first dedicated resource for offering structured post-incident staff support. In January 1991, 15 self-selected staff from all the participating emergency services attended a 2-day Psychological Debriefing (PD) training workshop facilitated by Dr A. Dyregrov (Mitchell, 1983; Dyregrov, 1989). In the course of the following 5 years those who had been given this training and had experience of facilitating PD meetings used their expertise to train more staff. This ensured a greater number of staff had the required level of competence to be members of the three-person teams advocated for use in group debriefings. By the summer of 1997 the Initiative had 31 trained staff available who could be mobilized to lead and support PD meetings. This operational group consisted of 11 staff from the health service, some of whom were clinical psychologists with extensive experience in providing psychological therapies, seven from social services, five from the police, and four each from the fire and ambulance services.

Several advantages accrued from having a debriefing team comprising of staff from all participating emergency services. Principal amongst these was the fact that the new debriefers had, during their own careers been called to critical and traumatic incidents. This bestowed not only a sense of personal credibility when facilitating a group meeting, but also helped to promote a greater understanding of factual events that had unfolded plus their impact over time. It also meant that officers' concerns about confidentiality could be addressed. For instance, whenever the police force requested a PD meeting be held the debriefing team mobilized for this response could be constituted by staff from other emergency services. This added to the sense of user friendliness and acceptability of the early intervention services provided.

A postal questionnaire survey carried out amongst members of the debriefing team determined the level of their activity between 1991 and April 1997. During this 6-year period 25 incidents had occurred within the county of Lincolnshire that, in turn, had prompted at least one emergency service to call for a PD meeting to be held. Some of these incidents involved more than one emergency service and, therefore, the number of requests received for such meetings totalled 35. This averages at nearly six requests per year. Further analysis of survey returns revealed the critical events in question comprised of six fatal road traffic accidents, six incidents involving fatalities and serious injury to emergency responders, and a further six where serious threat to officers had occurred. In addition, there was a cluster of five less frequently occurring events such as homicide and suicide. Two exceptional incidents in the community at large had also occasioned requests for an early intervention with members of the general public. Only one in four of these incidents were followed up with more than one group PD meeting to review consequences of a particular event over a longer period of time. Hence, the total number of PD meetings held during this 6-year period is estimated to have been 40. Although the constituency of each PD meeting was not formally investigated in the survey an informed estimate is that an overwhelming majority of meetings had multi-agency representation. This is, of course, consistent with call-out practices for critical and traumatic incidents that unfold in the community. Single service meetings were indicated for some events that had taken place within hospitals or social services residential facilities.

The Initiative was also asked to set in place arrangements for a hospital-based psychosocial support service for relatives and friends of military personnel involved in the Gulf War. This became an integral part of local contingency plans for hospitals in Lincolnshire to admit and treat medically-evacuated personnel from the battlefront. Although arrangements were put in place for the Initiative to provide such early psychosocial care, its services were never required.

Reviews of the early intervention service

Informal monitoring and review of services provided was a feature of the Initiative from the start. The teams called out to facilitate early interventions were under instruction to meet informally immediately after a PD session to share their own impressions and reactions to what they had just done and observed. The team leader could also form a view as to whether support for the helpers was indicated. Only on one occasion, following a multiple murder of children, were special arrangements made to provide additional follow-up and review for members of all PD responder teams. The Steering Group of the Initiative (its management group) would also receive reports of debriefing meetings held along with assessments of their impact on participants, as well as senior managers' views about their value to the emergency service generally.

A more systematic retrospective examination of the impact of PD meetings and service users evaluation of help provided was eventually undertaken by Hutt (1994). His study period spanned from 1991 to 1994 and the methodology allowed for a small-scale comparison of the course and development of event-related reactions amongst emergency services officers who, after specific critical incidents, had either participated in PD meetings or had chosen not to do so. In total, the survey sample comprised 54 volunteers from all the above-mentioned emergency services. Of these, 38 were male and 16 female. Thirty-five subjects had participated in debriefing meetings and 19 had not. Reasons given for not attending PDs included inconvenient timing due to shift patterns, being at work, distance to travel to the identified venue and also not feeling a need of the type of early intervention offered. All volunteers agreed to participate in a one-to-one structured interview to establish demographic variables, details of the critical incidents they had been involved in and their subjective appraisals of PD meetings and their impact over time. As part of the interview they completed the Impact of Events Scale (IES; Horowitz *et al.*, 1979) and the 90-item symptom check list (SCL-90-R; Derogatis, 1983) to furnish a guide as to their current adjustment relative to what had happened. Using the same symptom report measures all subjects also provided a retrospective assessment of the immediate impact of the critical event. The Coping Responses Questionnaire (Billings and Moos, 1981) and the Interpersonal Support Evaluation List (Cohen *et al.*, 1985) were also administered. Survey results revealed no differences in the PD and non-PD groups as regards the duration or intensity of reactions evoked by critical incidents. No one rated PD meetings they had attended as 'unhelpful', although only one in eight rated the meetings as 'very helpful'. Scores on the IES and the SCL-90-R indicated that officers with lowest retrospective scores for the period immediately after the index event tended to be those who rated PD meetings as most helpful. Rated helpfulness of debriefings had no consistent relationship to reported reductions in distress levels over time. Most marked reductions in event-induced distress scores was achieved by those emergency responders who reported having had access to and made active use of the various forms of social support available at the time in their work settings or in their lives generally. The extent of these changes proved to be independent of whether or not officers had attended PD meetings.

The implications of these results for the Initiative were scrutinized by a subcommittee of the Initiative Steering Group during the latter part of 1995. It was felt that at best the outcome of the retrospective evaluation of PD offered only qualified support for the view that this form of early intervention had a distinct beneficial effect upon the course and development of reactions and impressions evoked by critical incidents. Results also suggested that highest satisfaction ratings were reported by those who were least distressed and who also indicated having access to the highest levels of social support. With these considerations in mind the subcommittee recommended PD should no longer be offered as an early intervention for emergency services officers in Lincolnshire. When making this recommendation in 1995, the committee noted that the findings of Hutt's (1994) survey, and its implications, were broadly consistent with other, more methodologically sophisticated studies that linked reductions in event-evoked distress to levels of social support (Leavy, 1983) and having access to at least one significant confiding relationship (Cohen and Wills, 1985; Schwarzer and Jerusalem, 1995).

In addition, the debate about PD and CISD efficacy, engendered by an apparent lack of reliable evidence of their distinctive impact on event-related symptomatology, had been followed by members of the LJESI with growing concern. This was because no reasoned case could be made in favour of convening PD or CISD meetings if the evidence was not at hand that demonstrated a consistent, and distinctly positive influence upon adjustment after major work-related trauma and critical incidents. After much discussion, the working group eventually accepted it had to confront the possibility of there being some fundamental flaws in the theory and techniques that underpin these forms of early intervention after trauma, and that they might result in potentially harmful outcomes (e.g. Bisson and Deahl, 1994; Raphael *et al.*, 1995). These considerations apart, there was also the spectre for all participating emergency services in Lincolnshire, of possible financial ramifications arising from personal or group litigations, of advocating early intervention practices for emergency services officers without a sound evidence base for their therapeutic impact.

After carefully evaluating the implications of all the evidence at hand the working group reached the pragmatic conclusion it would advise the Steering Group of the Initiative of its conclusion there was insufficient evidence to justify retaining PD as the early intervention of choice for emergency services staff mobilized for traumatic and critical incident response. In turn, the Steering Group formally sanctioned a decision to abandon PD and declared as unsafe any claim that one-off early intervention will consistently prevent the development of post-traumatic symptomatology (Avery and Ørner, 1998). On the basis of available evidence, the LJESI accepted that the aims of its future provision should be less focused on event-related symptomatology. Its declared alternative is to seek to achieve the more modest, and possibly realisable aim of enhancing the quality of the recovery environment for emergency services staff in the aftermath of trauma and critical events.

Current structure of the service

The key consideration that informs the continued provision of early intervention services for emergency services staff in Lincolnshire is that, although most personnel report having some acute stress reactions after a critical incident, they do not typically go on to develop PTSD. This is confirmed by more systematic studies, which suggest that the incidence of PTSD in emergency services personnel varies according to the nature of incidents to which they are exposed and the deployment procedures used (Clohessy and Ehlers, 1999; Alexander and Klein, 2001). The norm for populations of professional responders is to experience a measure of distress after major or disastrous events, and that through their own coping and adjustment strategies these reactions resolve in time without necessarily involving outside helpers. Given these considerations the LJESI has reformulated its aims. Rather than specifically preventing the development of PTSD its aims are to facilitate naturally occurring recovery processes for staff by influencing the quality of the recovery environment. A key objective in this regard is to implement the Initiative's educational strategy, which seeks to disseminate up-to-date information about post-incident staff care practices through conferences and awareness days. Thus, within emergency services there is no reason why staff support should not begin well before traumatic and critical incidents actually occur and evoke staff reactions that need to be addressed.

Conferences and awareness days

At 6-monthly intervals the LJESI offers two 'awareness days' to all personnel in the five contributing services. When held, attendance averages about 30 on each day. Initially, front line staff were targeted for attending these conferences, but since the recent review of the Initiative's operational practices, special efforts have been made to ensure delegates are selected from the ranks of supervisors and line managers. These personnel have responsibility for staff in the immediate aftermath of incidents, and are best placed to identify reactions and staff needs evoked by what has happened. During the conferences much emphasis is placed on facilitating group discussions about participants' own reactions to unusual work-related events so as to normalize these reactions and highlight which effective coping strategies can be used to mitigate these reactions. Consideration is also given to circumstances and factors that place particular individuals at risk of developing more enduring reactions (Alexander and Klein, 2001), and how to access help and support services, if these are required.

As part of the Initiative's educational strategy a booklet titled *Your Reactions to Extremely Stressful Events: coping and mastery* has been produced for general distribution to staff and used during training events. It describes common physical and somatic reactions to extreme stressors, as well as detailing psychological reactions that may be experienced in their aftermath. The booklet also describes self-help and coping strategies known to be commonly used by emergency services personnel. By listing the physiological arousal items of the Revised Impact of Events Scale (Weiss and Marmar, 1997), that have predictive validity for longer term adjustment difficulties, officers are invited to assess and monitor the nature and course of their reactions over time. Names and telephone numbers of LJESI contacts are also included in the information booklet.

Also for use both at conferences and other awareness raising events Lincolnshire Police has financed the production of a 15-minute video programme titled, 'A Duty of Care'. It describes the Initiative, the services it offers and features personal statements from those who, in the past, have accessed its provisions.

Post-incident support services

The previous protocol-driven PD early intervention provision has been abandoned in favour of flexible options for post-incident help and support. Each emergency service that participates in the LJESI has a designated 'in house' representative to whom front line incident managers or supervisors can turn for immediate advice and guidance about informed staff care provision if this is indicated. The underlying principle of the Initiative's provisions is that staff support should progress through stages of response. These range, in the first instance from reliance on officers' own coping and adjustment strategies through to an option for convening group meetings to discuss the impact of particular events, and even individual assessments for possible clinical interventions. These stages of response are described below and summarized in Table 20.1.

Table 20.1 Summary of current LJESI post-incident support services

Levels	Core process	Support for:
Level 1	Education	Line manager in making informed choices
Level 2	Individual assessment	Formal and informal investigations into endurance of after effects and intervention of choice, if any
Level 3	Group meeting	Social support from the work group, family or social network

Level 1: education and support for the line manager

This level of response is aimed at supporting managers or supervisors who are most directly accountable for making informed decisions about help for their front line colleagues. Front line managers' and supervisors' responsibilities are encompassed in 'duty of care' legislation, but effective implementation requires appropriate knowledge and access to information upon which to take action when psychological distress is evident. This is especially so in the aftermath of critical and traumatic events. Thus, it is essential to keep up the rolling programme of 'awareness days' not only to account for staff promotion and turnover, but also to provide continuing education for staff responsible for implementing policies. At Level 1, therefore, a typical response may be to ensure the information booklet titled *Your Reactions to Extreme Stress: coping with trauma* is made available to all staff involved in a particular incident. Details of the incident may be discussed with the designated 'in house' representative of the Initiative to ascertain what level of support is warranted. Advice may be offered to staff to informally share their thoughts and reactions evoked by the incident or it may be decided to do nothing other than monitor developments and formally review the impact of the incident after 1 week.

Level 2: individual risk assessment, both informal and formal

The focus of response at this level is to identify individuals who may be at risk for developing longer-term psychological distress. Trained emergency services officers, who expect to encounter traumatic events as part of their operational duties, are usually well placed to assess colleagues reactions. The booklet features a short list of questions that may be used to monitor hyper-vigilance and hyper-arousal reactions over time. Their persistence over time is a reliable predictor of continuing adjustment difficulties so the booklet offers advice about further formal and informal steps that may be taken to reduce risk. The former may be to seek a consultation with a family doctor who, in turn, may wish to make an onward clinical referral to a therapist. The latter more informal option would be to seek confidential help through the Initiative. It is emphasized to line managers that staff should be consulted about options for post-incident support and their agreement sought before taking further action. The key considerations at Level 2 are to ensure that staff are made aware of possible needs and choices at the point of service delivery, to encourage a culture of informed care, and provide useable and practical assistance according to identified need.

Level 3: group support

Within our own audit (Hutt, 1994) and elsewhere (e.g. Leavy, 1983) it has been noted that access to social support is especially important in helping individuals cope with psychological reactions after critical and traumatic events. Therefore, the Initiative considers situations may arise when a group meeting may be a useful component of staff support. They are referred to as 'Incident Review and Follow-up Meetings' (IReFs), and can be convened at the request of managers or front line staff. It is a specific point of policy not to make IReFs mandatory after all critical incidents, since this tends to imply treating emergency personnel as potential patients and pathologizes their reactions. Turning away from a 'pathologizing' model implies the recognition that emergency services staff typically cope well and adjust to work-related stressors. Thus, the Initiative has sought to embrace a 'wellness model' that emphasizes the salutary learning opportunities available to those involved in traumatic incidents (Dunning and Dunning, 1997).

Incident review and follow-up meetings (IReF) are called at the specific request of responder staff or their managers, and are not conducted within a specified period of time. Some have been held within weeks of an event, others after several months. Participation in IReFs is voluntary and meetings follow a semi-structured protocol that seeks to elicit comments about the meaning made of the event, fosters a positive perception of officers' incident response, and points to the appropriate coping and adjustment strategies used since its occurrence. Experience suggests it is essential to foster and build upon group cohesiveness to facilitate continued coping, and that a salutogenic framework is helpful for promoting this objective.

Reflections

Since the Initiative was established during the late 1980s experience suggests that emergency services staff are typically resilient to the effects of critical and traumatic events. Through training and 'hands on experience' they become competent in adjusting to emergency stressors inherent in their work. All the same it is necessary to acknowledge they are, more than most professions, at risk for developing PTSD and other debilitating adjustment difficulties. It should be noted that resilience is a complex phenomenon and does not necessarily rest exclusively upon the psychological strengths of an individual or the perceived nature of particular events (Rutter, 2000). Rather it is the result of interaction between event, individual and environmental characteristics. A prerequisite for informed early intervention policies and practices with emergency services organization is to acknowledge this inherent complexity. From this premise it is possible to approach the challenge of providing informed staff support in a flexible manner that incorporates the essential principle of consultation with possible service users.

References

Alexander, D.A. and Klein, S. (2001) Ambulance personnel and critical incidents. Impact of accident and emergency work on mental health and emotional well-being. *Br J Psychiat* **178**, 76–81.

American Psychiatric Association (1980) *Diagnostic and Statistical Manual of Mental Disorders III*. Washington DC: APA.

Avery, A. and Ørner, R. (1998) First report of psychological debriefing abandoned – the end of an era? *Traum Stresspoints (ISTSS)* **12**(3), 3–4.

Billings, A.G. and Moos, R.H. (1981) The role of coping responses and social resources in attenuating the stress of life events. *J Behav Med* **4**, 139–57.

Bisson, J.I. and Deahl, M.P. (1994) Psychological debriefing and prevention of post-traumatic stress. *Br J Psychiat* **165**, 717–20.

Clohessy, S. and Ehlers, A. (1999) PTSD symptoms, response to intrusive memories and coping in ambulance service workers. *Br J Clin Psychol* **38**, 251–65.

Cohen, S., Mermelstein, R., Kamarck, T. and Hoberman, H.M. (1985) Measuring the functional components of social support. In Sarason, I.G. and Sarason, B.R. (eds) *Social Support: theory, research and applications*. Lancaster: NATO Advanced Science Series.

Cohen, S. and Wills, T.A. (1985) Stress, social support and the buffering hypothesis. *Psycholog Bull* **98**, 310–57.

Derogatis, L.R. (1983) *The Symptom Checklist—90 Revised (SCL-90-R Manual II*. Towson: Clinical Psychometric Research.

Dunning, C.M. and Dunning, D.A. (29 June–3 July 1997) *Beyond Debriefing: a salutogenic model based on cognitive theory*. Paper presented at the 1997 Conference of the ESTSS, Maastricht, The Netherlands.

Dyregrov, A. (1989) Caring for helpers in disaster situations: psychological debriefing. *Disaster Manag* **2**, 25–30.

Figley, C.R. (1995) *Compassion Fatigue: coping with secondary traumatic stress disorder in those who treat the traumatised*. New York: Brunner-Mazel.

Horowitz, M., Wilner, N. and Alvarez, W. (1979) The impact of event scale: a measure of subjective stress. *Psychosom Med* **41**, 209–18.

Hutt, M.J. (1994) *Post Traumatic Stress and Debriefing in the Emergency Services*. Thesis for Doctor of Clinical Psychology, University of Sheffield.

Leavy, R.L. (1983) Social support and psychological disorder: a review. *J Comm Psychol* **11**, January, 3–21.

Mitchell, J.T. (1983) When disaster strikes … the critical incident debriefing process. *J Emerg Med Serv* **8**, 36–9.

Raphael, B., Meldrum, L. and McFarlane, A.C. (1995) Does debriefing after psychological trauma work? *Br Med J* **310**, 1479–80.

Rutter, M. (1985) Resilience in the face of adversity. *Br J Psychiat* **147**, 598–611.

Schwarzer, R. and Jerusalem, M. (1995) Optimistic self-beliefs as a resource factor in coping with stress. In Hobfoll, S.E. and de Vries, M.W. (eds) *Extreme Stress and Communities: impact and intervention*. Dordrecht: Kluwer.

Weiss, D.S. and Marmar, C.R. (1997) The impact of event scale-revised. In Wilson, J.P. and Keane, T.M. (eds) *Assessing Psychological Trauma and PTSD*, pp. 399–441. New York: Guilford Press.

21 Strategies for early intervention after trauma adopted by the Norwegian Armed Forces

Lars Mehlum

Introduction

Acute traumatic stress reactions, in the military typically referred to as 'combat stress reactions' (CSR) account for 20–30% of battle losses in modern warfare (Noy, 1991). Soldiers with CSR run a considerable risk of developing chronic post-traumatic stress disorder (PTSD; Solomon and Kleinhauz, 1996). In many nations, therefore, large groups of psychiatrically disabled war veterans are to be found (Kulka *et al.*, 1990; Ørner, 1992). In less severe cases, the clinical course of CSR ends in full or partial remission, although vulnerability to repeated trauma (Solomon *et al.*, 1987) or to emotional problems in later life may persist. These are some of the reasons why prevention of and early intervention in CSR have been given such a high priority in armed forces in many countries.

In the Norwegian Army, as in those of many other countries (COMEDS, 1999), intervention procedures follow the principles of the so-called 'forward combat psychiatry'. This is perhaps one of the most potent psychiatric treatment methods available for implementation. Most authors in this field claim it results in 80–90% recovery and subsequent resumption of combat ability within 72 hours. As shown in Chapter 1 by Weisæth, clinical experiences from past wars indicate that the forward psychiatry concept has clear advantages over available alternatives, such as routine evacuation of psychiatric casualties, which is characterized by a tendency to cause highly prevalent morbidity and long-term disability. For instance, a quasi-experimental study from the Israeli Defence Forces showed that the more front-line treatment principles were administered to soldiers, the more likely they were to return to their units and the less likely they were to have developed PTSD at 1 year follow-up (Solomon and Benbenishty, 1986).

To reduce the number of psychiatric casualties and minimize long-term damage to health are important objectives, not only to the individual and to the civil society. For military units there is, in addition, the crucial aspect of rapidly restoring a potentially resource demanding patient populations back to the operational duties and responsibilities of well-trained and fully functioning soldiers in active service. This helps conserve as much combat capacity as possible. It is basic considerations such as these and actual field experience that has furnished a rationale for the doctrine of combat psychiatry adopted by several NATO countries. In turn, this is reflected in the Norwegian concept of forward psychiatry and early intervention after trauma, which will be described in this chapter (Director General of Joint Medical Services 1987).

Risk factors for CSR

It is well documented that the more intense and prolonged the battle, or the higher the number of killed and wounded in action, the higher the rates of CSR are likely to be (Levav *et al.*, 1979; Noy, 1991). The common denominator for these observed phenomena is the threat of annihilation to which individual soldiers are exposed. Of all CSR predictive factors this is the strongest and most widely endorsed. An individual's capacity to deal with this threat depends on a number of internal and external resources. Paramount amongst these are quality of training, degree of combat readiness, strength and type of motivation for combat, level of unit cohesion and social support, trust in leadership and the availability of medical support.

However, even the best of all soldiers may eventually or under certain circumstances suffer depletion of internal coping resources. This reduces capacity to deal with basic threats of annihilation, and increases risks of becoming helpless, anxious and developing CSR. Furthermore, when a unit's social support disintegrates under the stress of combat soldiers will be much more vulnerable to the horrors of war. In many instances, a conflict emerges between the basic need for survival and higher order needs, such as compliance with demands of active duty and considerations of loyalty (Kardiner and Spiegel, 1947). Furthermore, the ever-increasing complexities of modern, high-tech and continuous battle operations place personnel under almost unimaginable and unrelenting physical and mental strain.

Frontline management of CSR

Management of CSR is conducted at the front but removed from areas of actual combat. It is based on the well-known principles of 'proximity, immediacy, expectancy and simplicity' (PIES) (Salmon, 1919; Artiss, 1963). It builds on the explicit assumption that CSR are reactions in which previously healthy personnel become overwhelmed by extremes of stress, which in turn severely reduces functional capacity. Intervention principles imply that:

- Symptoms must be recognized and dealt with as soon as possible.
- Whenever possible, interventions are administered by comrades or leaders within soldiers own units. Not only will commanding officers, comrades and forward medical personnel tend to be better informed about difficulties experienced at a particular front line position, but will also be more aware of resources and strengths possessed by individual soldiers and their unit. Experience shows that these peers are far more likely to return soldiers to normal operational duties than therapists who often work in remote locations where they may under-estimate the strength of social support available within active units and soldiers capacity to effect a recovery within this context (Noy, 1991).
- Soldiers should be removed from the area of most intensive battle. Rest, food, drink and facilities for washing and cleaning up should be provided.
- Soldiers should be helped to interpret their reactions as transient and normal in the light of the highly abnormal situation in which they have been. Suggestions of their having developed an illness or personal failure are actively avoided. Personnel should be given opportunities to talk about battle experiences in an atmosphere of support, acceptance, reassurance and positive expectancy. In this situation, compassion shown by other persons who also engender a sense of physical and psychological closeness exert influences that are regarded as more essential factors for recovery than resorting to the administration of specific therapeutic techniques.
- Psychoactive drugs are not used unless gross mental disturbances are present.
- If management has to take place outside the soldiers unit this should occur at a dedicated mental health unit (MHU; also referred to as a 'Combat stress unit') located as close to the scene of combat as possible.

Whenever evacuation is necessary, soldiers should return to their units to resume normal functions as soon as possible. Large-scale controlled studies conducted in Israel demonstrate the effectiveness of this principle (Noy *et al.*, 1986).

- All evacuated soldiers must walk away from the combat zone and carry their own equipment. They should not be carried, and as far as possible the role of soldier is to be maintained by all keeping their weapons and packets. Throughout they should be given adequate tasks that ensure they are kept in continued activity. This also helps avoid passivity, hopelessness and role diffusion.

- Soldier's contact with their battle units should be maintained if at all possible, and they should be given information about the fate of comrades and friends. Other messages that are important to convey are that they will be accepted back into their units, which expect their return plus reassurance that their performance in the battle was good enough.

- All methods used should be simple and easy to learn. Brief interventions are preferred.

These intervention principles are adopted in most NATO countries and a number of other armies of the world. How the CSR management is conducted behind the lines may, however, vary. In the Norwegian Armed Forces soldiers suffering from CSR are kept in their own units up to 48 hours. If not recovered within this time, they will be evacuated to light field hospital areas at the rear of each brigade (a brigade generally consists of about 5000 soldiers). Such action may also be necessary in more serious cases of CSR if the clinical picture is dominated by confusion, psychosis, depression/apathy or panic anxiety. MHUs are usually mobile, but have their base at light field hospitals, which run CSR recovery units. At these locations soldiers are retained for up to 72 hours observation, and early intervention is offered before decisions are made about a possible return to combat units or further evacuation. MHUs are headed by a psychiatrist and will be staffed by clinical psychologists and mental health nurses. The principal tasks of MHUs are to observe, diagnose and treat more serious CSR cases, to make decisions concerning evacuation of personnel and to advise other medical personnel and military leaders on matters relevant to staff management and good leadership practices.

Group interventions

Group cohesion is a crucial resource for those who have to cope with extremely stressful situations such as those that occur during combat. When an individual's natural defences are disrupted through threat, a state of internal emotional chaos may ensue. It is at such times that the small group becomes very important, not primarily as a place to communicate or integrate experiences, but as a place to re-establish order, trust and safety (Herlofsen, 1996). An aspect of this is to encourage soldiers to share their experiences and evoked emotions. This can happen both in groups and in one-to-one relationships.

Emotional abreaction or ventilation, cognitive processing of the traumatic material and social support are the three most important elements in such incident reviews. Of the three, it is only cognitive processing of traumatic experiences that is probably best taken care of in group meetings, rather than in a one-to-one relationship. In reality, military management of CSR emphasizes simple measures to be conducted in one-to-one relationship, and in the context of leader interventions, buddy-aid or spontaneous group abreaction. Group incident review meetings may serve several useful purposes other than to seek to counteract traumatic stress reactions. Particularly important aims are the promotion of a common understanding of what has happened so as to avoid cognitive distortions, misinterpretations and the formation of rumours. Learning and preparation for new challenges can be further aims of other early interventions, as are the tasks of strengthening group cohesion, improving communication, giving social and emotional support and facilitation of grief work.

Leaders' responsibilities

Management of CSR is based on self-help, buddy-aid and interventions from leaders or dedicated personnel from the MHU placed in forward positions. Due to the simplicity of the early interventions used their implementation can be delegated through appropriate training to all personnel groups so that it is not a prerogative of mental health workers only. It is however the responsibility of the line commanders to institute preventive measures that minimize risks of CSR as well as promote early recognition of its signs and symptoms plus initiate appropriate interventions and support. Leaders should seek to promote group cohesion and emphasize the importance for soldiers to stay together after experiencing traumatic events. They should also try to keep soldiers active, if appropriate continue training and preparing for combat, pass on adequate and honest information so as to counteract rumours, be caring and interested, and convey a sense of being in control of events. This will serve to strengthen confidence of junior ranks in officers who thus demonstrate important qualities of good leadership, which in turn has a preventive effect in respect of CSR. Control of stress is one of the responsibilities of commanding officers and at each echelon, unit leaders, medical personnel, chaplains, staff members and troops must be educated, trained through exercises, and supervised to maintain high standards in early intervention provision.

Education

Any nation's military defence system can be viewed as a very large disaster response organization characterized by an ability to maintain continuous, self-sustained military functionality and independent operational capacity. Whenever a national crisis occurs this resource is of paramount importance.

In keeping with this construction of national military organizations all its educational levels are primed and geared towards being prepared for crisis. The organizational setting is therefore very favourably disposed and accepting of knowledge about human behaviour under stress. In particular, it will seek to integrate evidence about psychological reactions to trauma with other types of knowledge that sustain operational readiness. As an example of this combat stress control and CSR management are subjects taught at all educational levels of the Norwegian Armed Forces. Naturally, course content is adjusted to take account of specific needs prevailing within each group (Director General of Joint Medical Service, 1987).

Lessons learned may soon be forgotten

History alerts us to a repeated tendency for lessons learned about management of CSR during a particular war to be forgotten before the next one (Artiss, 1963). What factors have contributed to the armed forces of our times continuing to act upon an awareness and knowledge base that is, in part, more than 50 years old to prevent combat stress reactions? In the case of Norway, particular importance appends to the challenges engendered by catastrophic events during peace-time and operations other than war.

Catastrophic events during peacetime

Armed forces are not exempt from involvement in disastrous events that occur during peacetime. Rather, their mode of operation presents risks to military personnel that are avoided by civilians.

Over the last decade or so several major events have occurred that directly implicated Norwegian military units. These have proved valuable object lessons for gaining new experience in providing early intervention services after trauma and were timely reminders of the usefulness of the historical knowledge base of the organization.

An investigation into the after-effects of a snow avalanche disaster that killed 55% of a Norwegian infantry platoon in 1986 confirmed the protective power of forward psychiatry models in preventing long-term post-traumatic stress disorders (Herlofsen, 1994). Early intervention strategies ensured surviving soldiers stayed together as a group the first few days after the disaster. During this time ample rest, warm clothes, food and social support were made available along with regular update information about matters relating to the disaster. Furthermore, survivors were encouraged to share their impressions, emotions and reactions. An early formal incident review and follow-up meeting was also held. All survivors were followed up on a number of occasions during the first 10 years after the disaster and, to date, none have developed PTSD (Herlofsen, 1994; P. Herlofsen, personal communication).

In retrospect, this incident and experiences gained during its aftermath clearly demonstrate how valuable unit cohesion is for military personnel and how much can be achieved through small group early interventions. Further crucial experience was gained in optimizing the efficiency of the consultative processes that must unfold between military leaders and the early intervention team mobilized to help with the situation.

Some military operations are carried out under extreme climatic, geographic and physical conditions involving use of dangerous equipment and weaponry. In Norway, this is the rule rather than an exception. Inevitably, accidents happen leading to situations that, in some instances, have their parallels in civilian disasters such as shipwrecks and avalanches (Eid *et al.*, 1995), environmental catastrophes (Weisæth, 1992) and when unexpected deaths occur due to homicide or suicide (Mehlum *et al.*, 2001). Taken together these serve as effective reminders for leaders and professional healthcare providers not to under-estimate the importance of having in place educational strategies and operational procedures that not only anticipate the psychosocial needs evoked by major incidents, but also address these in the wake of such events. Important resources that can be accessed during such situations are the Mental Health Units, which exist within military organization even in times of peace. These can serve as models for civilian providers, offer advice, facilitate developments and run training events about management of stress reactions evoked by traumatic events. A civilian-military interface is one of the ways of ensuring that evidence-based early intervention services are in place to give help and support following critical events, such as accidents, suicides and violent assault that involve one or two persons or families.

Operations other than war (OTW)

During the last half century the concept of 'peace-keeping' has gradually evolved through different painful experiences into a less pretentious, but no less ambitious concept of 'multinational military operations' under the flags of the United Nations and NATO. Not only has our understanding of the political problems inherent in multinational military operations increased, but fortunately so has also our awareness and understanding of the specific stresses endured by personnel engaged in such operations. It is now recognized that soldiers engaged in peace-keeping, peace-controlling or peace-enforcing operations often have more complex roles, and in some crucial respects difficult tasks to perform than those associated with traditional combat (Weisæth and Sund, 1982). Personnel on such missions will tend to be equipped for defence, whereas parties to be kept apart or be contained are usually better armed, are more numerous and are under less restrictive rules of engagement than the multinational force. Although often in less mortal danger than soldiers in regular combat peace-keepers may be exposed to numerous and seemingly irreconcilably difficult situations, humiliations and even occasional sudden attack. Such strains may evoke intense feelings of anger the mastery of which may be crucial for the overall course of a mission. Peacekeepers therefore have to suppress and control both their fight and flight impulses, as well as the basic behaviour associated with such reactions. Also to be contended with may be feelings of disillusionment and hopelessness that arise in conjunction with the bizarre political, human or ethical dilemmas that are a frequent feature of areas of unrest.

According to a number of studies there is an increased risk of PTSD in veterans from multinational missions other than war (Bache and Hommelgaard, 1994; Mehlum, 1995; Litz *et al.*, 1997). When 16,000 Norwegian peacekeeper veterans who had served with the UNIFIL force in South Lebanon between 1978 and 1991 were followed up at an average 6.6 years after demobilization, a PTSD prevalence rate of 5.2% was found (Mehlum and Weisæth, 2002). For the time period covered by the study the veteran population was also characterized by a significantly increased suicide rate compared with their same age and gender cohorts in the general population (Mehlum, 1995).

Many of the same predictors for PTSD that are known to apply in traditional warfare are also shared by OTW personnel. They include threats of annihilation, grotesque impressions, feeling helplessness or hopeless, frustration and loss of motivation (Bache and Hommelgaard, 1994; Stretch *et al.*, 1996; Mehlum and Weisæth, 2002). However, many protective factors, such as unit cohesion, confidence in the leadership and good morale are operative as well (Bache and Hommelgaard, 1994; Orsillo *et al.*, 1998, Litz *et al.*, 1997; Mehlum and Weisæth, 2002). All the same, some risk factors appear to be uniquely linked to OTW. In the Norwegian follow-up study post-traumatic stress reactions were predicted by reports of constant stress and tension, problems arising from not being able to act or retaliate in provoking situations or when witnessing atrocities in which innocent people were being hurt or killed, and associated feelings of meaninglessness (Mehlum and Weisæth, 2002).

Having documented increased risks of veterans from OTW developing PTSD the Norwegian Armed Forces adopted a series of preventive early intervention strategies. Improved personnel selection procedures, and expanded training and preparation for each mission are central to the new initiatives. So, in the pre-deployment period leaders are updated on combat stress management and on early intervention procedures. All personnel receive information about typical service-related stressors and the reactions that these can evoke, plus how to address these through self-help and buddy-aid. They are also made aware of where to get professional help when needed during and after their mission.

A dedicated stress management team, consisting of psychiatrists and psychologists, gives support to military units during deployment and provides follow-up services after mission closure. In respect of the latter, two risk groups are specifically targeted for routine follow-up. They are personnel who have been exposed to extraordinary critical events or severe traumatic stress, and those who were repatriated prematurely before the end of their 6 months service term because of severe emotional reactions, adjustment problems or disciplinary problems.

The four most common types of trauma in OTW settings seem to be threat to life, grotesque visual impressions (e.g. mass-graves, body handling), separation trauma (e.g. death of a comrade), and conflict or responsibility trauma (e.g. being responsible for decisions leading to disastrous consequences). Early interventions after trauma such as these are conducted locally and follow the PIES principles of forward psychiatry as described above. Leaders are thus expected to deal with critical incidents and consequent stress reactions as an integrated part of a mission. The same applies to ensuring information is passed back to base about which unit members have been most exposed to most severe trauma. This type of information is also acquired from each soldier through screening questions upon return to base after completion of missions. Our general experience, which has been more formally confirmed in a Danish study (Bache and Hommelgaaard, 1994), is that such service-related emotional reactions as will become manifest do so some months after home-coming. All personnel reporting severe traumatic exposure are therefore followed-up routinely by medical personnel. Contact is usually made by telephone 3–6 months after a mission and interviews are conducted to establish present adjustment, well being and health.

Repatriated personnel comprise the second group targeted for special follow-up. Immediately after return to military bases in Norway clinical evaluations take place to establish what further treatment or follow-up arrangements may be indicated. Traumatic stress reactions, clinical depression and suicide risk are some of the clinical presentations most frequently encountered with this group. There is often a need for crisis intervention measures, counselling and treatment under circumstances where repatriated personnel often harbour feelings of having failed, and are in need of support to be able to face their families, friends and colleagues at home. As far as is reasonable, this group of personnel will be followed-up through direct clinical consultations, telephone contacts and occasional home visits, especially during the first few weeks after repatriation.

Currently, all veterans included in these two early intervention after-care programmes have now been included in a follow-up study at approximately 3 years post deployment. Selected for examination are veterans' current mental health and well being, as well as their perception and degree of satisfaction with the various short-term support measures offered to date. The Norwegian Armed Forces have, so far, not accepted responsibility for providing long-term psychiatric treatment for veterans from international military operations who may need this level of care. It is therefore a matter of particular interest to establish the extent to which such treatment needs have not been formally detected or whether veterans find their problems have been adequately addressed within the general provisions of the Norwegian National Health Service.

Closing remarks

Experiences from a number of wars and peacetime operations have engendered a large body of evidence about short- and long-term consequences of traumatic stress in previously healthy individuals. Since war is such an unpleasant aspect of reality, however, politicians, professionals and members of the general public have, in the past, tended to 'forget' some of the essential lessons learned at times of conflict. However, in recent decades, Norway has been one of the leading nations seeking to protect and develop this very important knowledge. Most particularly, evidence relates to early intervention after trauma that is relevant not only for armed forces worldwide, but should also inform civilian research and practice in academic, clinical and policy-making organizations.

So, which are the essential points about early intervention after trauma that are now recognized within military settings, which these organizations should take particular note of? Most of all, it is to give credence to the capacity for self-healing evinced by most people and to place less emphasis on specific treatments provided by experts. In so doing, it is crucial never to forget or overlook the containing and supportive influences of social networks within which we do well, within reason, to help traumatized people maintain or resume their customary roles and functions. The earlier this can be effected, the greater the benefits are likely to be. Finally, it is also of the essence to try to give reassurance about early reactions evoked by trauma. This serves to enhance a person's self-acceptance and help develop tolerance for uncertainties inherent in awaiting natural developments over time.

References

Artiss, K.L. (1963) Human behaviour under stress: from combat to social psychiatry. *Mil Med* **128**, 1011–15.

Bache, M. and Hommelgaard, B. (1994) *Danske FN-soldater, Opplevelser og stressreaksjoner*. Copenhagen: Forsvarets Center for Lederskab.

COMEDS (1999) *Doctrine for the Management of Mental Conditions Generated by War and Operations Other Than War in Personnel in the Armed Forces*. Brussels: North Atlantic Treaty Organisation.

Director General of Joint Medical Services (1987) *Leadership. Mastering of Battle Reactions*, FSAN P-1–11. Head Quarters Defence Command Norway.

Eid, J., Johnsen, B.H., Lövstad, T. and Michelsen, L.T. (1995) Organisation of psychosocial support–experiences from two accidents in the Norwegian Armed Forces. *Tidssk Norske Laegeforen* **20**, 115: 959–61.

Herlofsen, P. (1994) Group reactions to trauma: an avalanche accident. In Ursano, R.J., McCaughey, B.G. and Fullerton, C.S. (eds) *Individual and Community Responses to Trauma and Disaster: the structure of human chaos*. Cambridge: Cambridge University Press.

Herlofsen, P. (1996) Group treatment in the aftermath of trauma. In Giller, E.L. and Weisath, L. (eds.) *Post-traumatic Stress Disorder*, Baillière's Clinical Psychiatry. International Practice and Research. Vol. 2, Number 2. London: Baillière Tindall, pp. 315–28.

Kardiner, A. and Spiegel, H. (1947) *War, stress and neurotic illness*. Hoeber, New York.

Kulka, R.A., Schlenger, W., Fairbank J., Hough, R., Jordan K., Marmar, C. and Weiss, D. (1990) *Trauma and the Vietnam War Generation: the findings from the National Vietnam Veterans Readjustment Study*. New York: Brunner/Mazel.

Levav, I., Greenfeld, H. and Baruch, E. (1979) Psychiatric combat reactions during the Yom Kippur war. *Am J Psychiat* **136**, 637–41.

Litz, B.T., Orsillo, S.M., Friedman, M., Ehlich, P. and Batres, A. (1997) Posttraumatic stress disorder associated with peacekeeping duty in Somalia for U.S. military personnel. *Am J Psychiat* **154**, 178–84.

Mehlum, L. (1995) Positive and negative consequences of serving in a UN peace-keeping mission. A follow-up study. *Int Rev Armed Forces Med Serv* **68**, 289–95.

Mehlum, L. and Schwebs, R.G. (2001) Suicide prevention in the military—recent experiences from the Norwegian Armed Forces. *Int Rev Armed Forces Med Serv* **74**, 71–4.

Mehlum, L. and Weisæth, L. (2002) Predictors of post-traumatic reactions in Norwegian UN peace-keepers seven years after service. *J Traum Stress* **15**, **1**, 17–26.

Noy, S. (1991) Combat stress reactions. In Gal, R. and Mangelsdorff, A.D. (eds) *Handbook of Military Psychology*. Chichester: J. Wiley & Sons Ltd, pp. 507–30.

Noy, S., Solomon, Z. and Benbenishti, R. (1986) The forward treatment of combat stress reactions: a test case in the 1982 conflict in Lebanon. In N.A. Milgram (ed.) *Stress and Coping in Time of War. Generalizations from the Israeli Experience*, Psychological Stress Series. New York: Brunner/Mazel Publishers.

Ørner, R. (1992) Post-traumatic stress disorders and European war veterans. *Br J Clin Psychol* **1**, 387–403.

Orsillo, S., Roemer, L., Litz, B.T., Ehlich, P. and Friedman, M.J. (1998) Psychiatric symptomatology associated with contemporary peace-keeping: an examination of post-mission functioning among peace-keepers of Somalia. *J Traum Stress* **11**, 611–25.

Salmon, T.W. (1919) The war neurosis and their lesson. *NY J Med* **59**, 993–4.

Solomon, Z. and Benbenishty, R. (1986) The role of proximity, immediacy and expectancy in frontline treatment of combat stress reaction among Israelis in the Lebanon War. *Am J Psychiat* **143**, 613–17.

Solomon, Z. and Kleinhauz, M. (1996) War-induced psychic trauma: an 18-year follow-up of Israeli veterans. *Am J Ortho Psychiatry* **66**, 152–60.

Solomon, Z., Mikulincer, M. and Jakob, B.R. (1987) Exposure to recurrent combat stress: combat stress reactions among Israeli soldiers in the Lebanon War. *Psycholog Med* **17**, 433–40.

Stretch, R.H., Marlowe, D.H., Wright, K.M., Bliese, P.D., Knudson, K.H. and Hoover, C.H. (1996) Post-traumatic Stress Disorder Symptoms among Gulf War Veterans. *Mil Med* **161**, 407–10.

Weisæth, L. and Sund, A. (1982) Psychiatric problems in UNIFIL and the UN soldiers stress syndrome. *Int Rev Army Navy Air Force Med Serv* **55**, 109–16.

Weisæth, L. (1992) Psychosocial reactions in Norway to nuclear fallout from the Chernobyl disaster. In Baarli, J. (ed.) *Proceedings from the Conference on Radiological and Radiation Protection Problems in Nordic Regions*, Tromsø 21–22 November 1991. Oslo: Nordic Society for Radiation Protection.

22 The role of hospitals in delivering early intervention services following traumatic events

Josef I. Ruzek and Matthew J. Cordova

Any attempt to reconstruct early psychological intervention services after traumatic events must include a consideration of how hospitals might provide this essential service. Many of the injuries for which patients seek hospital care result from events (e.g., assault, motor vehicle collisions, other accidents) that may be experienced as life threatening and may elicit significant emotional distress. Other medical stressors (e.g. life-threatening illness, myocardial infarction, burns, invasive procedures) may also exact a serious psychological toll. In short, hospitals are full of patients whose experiences can be conceptualized as psychological trauma, making this setting a vital 'capture site' for those at risk for a broad range of trauma-related psychosocial problems. In this chapter, we specifically focus on traumatic injury as an example of a traumatic medical stressor for which early intervention may be efficacious. We discuss the negative outcomes associated with traumatic injury, note limitations of psychosocial care in most emergency medical settings and propose a model of hospital-based early intervention services following traumatic events.

Negative sequelae of traumatic injury

Traumatic events commonly associated with injury may lead to a variety of negative psychological and behavioural outcomes. In general, high rates of PTSD (Talbert *et al.*, 1995) and depression (Shalev *et al.*, 1998) are found among trauma victims in emergency medical settings. PTSD is highly prevalent in survivors of general criminal assault (Brewin *et al.*, 1999), sexual assault (Rothbaum *et al.*, 1992; Resnick *et al.*, 1999), domestic violence (Astin *et al.*, 1993), accidental injury (Scotti *et al.*, 1995), motor vehicle accidents (MVA; Blanchard and Hickling, 1997), and sudden unexpected bereavement (Zisook *et al.*, 1998). Survivors of MVA and interpersonal violence also commonly experience other anxiety disorders, depression and substance abuse (Resnick *et al.*, 1993; Taylor and Koch, 1995). In addition, many individuals receiving injury-related medical care have psychological problems that predate their hospital visit (Whetsell *et al.*, 1989), including substance abuse and depression (Shalev *et al.*, 1998).

Trauma-related psychological symptoms are likely to have broad effects on ability to function post-trauma. Return to productive roles is not definitively predicted by severity of injury or physical disability, suggesting that psychological factors play a significant role (Holbrook *et al.*, 1994; MacKenzie *et al.*, 1998; Schnyder *et al.*, 1999). Indeed, psychological problems in the aftermath of traumatic injury have been related to functional impairments and diminished quality of life

(Landsman *et al.*, 1990). It is also important to note that trauma victims seen in emergency medical settings may be at risk for future re-traumatization (Sims *et al.*, 1989; Cobb *et al.*, 1992). Finally, traumatic events precipitating emergency medical care may also adversely affect social functioning of patients and their families (Solursh, 1990; Watkins *et al.*, 1996).

Limitations of existing services

Post-injury psychological care is limited in most emergency medical settings in the USA and other countries worldwide, although there may be more incentives to develop such services in countries with publicly-funded healthcare systems. In general, systematic screening for psychosocial problems is not standard practice thus limiting recognition of impaired patients (Whetsell *et al.*, 1989). For example, rates of identification and referral for substance abuse are low compared with prevalence rates (Lowenstein *et al.*, 1990). Opportunities are missed to identify and treat those at risk for later traumatic stress-related impairment (Green *et al.*, 1993). For instance, patients are not currently screened for acute stress disorder (ASD) and receive little information about the trajectory of emotional recovery. Physicians and nurses have little time to provide health education and, although they are a critical source of support their services are usually terminated upon hospital discharge. Psychiatric and social work support is provided to a small minority of patients, and is usually limited to acute care. Few hospitals offer trauma survivor support groups, leaving patients largely on their own once actual life threat has been averted.

Toward a model of psychosocial trauma care in the hospital setting

Many patients seen in hospital emergency medicine settings will develop PTSD, and other psychological and behavioural problems, with real impact on their ability to lead productive lives. In this context, what is required is a 'population-based' model of care. In such a model, all patients receive some level of psychological assessment and intervention, however brief, with the goals of prevention and matching level of care with level of need. While further research is needed to assess the utility of a population-based model, this approach is consistent with common sense, practical patient care.

Provision of population-based preventive psychological care places design constraints on these services. Such services must be *brief*, so that they can be delivered to large numbers of patients. Brevity is also warranted given that immediate post-trauma distress will remit naturally for many patients and may not require more than limited formal help (Blanchard *et al.*, 1995). Many brief interventions may need to be delivered by health care providers indigenous to hospital settings (e.g. nurses, physicians), rather than mental health specialists. Health care professionals provide much emotional support and advice, and their methods may be improved in ways that fit within existing roles. More intensive preventive services, delivered by specially-trained personnel, will need to be made available to patients based upon level of risk for continuing adjustment and coping difficulties. The financial and staffing constraints under which most hospital emergency departments operate will necessitate a staged, multi-modal approach. Below, we describe the key components of such a service, including screening, education, referral and outreach, and targeted treatment modules, and suggest clinical pathways for combining these elements of care.

Screening

Early identification of those at risk for negative outcomes following trauma can facilitate prevention, referral and treatment. Screening for current psychopathology and risk factors for future impairment can be accomplished via brief semi-structured interviews and standardized assessment questionnaires (see Brewin *et al.*, Chapter 12). For example, acute stress symptoms and disorder can be assessed via the Stanford Acute Stress Reaction Questionnaire (SASRQ, Cardeña *et al.*, 2000) or the Acute Stress Disorder Interview/Scale (Bryant *et al.*, 1998b, 2000). The Alcohol Use Disorders Identification Test (Saunders *et al.*, 1993; Cherpitel, 1998) can be used to screen for alcohol problems. Screening should also address past and current psychiatric and substance use problems and treatment, prior trauma exposure, pre-injury psychosocial stressors (Schnyder *et al.*, 2000) and existing social support. Event-related risk factors should also be assessed, including exposure to death, perception of life-threat and peri-traumatic dissociation. Especially important are acute levels of traumatic stress symptoms, which predict chronic problems; for example, more than three-quarters of MVA patients diagnosed with ASD will have chronic PTSD at 6 months post-trauma (Bryant and Harvey, 2000).

Patient education

Education for patients and their families may help normalize common reactions to trauma, improve coping, enhance self-care, facilitate recognition of significant problems, and increase knowledge of and access to services. First, patients should be reassured about common reactions to traumatic experiences, and advised regarding positive and problematic forms of coping with these. Information about social support and stress management is particularly important. Secondly, opportunities to discuss emotional concerns in individual, family or group meetings can enable patients to reflect on what has happened. Thirdly, patients may benefit from increased knowledge of health issues, including health care behaviour, medications and their side effects, pain management, wound care and relevant medical procedures. Fourthly, education regarding indicators of clinical impairment is vital; signs and symptoms of PTSD, anxiety, depression, substance use disorders, and other difficulties should be explained. Finally, patients will need information about financial, mental health, rehabilitation, legal and other services that may be available, as well as education about common obstacles to pursuing needed services (see below).

Referral and outreach

Emergency medical settings are in an excellent position to make referrals for appropriate follow-up services. Often, this opportunity is lost due to a number of obstacles. First, health care providers do little to assess patients' attitudes about actively seeking other forms of help than those that are routinely offered. Embarrassment, fear of stigmatization and cultural norms may all limit motivation to pursue a referral. Discussing these attitudes and employing motivational interviewing techniques (Rollnick *et al.*, 1992) may enable health care providers to increase rates of referral acceptance. Secondly, patients may not pursue a mental health referral early in the recovery process because they are coping with the practical problems caused by the experience, do not feel ready to face the trauma, do not recognize the need for services or are not yet experiencing significant impairment. Follow-up, re-screening and repeated referral may help ensure delivery of referral information at a time when patients may be better able to take advantage of it.

Brief problem-specific treatments

Relatively brief interventions targeting specific post-trauma problems may significantly improve outcomes of emergency medical treatment. Many problems (e.g., substance abuse, depression) are co-morbid with PTSD and may remit once PTSD is successfully treated (Foa *et al.*, 1995; Bryant *et al.*, 1998a). However, these problems may also occur independently of PTSD, suggesting that help and treatment targeting multiple problem areas is sometimes indicated.

It is a challenge to develop empirically supported brief interventions and systems of matching patient to preventive treatment (Bisson *et al.*, 2000; Raphael and Wilson, 2000). Research suggests that relatively brief hospital-based interventions may effectively prevent PTSD in some subgroups of trauma patients. Several controlled trials have suggested that brief (i.e. four or five sessions) cognitive behavioural treatments, comprised of education, breathing training/relaxation, imaginal and *in vivo* exposure, and cognitive restructuring, delivered within weeks of the traumatic event, can prevent PTSD in a number of survivors of sexual and non-sexual assault (Foa *et al.*, 1995) MVAs, and industrial accidents (Bryant *et al.*, 1998a, 1999). Studies have also demonstrated the utility of alcohol consultation and referral services for trauma centre patients (Chafetz *et al.*, 1962, Fuller *et al.*, 1995). Brief intervention with patients hospitalized for injury has been found to reduce alcohol consumption in those with existing alcohol problems (Gentilello *et al.*, 1999). Controlled trials of brief early intervention services targeted at other important trauma sequelae (e.g. problems returning to work, depression, family problems, trauma recidivism, bereavement-related problems) remain to be conducted.

Matching patient to level of care

Services will need to be delivered in a stepped form, whereby patients are matched to type and level of care, depending on initial distress and risk for developing chronic problems. Treatment matching is complicated by the fact that there are various clinical pathways through the emergency medical care setting. Some patients are treated in the emergency room (ER) and released within hours. Others are seen in the ER and admitted to an in-patient trauma ward for acute treatment and recovery. In either case, patients may or may not be followed up by a specialist or primary care physician as physical recovery proceeds. Given that each contact with the health care system affords an opportunity to screen for impairment and intervene appropriately, co-ordinating assessment, referral and treatment services across settings is a necessity.

For patients treated and released from the ER, brief services are essential. Such services should include screening for existing psychopathology and for risk factors for future impairment, education and provision of referral information. Depending on data collected during screening, targeted brief intervention for existing problems (e.g. alcohol abuse) may be delivered in the ER setting. Priming patients to follow-up on referrals may be accomplished via motivational interviewing and attempts to pre-empt avoidance of needed services. Obtaining detailed contact information may facilitate follow-up and outreach. For patients admitted to the in-patient trauma ward, there is an opportunity for more systematic assessment and for introduction of more comprehensive educational and intervention modules.

For both 'treat and release', and hospitalized patients, follow-up appointments represent opportunities for reassessment, referral and treatment. Therefore, communication among emergency care providers, specialists and primary care providers is imperative. ER and trauma ward providers can share concerns regarding existing problems and/or risk factors for future impairment with providers of follow-up care to facilitate continuity of assessment. During follow-up appointments it will be important to screen for PTSD and other anxiety disorders, depression, alcohol and substance abuse, problems with return to work and other productive roles, adherence to medication regimens and other appointments, and potential for re-traumatization. At this point, referral to appropriate treatment may be indicated.

System change

Traditionally, medical treatment and psychological services have been delivered separately, in different settings and by helpers of different disciplines. A rethinking of this institutional form of mind-body dualism is warranted (Strosahl, 1996). Furthermore, both medical and psychological services are characterized by a relatively limited focus on prevention, despite the obvious potential benefits. System change is necessary if population-based integrated, preventive trauma services are to be implemented.

Those developing early interventions should think ahead about the issue of system influence and dissemination. It will be important that interventions focusing on prevention of PTSD be designed in such a way that they can be easily integrated with services targeting other key problems encountered in the hospital setting. Furthermore, they should be developed in partnership with medical professionals and other members of multidisciplinary care teams. Collaborative design will be important if innovative services are to be adopted by the practitioners who must deliver them.

In order to shape development of evidence-based early intervention services in the hospital setting, a number of crucial issues must be investigated. First, more prospective studies following emergency medicine patients are required to better establish rates of a range of chronic trauma-related problems. Secondly, effective interventions must be developed to treat those problems. Thirdly, there must be a focus on the large number of patients with sub-threshold traumatic stress symptoms, many of whom experience significant impairment in occupational and social functioning. Fourthly, it is important to learn more about patients' primary concerns over the recovery trajectory and their openness to various potential services. Preliminary work suggests that the majority of injured patients value the opportunity to undergo a comprehensive psychosocial assessment during hospitalization, despite any inconvenience or distress caused by the process (Ruzek and Zatzick, 2000). Fifthly, it is vital to determine what hospital-based health care providers consider to be the important issues related to development and delivery of preventive psychosocial services.

Finally, it must be determined whether interventions delivered by clinical research teams in carefully controlled efficacy studies can be generalized to hospital settings. While such studies are necessary in developing early interventions, they will not establish the effectiveness of such services when they are delivered to the unselected population seeking care in busy, understaffed hospitals. For example, evaluations of early intervention should be developed that address the co-morbidity of problems encountered in the emergency medicine setting. Studies of prevention of PTSD that exclude substance abusers will be importantly limited in terms of their generalizability. Alcohol and substance abuse are highly prevalent among patients admitted to surgical trauma units (Soderstrom et al., 1997). Many patients requiring early intervention to prevent development of PTSD will have established patterns of substance abuse, so that early intervention services must tackle both sets of problems, in serial or integrated fashion.

Conclusions

Current evidence supports the following propositions:

- significant numbers of trauma survivors seek hospital medical services;
- many hospital patients will develop PTSD or other post-trauma problems;
- little systematic preventive care is delivered to these patients;
- it is possible to identify patients who are at risk for psychological problems.

Evidence, although limited, also supports the efficacy of early intervention in preventing PTSD, reducing alcohol consumption and increasing participation in substance abuse counselling. Studies are needed to investigate the role of early intervention in reducing other trauma-related difficulties.

Psychosocial trauma care in the hospital setting will need to be brief and largely capable of implementation by non-specialists. It will need to combine identification of patients at risk for PTSD and other problems, education of patient and family, delivery of brief interventions for trauma-related problems, referral and outreach. Research is necessary to design and evaluate these components of care. Methods of prevention of PTSD must be developed that are compatible with the need in hospitals to also intervene with other psychosocial problems, such as substance abuse, depression and problems with return to work, and that address the co-morbid nature of many post-trauma problems. Helping approaches must also be acceptable to patients and their families, which means that research investigating their needs and preferences will be important. Finally, if the prevailing cultures of hospital care are to be modified to include early intervention services for trauma survivors, it will be important that traumatic stress specialists form collaborative working relationships with emergency medicine practitioners sensitive to these issues.

References

Astin, M.C., Lawrence, K.J. and Foy, D. W. (1993) Posttraumatic stress disorder among battered women: risk and resiliency factors. *Violence Victims*, **8**, 17–28.

Bisson, J.I., McFarlane, A.C. and Rose, S. (2000) Psychological debriefing. In Foa, E.B., Keane, T.M. and Friedman, M.J. (eds) *Effective Treatments for PTSD*. New York: Guilford Press, pp. 39 59.

Blanchard, E.B. and Hickling, E.J. (1997) *After the Crash: assessment and treatment of motor vehicle accident survivors*. Washington D.C: American Psychological Association.

Blanchard, E.B., Hickling, E.J., Vollmer, A.J., Loos, W.R., Buckley, T.C. and Jaccard, J. (1995) Short-term follow-up of post-traumatic stress symptoms in motor vehicle accident victims. *Behav Res Ther* **33**, 369–77.

Brewin, C.R. Andrews, B., Rose, S. and Kirk, M. (1999) Acute stress disorder and posttraumatic stress disorder in victims of violent crime. *Am J Psychiat* **156**, 360–6.

Bryant, R.A. and Harvey, A.G. (2000) *Acute Stress Disorder: a handbook of theory, assessment and treatment*. Washington D.C: American Psychological Association.

Bryant, R.A., Harvey, A.G., Dang, S.T., Sackville, T. and Basten, C. (1998a) Treatment of acute stress disorder: a comparison of cognitive-behavioural therapy and supportive counseling. *J Consult Clin Psychol* **66**, 862–6.

Bryant, R.A., Harvey, A.G., Dang, S.T. and Sackville, T. (1998b) Assessing acute stress disorder: psychometric properties of a structured clinical interview. *Psycholog Assess* **10**, 215–20.

Bryant, R.A., Sackville, T., Dang, S.T., Moulds, M. and Guthrie, R. (1999) Treating acute stress disorder: an evaluation of cognitive behaviour therapy and supportive counseling techniques. *Am J Psychiat* **156**, 1780–6.

Bryant, R.A., Moulds, M.L. and Guthrie, R.M. (2000) Acute stress disorder scale: a self-report measure of acute stress disorder. *Psycholog Assess* **12**, 61–8.

Cardeña, E., Koopman, C., Classen, C., Waelde, L.C. and Spiegel, D. (2000) Psychometric properties of the Stanford Acute Stress Reaction Questionnaire (SASRQ): a valid and reliable measure of acute stress. *J Traum Stress* **13**, 719–34.

Chafetz, M.E., Blane, H.T., Abram, H.S., Golner, J.H., Lacy, E., McCourt, W.F., Clark, E. and Myers, W. (1962) Establishing treatment relations with alcoholics. *J Nerv Ment Dis* **134**, 395–409.

Cherpitel, C.J. (1998) Differences in performance of screening instruments for problem drinking among Blacks, Whites and Hispanics in an emergency room population. *J Stud Alc* **59**, 420–6.

Cobb, N., Maxwell, G. and Silverstein, P. (1992) 'Burn repeaters' and injury control. *J Burn Care Rehab* **13**, 382–7.

Foa, E.B., Hearst-Ikeda, D. and Perry, K.J. (1995) Evaluation of a brief cognitive-behavioural program for the prevention of chronic PTSD in recent assault victims. *J Consult Clin Psychol* **63**, 948–55.

Fuller, M.G., Diamond, D.L., Jordan, M.L. and Walters, M.C. (1995) The role of a substance abuse consultation team in a trauma center. *J Stud Alc* **56**, 267–71.

Gentilello, L.M., Rivara, F.P., Donovan, D.M., Jurkovich, G.J., Daranciang, E., Dunn, C.W., Villaveces, A., Copass, M. and Ries, R.R. (1999) Alcohol interventions in a trauma center as a means of reducing the risk of injury recurrence. *Annl Surg* **230**, 473–83.

Green, M.M., McFarlane, A.C., Hunter, C.E. and Griggs, W.M. (1993) Undiagnosed post-traumatic stress disorder following motor vehicle accidents. *Med J Austr* **159**, 529–34.

Holbrook, T.L., Hoyt, D.B. Anderson, J.P., Hollingsworth-Fridlund, P. and Shackford, S.R. (1994) Functional limitation after major trauma: a more sensitive assessment using the quality of well-being scale—the trauma recovery pilot project. *J Trauma* **36**, 74–8.

Landsman, I.S., Baum, C.G., Arnkoff, D.B., Craig, M.J., Lynch, I., Copes, W.S. and Champion, H.R. (1990) The psychosocial consequences of traumatic injury. *J Behav Med* **13**, 561–8.

Lowenstein, S.R., Weissberg, M.P. and Terry, D. (1990) Alcohol intoxication, injuries and dangerous behaviours – and the revolving emergency department door. *J Trauma* **30**, 1252–8.

MacKenzie, E.J., Morris, Jr, J.A., Jurkovich, G.J., Yasui, Y., Cushing, B.M., Burgess, A.R., deLateur, B.J., McAndrew, M.P. and Swiontkowski, M.F. (1998) Return to work following injury: the role of economic, social and job-related factors. *Am J Publ Hlth* **88**, 1630–7.

Raphael, B. and Wilson, J.P. (2000) *Psychological Debriefing: theory, practice and evidence.* Cambridge: Cambridge University Press.

Resnick, H.S., Kilpatrick, D.G., Dansky, B.S., Saunders, B.E. and Best, C. (1993) Prevalence of civilian trauma and post-traumatic stress disorder in a representative national sample of women. *J Consult Clin Psychol* **61**, 984–91.

Resnick, H., Acierno, R., Holmes, M., Kilpatrick, D.G. and Jager, N. (1999) Prevention of post-rape psychopathology: Preliminary findings of a controlled acute rape treatment study. *J Anx Disord* **13**, 359–70.

Rollnick, S., Heather, N. and Bell, A. (1992) Negotiating behaviour change in medical settings: the development of brief motivational interviewing. *J Ment Hlth*, **1**, 25–37.

Rothbaum, B.O., Foa, E.B., Riggs, D.S., Murdock, T. and Walsh, W. (1992) A prospective examination of post-traumatic stress disorder in rape victims. *J Traum Stress* **5**, 455–75.

Ruzek, J.I. and Zatzick, D.F. (2000) Ethical considerations in research participation among acutely injured trauma survivors: an empirical investigation. *Gen Hosp Psychiat* **22**, 27–36.

Saunders, J.B., Aasland, O.G., Babor, T.F., de la Puente, J.R. and Grant, M. (1993) Development of the Alcohol Use Disorders Screening Test (AUDIT): WHO collaborative project on early detection of persons with harmful alcohol consumption. II. Addiction **88**, 791–804.

Schnyder, U., Buchi, S., Morgeli, H., Sensky, T. and Klaghofer, R. (1999) Sense of coherence—a mediator between disability and handicap? *Psychother Psychosom* **68**, 102–10.

Schnyder, U., Morgeli, H., Nigg, C., Klaghofer, R., Renner, N., Trentz, O. and Buddeberg, C. (2000) Early psychological reactions to life-threatening injuries. *Crit Care Med* **28**, 86–92.

Scotti, J.R., Beach, B.K., Northrop, L.M.E., Rode, C.A. and Forsyth, J.P. (1995) The psychological impact of accidental injury: a conceptual model for clinicians and researchers. In Freedy, J.R. and Hobfoll, S.E. (eds) *Traumatic Stress: from theory to practice.* New York: Plenum Press, pp. 181–212.

Shalev, A.Y., Freedman, S., Peri, T., Brandes, D., Sahar, T., Orr, S.P. and Pitman, R.K. (1998) Prospective study of posttraumatic stress disorder and depression following trauma. *Am J Psychiat* **155**, 630–7.

Sims, D.W., Bivins, B.A., Obeid, F.N., Horst, H.M., Sorensen, V.J. and Fath, J.J. (1989) Urban trauma: a chronic recurrent disease. *J Trauma* **29**, 940–6.

Soderstrom, C.A., Smith, G.S., Dischinger, P.C., McDuff, D.R., Hebel, J.R., Gorelick, D.A., Kerns, T.J., Ho, S.M. and Read, K.M. (1997) Psychoactive substance abuse disorders among seriously injured trauma center patients. *J Am Med Ass* **277**, 1769–74.

Solursh, D.S. (1990) The family of the trauma victim. *Nurs Clin N Am* **25**, 155–62.

Strosahl, K. (1996) Mind and body primary mental healthcare: new model for integrated services. *Behav Hlthcare Tomorrow* **5**, 93–5.

Talbert, F.S., Wagner, P.J., Braswell, L.C. and Husein, S. (1995) Analysis of long-term stress reactions in emergency room patients: an initial study. *J Clin Psychol Med Sett* **2**, 133–48.

Taylor, S. and Koch, W.J. (1995) Anxiety disorders due to motor vehicle accidents: nature and treatment. *Clin Psychol Rev* **15**, 721–38.

Watkins, P.N., Cook, E.L., May, S.R., Still, J.M., Luterman, A. and Purvis, R.J. (1996) Postburn psychologic adaptation of family members of patients with burns. *J Burn Care Rehab* **17**, 78–92.

Whetsell, L.A., Patterson, C.M., Young, D.H. and Schiller, W.R. (1989) Preinjury psychopathology in trauma patients. *J Trauma* **29**, 1158–61.

Zisook, S., Chentsova-Dutton, Y. and Shuchter, S.R. (1998) PTSD following bereavement. *Annl Clin Psychiat* **10**, 157–63.

23 Training programmes for building competence in early intervention skills

Søren Buus Jensen and Nancy Baron

Introduction

Each disaster requires emergency response specifically for its survivors. Early interventions that seek to prevent or minimize psychosocial and mental health consequences of exposure to potentially traumatic events do so by promoting resilience and coping. This chapter offers a plan for training groups of helpers to integrate this perspective into early interventions following trauma. Three vignettes are used to exemplify the training processes and interventions that may follow from this new competency.

Vignettes: the events

A coach accident in Scandinavia

One dark and rainy evening a coach with 32 football fans was returning from a sports event and was hit by a car heading in the opposite direction. The coach slid off the road and tipped over. Although all the coach passengers were thrown out of their seats none, incurred serious injuries. However, three passengers in the car were killed instantly. Police and a crisis team from the local hospital emergency unit arrived on the scene within 10 minutes.

War in a Bosnian town

In the midst of war, a group of Bosnian mental health professionals attended a 2-day course on crisis intervention and disaster preparedness. Delegates complained their work was tiresome and they felt exhausted. Although no shelling of the town had taken place for 3 weeks, most of the helpers, their families and clients struggled with the ongoing psychosocial consequences of war. They lived with an unrelenting fear that the violence could start again at any time. Indeed, 2 days later a bomb killed a group of teenagers and injured others. The group of mental health professionals who joined the course hurried to assist survivors.

Abduction in a Sudanese refugee camp

Sudanese refugees have lived in camps inside Uganda for more than 17 years under constant threat from rebels. A community-based mental health programme trained paraprofessional refugee counsellors to assist in their own communities. One night a settlement was attacked and a group of 12 children abducted. From previous experiences, the refugees knew these boys would be forced to become child soldiers and the girls taken as 'wives' for the rebels. Community leaders tried to console the families of the abducted and called the counsellor for assistance.

Training early intervention skills

Our global media reports traumatic events daily. Although there is a need for research to prove effectiveness, the knowledge of how to provide mental health assistance to those involved has grown exponentially in recent years (Ursano *et al.*, 1996). It is already a significant task to integrate the existing new knowledge into daily best practice and into training programmes to build the competence of helpers in early intervention skills.

Implementing a training programme requires numerous dimensions. Consideration for who should be trained, what should be the content of the training and how do we ensure the quality, sustainability and continuity after the training is essential. Different resources in the 'developed', 'developing' and so-called 'countries in transition' define different possibilities. Essential is the level of sustainability and continuity of the competence achieved after the training. Therefore, each training programme from the beginning must build capacity to sustain helping efforts though the existing crisis and for future crises. This is effectively done through a 'cascading approach' (de Jong, 1995, 2002; Baron *et al.* 2002; Fairbanks *et al.*, 2002). In this approach, each trained group has its capacity raised to the point where it can train another group and multiple trained groups cascade together to provide comprehensive help. This is especially important due to the extensive needs for training in large-scale disasters.

Within this chapter, the design of training courses and curriculum are outlined through the use of three phases of early intervention.

Three phases of early intervention

Practical early interventions can be organized into three phases:

- Phase 1: Needs assessment leading to emergency response;
- Phase 2: Preventive brief interventions;
- Phase 3: Early clinical interventions.

The training curriculum is then adapted to the specific skills needed to provide assistance in each phase.

Phase 1: needs assessment leading to emergency response

It is essential to make a correct assessment of individual and group needs before initiating any intervention in any context. This can be done quickly and is crucial to ensuring that from the onset interventions address the actual needs of service users. To collect the needed information and create an immediate overview of the priorities, helpers compassionately interact with the survivors and offer emotional support as they collate the needed information. Based on the needs assessment, they co-ordinate the 'here and now' efforts, and begin to meet the practical needs of the current emergency. As this is happening, plans can be formulated to deliver other early intervention services at later phases of the crisis.

Phase 2: preventive brief interventions

The goals of preventive brief interventions are to minimize exacerbation of emotional and practical problems caused by crisis situations. Target populations served can be survivors and their families, witnesses, emergency workers and whole communities. These early interventions comprise of activities intended to be in place within days of completing an initial needs assessment and are provided once or over an extended time.

During these early brief interventions, participants are encouraged to openly share information, experiences and feelings evoked by the traumatic events. Early intervention activities seek to reduce or dissipate emotional distress, advise participants about how to cope emotionally and practically with crises, and promote resiliency through family and community support. During these early interventions, helpers try to identify survivors who are more deeply distressed and require onward referral for additional care.

Phase 3: early clinical interventions

Early clinical interventions target individuals, families or small groups in need of more specialized assistance than provided in the preventive brief interventions phase. They seek to address the needs of survivors who are extremely distressed or are so emotionally disorganized that they have been unable to return to normal functioning. Early clinical interventions help participants understand their reactions and promote adaptive coping strategies, in order to prevent escalation of adjustment difficulties into longstanding or chronic problems.

Whereas preventive brief interventions comprise of activities that seek to resolve distress and promote resiliency, early clinical interventions are like short-term counselling sessions with a 'here and now' focus on reactions evoked by the traumatic event.

Additionally, a small number of survivors may need more help than can be provided through these three levels of early intervention. Some may require long-term psychotherapy, especially if a recent event has revived memories and reactions to previous traumatic experiences.

In practice, these levels of early intervention may overlap, but the framework is useful for systematizing and planning. This framework is used to outline the main themes in the training curriculum to prepare helpers to intervene at each phase. These themes for training are then illustrated through the development of events in each of the three vignettes.

Who should be trained to provide early interventions?

In the vignettes the traumatic events occurred in three distinct cultural contexts, each characterized by significant differences in accessible economic and professional resources. It is therefore essential to begin by addressing the question of who should be trained when seeking to develop early intervention skills appropriate for a particular cultural context:

In 'Developed' countries

The first vignette of a traffic accident in a developed and peaceful country demonstrates how early intervention can be provided with the resources of a well functioning health care system staffed by sufficient numbers of trained professionals who can be mobilized at short notice. In developed countries, survivors and members of the general population expect local professionals to be available to address social, psychological, psychiatric and physical needs that arise after major events. In this context, all potential helpers including police, fire fighters, health professionals, psychiatrists, psychologists, social workers and other emergency volunteers need specialized training in mental health service.

In 'Countries in Transition'

A traumatic event in the midst of a war-affected 'country in transition' is described in the second vignette. Although some trained professionals are available to provide health, social, psychological and psychiatric care, the health care system is not prepared to handle the overwhelming consequences of war. In such situations, often only a few national professionals have specialized knowledge about how to assist communities with traumatic experiences. The target group for training in this context is similar to that of a developed country, but because of the severity and magnitude of the crisis these professionals can be complemented by local police, government officials, community and religious leaders, human rights workers and emergency volunteers. Expertise available within United Nations organizations and international non-governmental organizations (NGOs), soldiers or peacekeepers can also be used.

In 'Developing' countries

The third vignette is set in the context of a refugee camp in a developing country. Community and religious leaders, healers and families are expected to assist those in need by providing emotional and physical support, ritual and prayer. Only a small number of trained mental health professionals are available within most countries, and they typically provide services to the national population and are unavailable to refugees. In the developing countries, the target group for training is similar to that for countries in transition. One main difference is that the number of mental health professionals is often limited so the establishment of a trained paraprofessional team is helpful. Co-operative work with community elders, leaders and traditional healers is essential.

Training curriculum for Phase 1: building skills for needs assessment and emergency response

Training given to develop competence in needs assessment and emergency response encourages participants to take a pragmatic, common sense perspective on acute and early interventions after trauma. In the very early aftermath of an emergency, the imperative is to offer practical intervention at individual, family, group and community levels. Learning how to do a needs assessment is essential to all helpers, since the appropriate practical emergency response will differ as illustrated through the continuation of the vignettes.

Vignettes of Phase 1 interventions

The Scandinavian coach accident

A crisis team arrived to assess the situation and the police organized a simple shelter for survivors in which refreshments were served. Brief interviews were conducted with all coach passengers and its driver, while immediate needs were addressed. Special attention was given to anyone appearing physically hurt or severely affected emotionally. Relatives were contacted. The team addressed the whole group and expressed the hope that all would cope fine, but also explained that nightmares, flashbacks, and feelings of anxiety during coming days and nights might be anticipated as natural transitional reactions. They were advised that if these reactions persisted or interfered with daily functioning they could find help at a local psychiatric emergency unit. Details of a follow-up meeting to be held within a week of the accident were circulated. After a brief questions and discussion session all passengers decided to go home to their families and friends. Transport was organized. The team agreed to meet the next day for an operational review.

War in a Bosnian town

The blast was heard all over town. A social worker who lived near the site of the incident contacted members of her previous training group and within minutes they arrived at the scene to form a crisis team. They assessed the needs of survivors and ensured that the injured were transported to the medical emergency room. The team established a focal point for information and made themselves available the next day to offer assistance in a community mental health centre. They prepared a list of the families most directly affected by the attack and sought permission to contact them within a week for follow-up.

Abduction in a Sudanese refugee camp

The refugee counsellor visited all families whose children were abducted and discussed details of the incident, while also assessing the immediate needs of those involved. She educated them about normal psychological reactions they might expect from this traumatic event and established the extent to which support was available from family, elders, community leaders and healers. All were encouraged to seek help if needed. She explained where she could be contacted should they become overwhelmed by distress and promised a follow-up visit within a week. She asked to be informed should the abducted children return, and discussed the potential physical and emotional effects for returning children. Since all families lived in fear due to lack of safety in the camp, she met with officials to advocate improved security on their behalf.

Content of training

Each vignette illustrates different emergency interventions appropriate for the three different cultural and situational contexts. Some of the main skills to be included in a training curriculum to prepare helpers for appropriate emergency response are listed below.

Fostering good helper–survivor dialogues

Helpers are trained in key skills required to initiate brief, focused and comprehensive dialogues with survivors, which foster comfort and trust. These skills build on inherent helping abilities and natural compassion. From the start, helpers need to convey confidence to engender trust and show that they are responsible people able to provide immediate practical help.

Knowing how to share information

Helpers are taught practical methods for collecting and expediently passing on important information including details of the available sources of further help.

Coordination skills

Trainees are taught how to establish a comprehensive action plan and a structured scheme for its co-ordination so as to decrease fears and misunderstandings among survivors, relatives and the public.

Meeting survival needs

Techniques for assessing and problem solving basic survival needs are taught.

Upholding human rights

Helpers are familiarized with basic principles of human rights and to identify human rights violations. They learn when and where to advocate on behalf of survivors, register formal complaints and ask for specialist human rights assistance (Jensen, 1998).

Mental health education

Training is provided to promote understanding of normal reactions to abnormal situations and how to educate survivors about these to minimize fears evoked by their occurrence. Helpers are taught techniques that identify those in need of immediate care or onward referral. They are taught to encourage survivors to ask for support from their families or social networks, health care systems, religious organizations or other natural sources of help.

Follow-up to explore latent problems or needs

Helpers learn that some people appear untroubled immediately after the traumatic event only to require assistance at a later date. They learn follow-up skills to prepare them to contact people days, weeks or months after an event in a respectful way, honouring privacy and offering help only if needed.

Taking care of caretakers

Helpers are trained to recognize risks and signs of vicarious traumatization, and are made aware of the imperative of establishing appropriate self-support provision and supervision (Saakvitne and Pearlman, 1996; Jensen, 1996; Friedman *et al.* 2002). Information is also given about where they can get specialist help if required.

The training curriculum for Phase 2: preventive brief interventions

Preventive brief interventions go beyond the needs assessment and emergency response to introduce help for individuals, families, groups and communities. Examples of such interventions are given in the following vignettes.

Vignettes of Phase 2 interventions

A Scandinavian coach accident

A follow-up meeting was held for some of the survivors a few days after the accident. Such incident review meetings for survivors and their families foster discussion, exchange of information, processing of experiences and feelings, plus problem resolution. For many, these early interventions will be sufficient to close the experience so that normal routines can be re-established. Those requiring more intensive help can also be identified.

War in a Bosnian town

A few days after the bombing a memorial service was organized to mourn its victims. Such community events and collective rituals may have a strong personal impact due to allowing the survivors' pain and suffering to be symbolically communally recognized and shared.

Abduction in a Sudanese refugee camp

Meetings with the extended families of abducted children were held in the family's homes the day after the incident. The family members shared their fears and actual knowledge about the situation with each other and the counsellor. Time was given to mourn their loss, share hopes and mobilize coping resources.

Content of Phase 2 training

Training for Phase 2 early interventions concentrates on skills needed by helpers to assist survivors to process traumatic experiences and provide support, reassurance and problem resolution caused by or exacerbated by the 'here and now' situation. Trainees also learn to identify signs, symptoms and reactions for people requiring referral and more intensive follow-up. The more therapeutic the aim of these early interventions the more important it is for providers to be trained in mental health work. However, adequate skills for Phase 1 and 2 can be taught to all selected helper groups as follows:

Crisis response in Phase 2

Helpers learn skills for immediate crisis response including how to assess, respond and refer people at risk of suicide, homicide or mental decompensation. They are taught to take a 'here and now' practical focus and to choose the most relevant target group for intervention: individual, family, group or community.

Basic counselling skills

Basic counselling skills of listening, support, attending and questioning are taught, together with problem-solving and group facilitation skills. Much emphasis is placed on learning how to structure the immediate emotional chaos evoked by disasters and assist survivors in creating a comprehensive narrative of events (Jensen, 2001). To avoid unnecessary pathologizing, more is taught about normal versus abnormal responses to traumatic events, and about how to promote natural coping and foster resiliency.

Taking care of the caretakers

Helpers are made aware of the importance of attending to their own needs, feelings and stress reactions evoked by listening to survivors repeated narratives or by being a participant observer of unfolding events.

Networking

Training is given in how to mobilize natural helping systems available to survivors with particular emphasis being placed on actively encouraging the organization of collective healing rituals.

The training curriculum for Phase 3: clinical interventions

After trauma, most survivors cope by drawing on personal resilience and support available through their immediate family or social networks. Early intervention may therefore be limited to providing some support to those in immediate need, distributing relevant information or practical problem-solving, and the interventions offered in Phases 1 and 2. Only small numbers of survivors are likely to need Phase 3 early interventions in the form of clinical interventions to promote healing (Baron *et al.*, 2002).

Vignettes with Phase 3 interventions

The Scandinavian coach accident

The coach driver developed nightmares and became afraid of sleeping, since he would relive the accident in dreams that woke him up in an anxious state. He was unable to return to work due to flashbacks and anxiety attacks evoked by thoughts of once again driving a coach.

Preventive brief interventions proved insufficient to resolve these reactions, so a referral to a psychiatrist trained in the treatment of trauma survivors was arranged. A clinical management plan involving individual short-term psychotherapy combined with medication was implemented.

War in a Bosnian town

Some of the surviving teenage girls developed fainting spells, which intensified after they participated in the community mourning rituals. In response, a psychologist set up a support group for these teenage girls that met once a week for 10 sessions.

Abduction in a Sudanese refugee camp

The father of one of the abducted children started drinking to excess and was abusive to members of his family. He had previously participated in a preventive brief intervention in which the extended family discussed the abduction, but symptoms persisted. The counsellor made regular visits to the man and his family to encourage him to recognize his drinking problem, while offering protection and support to other members of this family.

Content of Phase 3 training

Professionals with expertise in mental health work are obvious candidates for training in early clinical interventions, since these draw upon the same skills and knowledge used in general mental health counselling and therapy. Special elements in the training curriculum for Phase 3 are outlined below.

Clinical skills

A variety of clinical skills can be taught ranging from conducting critical incident stress debriefing meetings (Mitchell and Everly, 1995), short-term crisis intervention and therapeutic approaches that focus on the subjective meanings of the present trauma as rooted in past formative life experiences.

Helpers are also trained in techniques of narrative therapy. This technique seeks to bring order to chaos by assisting survivors to reconstruct their immediate trauma story. Examples include the testimony method developed for individuals, families and groups (Cienfuegos and Monelli, 1983) or family-orientated narrative methods (White and Epson, 1990).

Special training in the use of EMDR (Shapiro, 1995) and related techniques are offered if special situations call for it. Use of body-orientated therapies are advocated only if therapists have previously acquired skills and experience (Levine, 1997).

Helpers are also made aware of the importance of self-care and supervision as means of minimizing risks of vicarious traumatization.

Some ways forward

To ensure continuity of high quality interventions, training programmes need to formally establish systems of evaluation that collate data about the success of training, acquisition of skills and resulting interventions (Jensen, 1998; Baron, 2002). Furthermore, supervision and follow-up of trainees is essential to building competence, since it is a rare situation in which someone learns the skills for needs assessment, brief preventive or clinical interventions in one easy lesson.

It is essential that training programmes achieve sustainability and continuity of high quality intervention after the training. The 'cascading approach' is recommended. This involves each trained group developing its resources and skills so that it can train and supervise other groups, thereby 'cascading' their competencies into the broader community.

Throughout this chapter, we have described the training needed to prepare helpers to carry out early interventions with a psychosocial and mental health focus. We have identified groups of potential trainees in different world contexts and outlined main elements in the content of training. In the practical world, these variations have to be translated into pragmatic training courses, which will target the specific group of trainees in their specific context. All courses crossing cultures and contexts will then prepare helpers to effectively deliver relevant interventions to minimize mental health suffering in the short and long term to any number of survivor groups, whatever the crisis situation.

References

Baron, N. (2002) Community based psychosocial and mental health services for southern Sudanese refugees in long-term exile in Uganda. In de Jong, J.T.V.M. (ed.) *War and Violence: public mental health in a socio-cultural context*. New York: Plenum Press (in press).

Baron, N., Jensen, S.B. and de Jong, J.T.V.M. (2002) Mental health of refugees and internally displaced people. In Fairbanks, J., Friedman, M., de Jong, J., Green, B. and Solomon, S. (eds) *Guidelines for Psychosocial Policy and Practice in Social and Humanitarian Crises: report to the United Nations*. New York: UN (in press).

Cienfuegos, J. and Monelli C. (1983) The testimony of political repression as a therapeutic instrument. *Am J Orthopsychiat* **53**, 43–51.

de Jong, J.V.T.M. (1995) Prevention of the consequences of man-made or natural disaster at the (inter) national, the community, the family and the individual level. In Hobfol, S.E. and de Vries, M.W. (eds) *Extreme Stress and Communities: impact and intervention*. Dordrecht: Kluwer Academic Publishers, pp. 207–28.

de Jong, J.V.T.M. (ed.) (2002) *War and Violence: public mental health in a socio-cultural context*. New York: Plenum Press.

Fairbanks, J.A., Friedman, M.J., de Jong, J.V.T.M., Green, B.L. and Solomon, S. (2002) Intervention strategies for populations, families and individuals exposed to traumatic stressors. In Fairbanks, J., Friedman, M., de Jong, J., Green, B. and Solomon, S. (eds) *Guidelines for Psychosocial Policy and Practice in Social and Humanitarian Crises: report to the United Nations*. New York: UN (in press).

Friedman, M., Warfe, P.G. and Mwiti, G.K. (2002) Mission-related stressors and their consequences among UN peacekeepers and civilian field personnel. In Fairbanks, J., Friedman, M., de Jong, J., Green, B. and Solomon, S. (eds) *Guidelines for Psychosocial Policy and Practice in Social and Humanitarian Crises: report to the United Nations*. New York: UN (in press).

Jensen, S.B. (1996) Mental health under war conditions during the 1991–1995 war in the former Yugoslavia. *Wld Hlth Statist Q* **49**, 213–17.

Jensen, S.B. (1998) *Psychosocial and Traumatic Stress: understanding, prevention and treatment. A Who Model Training Project on Mental Health in the Former Yugoslav Republic of Macedonia 1997–1998*. Copenhagen: WHO/EURO Report.

Jensen, S.B. (2001) Frontlines of mental health under war conditions. In Taipale. I. (ed.) *War and Health. A Reader*. London: Zed Books.

Levine, P. (1997) *Waking the Tiger—Healing Trauma*. California: North Atlantic Books.

Mitchell, J.T. and Everly, G.S. (1995) Critical incident stress debriefing (CISD) and the prevention of work related traumatic stress among high risk occupational groups. In Everly, G.S. and Lating, J.M. (eds) *Psychotraumatology: key papers and core concepts in post traumatic stress*. New York: Plenum Press, pp. 267–80.

Saakvitne, K.W. and Pearlman, L.A. (1996) *Transforming the Pain. A Workbook on Vicarious Traumatization*. New York: W. W. Norton and Co.

Shapiro, F. (1995) *Eye Movement Desensitization and Reprocessing: basic principles, protocols and procedures*. New York: Guilford Press.

Ursano, R.J., Grieger T.A. and McCarrol J.E. (1996) Prevention of posttraumatic stress. consultation, training and early treatment. In van der Kolk, B.A., MacFarlane, A.C. and Weisaeth, L. (eds) *Traumatic Stress. The Effects of Overwhelming Experience on Mind, Body and Society*. New York: Guilford Press, pp. 441–62.

White, M. and Epson D. (1990) *Narrative Means to Therapeutic Ends*. New York: Norton.

Section 5 Early intervention reconstructed

Looking back on all contributions made by a distinguished panel of expert chapter authors, it becomes apparent that everyone has added new pieces to a complex jigsaw of interconnected considerations about early intervention. With these in mind, readers will have been disabused of any notion that routine provision of mandatory 'one-off' group meetings is sufficient to address survivors' immediate psychological needs and prevent long-term adjustment difficulties.

Our concluding chapter seeks to put the pieces of the jigsaw together and define their relationship to one another. It details developments within psychotraumatology that have made a reconstruction of early intervention possible. New guidelines for informed practice mark, in several instances, a radical departure from past conventions. Confidence springs from the fact service innovations are rooted in evidence published and discussed in the public domain. As revealed in this book, evidence has not restricted or inhibited developments. Rather, it has inspired many practitioners to test their veracity in applied programmes of care for a range of disparate survivor populations exposed to many different types of traumas. Some of these may be single events, but others involve sequences of adversities spanning extended periods of time.

Reconstructed early intervention confronts the complexities of making comprehensive provision for trauma survivors. As a direct consequence of this, the concluding chapter is longer than all the others featured in this book. Readers may therefore welcome some guidance on how this section is structured so as to facilitate an integration of its many details.

The first part offers a brief and focused summary of each preceding chapter and relates its key points to the process of reconstructing early intervention. Not only does this lay a new foundation for informed practice in relevant and correctly applied theory, but it also incorporates evidence derived from systematic research and evaluation. Although the complexities of the emergent information base are undeniable, it is equally revealing to find the conglomerate of details are so organized as to comprise a cohesive whole. It is against this knowledge base that practitioners can establish the status of reconstructed early interventions that they intend to deliver and researchers may generate proposals for systematic evaluations to further develop this specialist field.

The second part of the concluding chapter moves beyond the details referred to above. It lists the main principles of practice that are, in effect, the benchmarks for reconstructed early intervention. That is, the text highlights some of the recurrent practical themes that emerge from an examination of recent experience of providing evidence-based early intervention. The significance of these themes is that they define service characteristics that are useful for assessing standards of current and future practice in this field.

The concluding chapter ends with a number of speculations about future directions for recon-structed early intervention. It also makes the point that credit conferred on this field of modern psychotraumatology by its capacity to radically review its practices will be further enhanced if it inspires other specialisms to do the same.

To retain a comprehensive overview of all matters raised in the two concluding chapters refer-ences are listed at the end of this section.

24 Progress made towards reconstructing early intervention after trauma: emergent themes

R.J. Ørner and U. Schnyder

Introductory remarks

Coincidence has it that the first paragraphs of the concluding chapters are being written during the weeks after the tumultuous upheavals of September 11 2001. Millions are in shock and fearful for their futures. Hardly anyone is likely to emerge unchanged from what is happening but the evidence supports optimism about most of those so affected making positive adaptations to unfolding events without accessing professional help. In this time of crisis a realization has dawned this is a special opportunity for developing some empathy for the predicament of survivors of a vast range of personal trauma.

Given the complexities of early post-trauma reactions, scant purpose is served by embarking on psychosocial interventions requiring high levels of abstraction. Simple help and support is called for. Little else will be appreciated or welcomed. So, voices are being heard calling for restraint, whilst pleading for letting more time pass lest further action proves precipitate.

At a moment of widely felt despair this book presents remarkable accounts of the many options that exist for providing help and support for survivors of recent traumas. Chapter authors set the stage for healing, reconstruction and reconciliation to commence. A more poignant time for reflecting on the current status of early intervention after trauma can hardly be imagined. For instance, recent events and reflections arising from a new world order lend strength to the conviction that early intervention is an imperative relevant to the lives of virtually all people. Appropriate provision is therefore an important humanitarian challenge and for those actively engaged in providing help and support this book is a manifesto of optimism. Early intervention marks the point where hope confronts survivors' despair. If only for this reason, responsibilities of providing appropriate and effective early intervention are of such magnitude they can no longer be championed or justified by subjective impressions or speculations about survivors' needs. To this end, therefore, chapter authors have laid new foundation for beginning the process of reconstructing early intervention after trauma. Through their contributions it is now, maybe for the first time, possible to root practice in theory and refer to a body of scientific evidence.

The book heralds a new era for this specialist field of survivor care. It also raises seminal questions with implications extending far beyond those of early intervention after trauma. For instance, how sound are the presumptions that inform diagnoses used for initial reactions evoked by trauma? To what extent are elicited signs and symptoms products of organic or environmental influences? How do evoked processes interact and what influence is exerted by either in effecting recovery?

Are some traumas so intense their impact cannot be reversed? Given the impact exerted by external events on neurobiological processes is it possible for healing and recovery to be effected by making planned changes in survivors' social and interpersonal environments? At an even broader level of generality, it is reasonable to speculate about the relevance of these same questions for functional disorders, such as depression, anxiety and panic reactions. In truth, these considerations touch upon the most basic assumptions on which psychiatric and psychological therapies are founded.

The evidence outlined in this book recommends itself for being pragmatic, practice based and unfettered by orthodoxy. It questions our most basic assumptions and offers radically different, but mainly complementary perspectives helpful for the process of reconstructing early intervention after trauma. In so doing, the book embodies several statements of basic principle that can inform future provision. Most important of these is the recognition that evidence-based practice is not an impediment to innovation. In fact, it confers on practitioners and researchers alike an unprecedented measure of informed freedom to think and act imaginatively in the interest of recent trauma survivors.

The relevance of history and theory

As explained by Weisæth in the introductory section, early intervention is not a recent innovation. It has a long legacy within military forces of many countries that have been mobilized for combat. Repeatedly and with predictable regularity the tangible consequences of psychological and psychosomatic reactions included impaired ability of soldiers to fight and win battles. Since psychological casualty rates are linked to the numbers killed and wounded there is a clear military imperative to minimize this particular type of attrition of the fighting force.

Reflecting cyclical changes in the preoccupations of senior military officers, early intervention has, at times, been viewed as a superfluous and unnecessary luxury for soldiers lacking in courage and moral fibre. According to this perspective, problems of psychological attrition in the battlefield could be eliminated by appropriate selection, training and competent leadership. Explanations for combat stress reactions (CSR) invoked notions of secondary gain and from this premise emerged cruel practices to change behavioural contingencies to favour a return to the front lines. Reflection on this phase of medical history engenders an impression of interventions that were, above all else, a product of the prevailing climate of violence. In this manifestation, early intervention seems to have achieved the singular feat of replicating core components of precipitating trauma, rather than soothe their effects.

History confirms that early intervention after trauma has typically sought to offer practical help in support of crucial operational imperatives. However, steps taken to care for traumatized soldiers were not informed by clinical theories about the nature of reactions to wartime trauma. Political and military expedience prevailed with the result that scant attention was paid to collating evidence against which theories could be tested and treatment effects documented. Not only do these procedural shortcomings help explain the proliferation of implausible intervention strategies, but they also carry a crucial message about the extent to which our views of acute stress reactions may be socially constructed, shaped by circumstance and time bound. The same may also be true for aims and objectives advocated for early intervention. Weisæth cautions against assuming future generations will not pass similar critical judgements on current practices.

However, significant lessons have been learned about how to minimize risks of doing harm. The best insurance comes from taking steps to ensure current practice derives from sound theory and collating data to gauge outcomes associated with early intervention. Practitioners should also be receptive to revising practice in the light of new evidence. It is therefore particularly helpful that Weisæth describes a model approach to quality assurance for military authorities based on an international infrastructure for pooling expertise, fostering co-operation and encouraging research. This has not resulted in uniform practices within participating armed services, but allegiance is owed to the principle of provision being subject to peer review. In this way, modern practice adheres to an explicit agenda of building upon lessons learned during past conflicts, linking current practice to relevant theoretical advances in medical and social sciences, and tailoring future provision to the demands inherent in new operational assignments, such as peacekeeping, emergency or disaster response. An example of generative power unleashed by this systematic approach is described in Mehlum's later chapter about services available to Norwegian military personnel.

With these considerations in mind it is informative to speculate about the extent to which developments of early intervention in non-military settings have been subject to similar impediments to informed progress. A key impetus for recent innovations came from claims made in 1983 about Critical Incident Stress Debriefing (CISD; Mitchell, 1983). Its beginnings were inauspicious because assurances were given this intervention protocol had roots in sound theory and research. CISD was pioneered as a one-off intervention for groups or individuals recently exposed to a critical or traumatic event, the rationales for which derived from crisis theory. Its aims were to normalize reactions evoked by the event, prevent onset of post-traumatic stress symptoms, foster group cohesion, identify individuals requiring further help, and engender a more complete or accurate narrative of what happened. Those being debriefed should have been guided through a phased agenda involving sharing thoughts, impressions and emotions evoked by the event, as well as reactions experienced in its aftermath.

Subsequent events suggest initial optimism about the veracity of this advocated practice was unfounded. There are clearly lessons to be learned from the above that should inform the current process of starting to reconstruct early intervention. Most especially about the importance of not championing idiosyncratic service innovations before their effectiveness has been proven, however pressing the need for effective intervention may be.

Gersons has shown how informative it is to consider if claimed links between crisis theory and the CISD protocol stand up to critical examination. He traces the roots of crisis theory and crisis intervention to Cannon (1932) and Selye (1956) who described the human body's dynamic capacity to maintain a steady state homeostatic equilibrium when confronted with environmental change. Later elaborations proved adjustments are evoked as much by changes in a person's social and interpersonal situation as by changes in physical environment. Taking Caplan's (1964, 1981) definition of 'stress' as a state other than equilibrium Gersons points out that, if this state is recognized at an early stage, prompt intervention should at least in theory prevent onset of physical and psychological complications associated with chronic homeostatic disequilibrium.

Based on clinical observations Lindeman (1944), and Klein and Lindemann (1961) put forward a model of crisis as a temporary process (not a state) lasting days or weeks. Symptoms engendered during crises are construed as being specifically related to the provoking and ongoing situation. Help delivered by individuals comprising the social network of those affected may be sufficient to exert a remedial influence on the processes in question. In support of this crisis intervention perspective Caplan and Kililea (1976) emphasized the healing power of mutual aid within committed groups.

To account for the therapeutic impact of crisis intervention Lindeman (1944) pointed to the restorative impact of practical actions that alter the balance of forces exerted by groups upon some of its individual members. Signs and symptoms of disequilibrium, whether expressed as a process or a state, can be reduced or minimized by interventions that help restore a healthier balance of forces in social orbits, redistribute role relationships within a group, or repopulate a person's social space. Over time, these rather abstract formulations have gained prominence as powerful rationales for crisis therapy interventions. This is so not only in family or systemic therapies, but also in other situations where patients present with recurrent or enduring psychiatric disorders (Schnyder, 1997; Datillio and Freeman, 2000).

Lindeman (1944) also claimed therapeutic effects derive from brief catharsis as previously proposed by Freud and Breuer (1893) for other patient groups. His rationale was that 'unfreezing' neurotic states engendered crisis processes that promote healing, through which healthy resolutions are achieved and homeostatic equilibrium is re-established. These ideas have survived into the present in the form of admonitions about the importance of developing comprehensive trauma narratives.

A further characteristic of the crisis process is its phased nature. Tyhurst (1957) distinguished three different phases that mediate 'transitional' states. During the *impact* phase the body is almost totally focused on the immediate here and now, whilst resources are mobilized to face dangers or threats. This is followed by a *recoil* phase, which allows emotional catharsis to occur as soon as danger has stopped. In the *post-traumatic* phase active steps can be taken to integrate recent distressing emotional experiences with other memories of critical events so that once again the dynamic steady state of normal life can be re-established. Gersons quotes the life events investigations of Holmes and Rahe (1964), Paykel (1969) and Dohrenwend and Dohrenwend (1981) as offering empirical support for this phased and dynamic perspective.

An important insight derived from crisis theory and life event research is that the risk of becoming overwhelmed in the aftermath of particularly adverse events is not exclusively a function of the multifactorial nature of stressors. Also to be considered are influences exerted by other recent or ongoing life events, availability of social support, etc.

A *prima facie* case may therefore exist for differentiating crises from trauma. Diagnostic and statistical manuals published before 1980 did not take a view of how a crisis may differ from a trauma. Both were merely viewed as events with a capacity to evoke reactive states. A turning point was reached in the late 1970's when social, political and military developments culminated in a new and distinct DSM-III classification of Post-traumatic Stress Disorder (PTSD; APA, 1980). Given the cardinal importance attributed to precipitating events, the diagnosis recognized the capacity of psychological trauma to evoke specific event-related reactions. However, these reactions differ from those provoked by and during a crises. With these considerations in mind, serious doubts have to be expressed about invoking crisis theory as a rationale for early intervention after trauma. Furthermore, whereas crisis intervention is explicitly championed as a form of therapy, CISD was championed as not being a therapeutic intervention at all. Finally, as explained by Gersons, some elements of the protocol prescriptions for CISD were not derived from crisis theory and may even be contraindicated by it.

Since such fundamental doubts exist about the wisdom of invoking crisis theory to rationalize early intervention after trauma, it is not surprising that outcome research engenders disappointing results, which, in turn, fuel controversy. Viewed from Gersons' perspective disagreements about the scope and limitations of one-off early interventions are not primarily a function of the relative methodological rigour of particular investigations, but the fact that such services have been championed on premises that pertain to entirely different types of interventions.

What can early intervention achieve?

The evidence submitted by Rose and her colleagues is particularly relevant to formulating an informed answer to this question. Having reported results from two Cochrane reviews of studies chosen for their methodological rigour, these authors conclude the strength of available evidence is at best neutral as to whether or not 'one-off' early interventions can deliver symptom outcomes as predicted for CISD. Their work highlights the importance of linking claims about what can be achieved to published evidence. This contrasts with past inclinations to foster impressionistic expectations of optimism only to see these dashed when systematic evaluations are carried out.

Another object lesson of both Cochrane reviews is the contrast between complexities pertaining to real life situations in which early intervention is indicated and the more controlled situations under which most outcome studies are conducted.

Of particular interest is the common discrepancy between initial subjective evaluations of services provided and longer-term symptom development. Carlier *et al.* (1998) found that police officers who had attended CISD meetings after a disaster were initially highly satisfied with this service. However, these same emergency responders were also the ones who at follow-up reported greatest symptom persistence in the longer term when compared with colleagues who had not attended CISD meetings. That the former group of police officers continued to regret not having participated in the meetings further amplifies this apparent paradox.

Gersons helps make sense of this phenomenon by drawing on crisis theory and accumulated experience about early intervention. In particular, he refers to some of the repercussions and consequences of the phased nature of human reactions to external events. Singled out for particular attention are the stages that follow in their immediate aftermath. Originally labelled the impact and recoil phases by Tyhurst (1957) and the honeymoon phase by Raphael (1986), these stages are characterized by psycho-physiological hyper-activation that engender powerful feelings of life being lived most intensely and with much more feeling than the 'dull' routines of daily life. Survivor attachments are formed based on presumptions of special bonds of loyalty, friendship and equality, as if by wishful thinking. Exactly as postulated by crisis theory, these descriptions highlight the importance of social support in the immediate aftermath of trauma. Group meetings may therefore be welcomed at this stage because survivors' preoccupations rightly focus on the here and now. It is no surprise, therefore, to find their statements have poor predictive power for eventual outcome. Providers of early intervention services must therefore be alert to the multitudes of influences that contribute to survivors' long-term adjustment. Whether positive or not, adaptations are a function of processes set in train by more than the influences exerted by psychological first aid.

Gersons also argues that recommendations for survivor group meetings to be facilitated by mental health professionals are ill advised. This is especially so if they use psychotherapeutic techniques for stimulating emotions as if in preparation for catharsis. The risk incurred is to further increase stimulation and emotional arousal in recent trauma survivors who, as a result of the trauma, are already in a hyper-aroused state. Because of the existing affect dysregulation, survivors may experience even stronger and more unwelcome feelings of being out of control if asked to focus on and express current feelings. This point also derives directly from crisis theory and explains why negative outcomes are reported from interventions that do not specifically seek to reduce arousal levels. Here again is another point of divergence between crisis theory and early intervention protocols championed during recent decades.

Survivors of recent trauma may be viewed as possibly being in a state of crisis. That is, they are living through an upset of a steady state that prevailed prior to the recent trauma. Care priorities should therefore include the re-establishment of a new steady state apposite for the current unfolding situation. Doing so is an essential precursor for taking steps to regaining control over emotions, re-asserting a sense of being able to actively determine the direction of one's life and re-establish routines of everyday living. Only when physical, psychological and social homeostasis are reported to be in place should consideration be given to introducing more complex forms of psychological therapy.

New conceptualizations of early reactions to trauma

Evidence presented in the opening section of this book highlights not only the timeliness of attempts to reconstruct early intervention, but also that past practices have been marred by weak theoretical, conceptual and empirical foundations. It is clear, therefore, that evidence-based practice will not be achieved by making cosmetic amendments to recently advocated practices. Rather, it will be achieved through detailed scrutiny of the nature of acute reactions to trauma and how best to conceptualize these so as to inform both clinical practice and research. Emergent perspectives can, in turn, be scrutinized in relation to a range of theoretical perspectives so as to highlight their implications for promoting, planning and providing early intervention after trauma.

Diagnostic formulations

As explained by McFarlane, descriptions of diagnostic criteria of acute stress disorder (ASD) in DSM-IV (APA, 1994) and acute stress reaction (ASR) in ICD-10 (WHO, 1992, 1993) have facilitated systematic research into the phenomenology of early reactions evoked by trauma. Current nosological terms were preceded by clinical formulations labelled 'gross stress reaction' in DSM-I (APA, 1952), and 'transient situational disturbance' in DSM-II (APA, 1968). However, as observed by Solomon *et al.* (1996), the basis on which informed decisions have been made about which early reactions to include or exclude for a given diagnosis lacks scientific rigour. This is a consequence of a historical poverty of systematic observation of these phenomena. With this in mind, watchfulness is called for in respect to the possibility that observational biases are being introduced by current diagnoses of early reactions to trauma.

McFarlane is right to warn against expectations of achieving a rigid nosology for reactions that are by their nature fluid, polymorphic and complex. Aspirations to formulate diagnostic markers for deciding which of any range of possible early interventions should be offered is therefore likely to be conceptually misguided. To be preoccupied with diagnostic formulations may carry a risk of presuming treatment need and, therewith, inadvertently interfering with natural healing processes.

A sounder basis for care planning is first to recognize survivors may want or need practical help or support in their personal efforts to cope with and adjust to recent events. Decisions about which forms of early intervention to offer, especially during the very early aftermath of trauma, should be based on a demonstrated need for practical assistance and not clinical diagnosis. Providers do well to recognize that survivors typically make adaptations conducive to improved control and mastery without professional assistance. On this basis, early intervention should incorporate the principle of consultation with possible service users to establish their individual and group preferences. At current standards of published evidence professionals might note the pitfalls of being prescriptive about survivors' service requirements. How can we know when interventions indicated after road traffic accident differ so markedly from those recommended after natural disasters, assaults, shipwrecks, combat, etc. McFarlane also stresses that provision must take account of the different population needs presented by children, adults, families, military staff, professional responder groups, and whether or not survivors live under conditions of continuing threat. By implication, therefore, it is highly unlikely that any single prescriptive intervention can possibly address all survivors' needs as these change through progressive stages of post-trauma adjustment.

Beyond diagnosis

Although problems associated with diagnosis of early reactions to trauma are legion, it is also recognized that such events can evoke dramatic survivor reactions. Because of their physical and psychological intensity the inclination of professional carers has been to construe reported effects as pathological and pathogenic. Such presumptions are difficult to reconcile with consistent findings of many survivors' early reactions resolving with time, even without access to professional help (Kessler *et al.*, 1995; Breslau *et al.*, 1998; Schnyder *et al.*, 2001a,b). The premises that inform emergent forms of early intervention after trauma should take a different view of evoked reactions. Namely, that early reactions tend to progress through phases that can be adaptive insofar they improve chances of survival and promote positive adjustment in the longer term. Shalev's review of recent advances in our knowledge of the psychobiology and neurochemical concomitants of early trauma reactions is extremely illuminating in this regard. He presents an evidence base on which new rationales for early intervention can be formulated.

Making sense of the inseparability of biology and environment

Immediate responses to traumatic events act as triggers for cascades of further psychobiological changes that, in the short term, may be conducive to their resolution, and positive learning or chronic expressions of distress. Under particularly adverse circumstances, where vulnerable individuals are repeatedly exposed to severe developmentally disruptive trauma, changes may be irreversible. On a more optimistic note, it is possible for soothing effects to be mediated during the early aftermath of trauma by the quality of survivors' social and interpersonal relationships. Shalev presents evidence in support of this period being characterized by enhanced neuronal plasticity during which psychological experiences become inseparable from the physiological processes by which they are mediated. He posits a dual process in which very early stress responses trigger a reflexive cascade of potentially adaptive mechanisms that are later followed by secondary biological responses. The latter relate mostly to past and current learning and are strongly influenced by the individual's unfolding environment. Together, these sets of responses have the potential to engender a sense of meaningfulness, adaptation and resilience, or kindle chronic stress disorders. So, while the processes that unfold during the early aftermath of trauma are experienced as highly subjective and personal, these reactions may have a common biological basis which, although crucial for eventual adjustment, are by no means predetermined.

A separate stream of evidence strengthens the rationale for early intervention. Meta-analyses of risk factors for PTSD reveal adversity during and after trauma to be the major determinants of subsequent disorder (Brewin *et al.*, 2000). At the point of being exposed to a trauma any number of possible outcomes are possible over time and early intervention should aim to shift the balance of probabilities towards successful coping and positive adaptation. It may usefully construe the process of doing so as effecting improvements in the quality of survivors' recovery environment.

It is clear from the above that aims and objectives of emergent forms of early intervention cannot be achieved through simplistic protocol prescriptions. Their innovative influence will be exerted, at least in part, by adopting principles of practice that accommodate a greater recognition of the many and complex psychological and physical mechanisms implicated in human responses to extreme events. By understanding and taking account of how these interact, it is also possible to increase the chances of favourable outcomes. This involves modifying processes related to bodily survival, learning, autobiographical memory-formation and complex socially modulated adaptations to change. All of these reactions should be examined in time frames that extend from fragments of seconds (for defence reflexes such as auditory startle), several seconds (for sympathetic activation), tens of minutes (for activation of the hypothalamic-pituitary-adrenal axis), hours (for early gene expression), days (for memory consolidation) and months (for permanent changes in the central nervous system; Post, 1992).

Learning and memory

Humans do not respond to trauma with a limited repertoire of bio-genetically predetermined reactions. One of the explanations offered to account for this fact is that through life we learn and events are imbued with what may be highly idiosyncratic meanings. Not only does this make us extremely sensitive to traumatic experiences, but it also creates conditions for evoked reactions to be modulated by other environmental influences exerted in their aftermath. Learning theory therefore provides one of the main platforms for deciding what is to be considered sensible practice in respect of early intervention. For instance, if survivors of recent trauma are in a psychobiological state that is adaptive for physical survival through the special focus it confers on actual threats there is no purpose in presenting them with complex new learning materials. At this particular stage of the phased trauma response, they will not retain this information and are unlikely to benefit from it.

Classical and operant conditioning paradigms are shown by Perrin to be particularly apposite for explanations of reactions observed in the early aftermath of trauma. Drawing in particular on Mowrer's two-factor theory (1960), he invokes both classical conditioning and operant learning paradigms to make sense of the extensive literature on learning processes elicited by aversive stimuli such as may be a feature of trauma. These stimuli evoke arousal, fear, startle and orientation reactions, as well as 'fight or flight' responses. How a survivor reacts when re-exposed to trauma is, according to learning theory, largely determined by whether or not other recently learned trauma-related responses increase or decrease in frequency. According to this perspective early intervention should primarily aim to increase the frequency of adaptive responses and also decrease the frequency of reactions that are not.

Learning theory posits that considerations of how this may be achieved should take account of the principle that extinction takes place via controlled re-exposures to eliciting stimuli and by changing their contingencies. As far as is feasible, therefore, care should be taken to ensure survivors are shielded from further exposures to stimuli that evoke intense aversive reactions. Readers should note learning theory is neutral in respect of the ideal or optimum timing for early intervention, but no controlled laboratory experiments have specifically addressed this point of theory.

Beyond conditioning theories

Conditioning theory accounts for some reactions evoked during the early aftermath of trauma and specifies parameters conducive to their elimination through contingency management. However, as argued by Shalev, human reactions to trauma also involve higher-level intellectual processes. These include memory, meaning and attributions that must be taken into account when trying to identify determinants of the nature and course of reactions to trauma (Beck and Emery, 1985). In recognition of this, Pilgrim has used cognitive theory to develop analysis and understanding beyond classical and operant conditioning paradigms.

Cognitive models are concerned with the personal significance of traumatic events and to this end focus on complex principles of information processing that occur in their aftermath. Of particular importance are existing cognitive structures, which incorporate the working beliefs and assumptions that survivors hold about themselves and the world in general. A characteristic of ordinary living is that new information is constantly registered and assimilated within existing, but modifiable structures. After trauma, however, incongruous reactions and impressions may be formed and assimilation of these is not so readily achieved (Janoff-Bulman, 1985). In Pilgrim's own study strong correlations were found between enduring symptoms and cognitions linked to themes of safety, trust, control, esteem, intimacy and self-blame (Pilgrim, 1999). Evidence is presented to suggest information processes may be compromised or avoided altogether by painful emotions or shattering of existing cognitive structures.

A number of possible objectives for early intervention after trauma are suggested by Pilgrim's review of cognitive theories. For instance, it is important to establish what beliefs and cognitions survivors hold about what has happened. This is because distorted beliefs become entrenched with the passing of time and seemingly irreconcilable cognitive structures can cause subjective distress. Beliefs deemed detrimental to cognitive information processing may be changed by improving understanding about what has happened and exploring cognitive structures that inform survivors' assessments of self and others. Discussion about event characteristics alone is unlikely to be helpful. Required help and support should ideally be phased to take account of the extent to which survivors are able to process new information. She also highlights how provision should be informed by more than one theory. For instance, cognitive-based interventions may not be effective unless time and care is taken to establish trust with trauma survivors. Mandatory instructions to participate in prescribed interventions are therefore contraindicated. Ideally, each individual should be consulted about their wish to access available services and the optimal timing for doing so.

Higher level processing

Practitioners in France have developed early intervention services rooted in psychoanalytic and psychodynamic theory. As explained by Bailly, provision aims to effect relief by group interventions that present opportunities to focus on specific aspects of trauma response. The purpose of doing so is to improve understanding of what happened, clarify subjective meanings of what happened and help develop more complete trauma narratives. Psychoanalytic and psychodynamic theories are advocated as a framework for understanding the most complex human reactions to trauma. Singled out for particular consideration is the way language is used during these critical times. Words are taken to be markers of the individual's post-trauma state and particular significance is attributed to survivor statements about there being no words to accurately describe what they have experienced.

In part, this perspective flows from the theory of Lacan (1966), which views the psyche as comprising of the Real, the Imaginary and the Symbolic. Raw and overwhelming sensory impressions evoked by trauma are assumed to offer a mirror on psychic realities manifest at the level of the Real. These may be un-symbolizable and cannot initially be expressed using words. Bailly takes the view that survivors have been confronted with their own death under circumstances where customary defences ceased to function (Briole et al., 1996). To remedy this situation therapists should rally the help of a group meeting of survivors to develop a trauma narrative. Healing will then take place through construction of an emergent group discourse. Theoretically, the aim of developing trauma narratives is to remove subjective impressions from the realm of the Real to the Symbolizable. In the process, survivors can assimilate more nuanced and subjectively meaningful perspectives on what happened (Daligand, 1997). Controlled clinical trials are required to verify these assumptions.

For this form of early intervention particular emphasis is given to the importance of keeping survivor groups intact, even if this means conducting meetings for up to 30 people. Psychoanalytic and psychodynamic theories also draw attention to the quality of the relationships that unfold between service providers and trauma survivors. For instance, at particularly troubled times it is important not to foster exaggerated expectations of early intervention or undermine each individual's capacity for coping and mastery. Because of the complexities emphasized by Bailly, he also raises the question about who is best qualified to deliver early intervention. Since this form of intervention is viewed as a highly complex and intricate form of therapy, a strong recommendation is made for group meetings to be facilitated by appropriately trained mental health professionals. Ideally, they should be psychotherapists, psychiatrists, psychologists and family therapists who are experienced in the management of strong emotional reactions expressed in a group context.

Considerations beyond those of the individual

Only passing references have so far been made to the importance of group processes and the broader social context for recovery. Ajducovic and Ajducovic illustrate how these considerations should not be peripheral to the challenge of reconstructing early intervention. Sound theoretical rationales exist for incorporating a host of contextual considerations beyond that of each individual survivor. Their perspective is particularly apposite under conditions of social upheaval provoked by wars or mass violence. However, to ignore its relevance for any survivor of recent trauma runs the risk of rendering both assessment and provision incomplete, culturally inappropriate and irrelevant to immediate needs (Wessells, 1999; Kleber, 2000). It may also impede recognition of strengths and resources that underpin empowerment of survivors, whole families, social networks and even entire communities.

The perspective advocated by Ajducovic and Ajducovic helps engender a sense of coping and mastery even when large-scale trauma results in grief, anger, aggression, fear, a sense of betrayal, despair, hopelessness and loss of control (Reichenberg and Friedman, 1996; Ayalon, 1998). Some of the restorative effects of social and community interventions can be immediate, but formulation of long-term aims and objectives is more appropriate. Fundamentally, early intervention along the lines suggested is primarily concerned with regenerating a sense of purpose and shared meaning, where recent events may have dramatically eroded most of the sense of community (Peddle *et al.*, 1999).

Systemic theory is one of the rationales for early social interventions. Its implementation should be strongly informed by sound practical considerations that are readily explainable to service users. For all its apparent simplicity, the complex challenges involved in delivering systemic interventions are legion. Why this should be so can be appreciated from a consideration of the types of practical initiatives called for when whole communities are traumatized. In unstable and volatile situations providers may endeavour to establish infrastructures for extended family and neighbour support, informal networking, parent groups, education, family reunification programmes, skills training, informal councils with community elders, *ad hoc* task groups, as well as ceremonies and rituals. Furthermore, under extremely disruptive circumstances one major trauma is likely to be followed by others (Allen, 1995; Terr, 1990, 1991). This is an entirely different survivor predicament from those experienced by victims of road traffic accidents or assault, and raises profound questions about how best to deliver early intervention under entirely different circumstances. Ajducovic and Ajducovic are clear in their recommendations. There is seldom justification for delaying offers of help. Practical considerations of safety and security must take precedence over promoting community coherence. In this respect, the 'Pyramid of Community Psychosocial Interventions' and its supporting narrative are useful guides for service providers.

Evidence

The complexities of early reactions to trauma

As argued above, the complexities of initial reactions to trauma are reflected in the historical legacy of early intervention and the various theoretical perspectives that inform the broad band of provision referred to as psychological first aid. As so eloquently demonstrated in the 'History and Theory' section of this book, all theories under consideration inform some or several aspects of reactions evoked by trauma and help that is indicated for survivors. When theories are supported by empirical findings, rationales can be invoked to account for the many forms of early intervention indicated at times of acute crises. By viewing reconstructed early intervention as a continuum of psychological first aid (Raphael, 1986), it becomes possible to assess service options in terms of their phase appropriateness. However, these suggestions should not distract from the inherent complexity of early reactions to trauma and, with it, the imperative of taking a flexible, staged and evidence-based approach to early intervention.

It is unlikely that any one of the theories reviewed in this book will ever suffice to account for the full diversity of reactions reported by trauma survivors. Nor is it realistic to expect that early intervention after trauma can be championed on the strength of a simple theory or universal protocol prescriptions with guaranteed outcomes. This is not to imply innovation should proceed without due regard to theory and evidence supporting its usefulness. Recent history has taught us how ill advised it can be not to balance imperatives of service innovation with evidence published in the public domain. Such complexities as have come to light are no reason to despair about or abandon the challenge of reconstructing early intervention. Rather, it engenders a stronger resolve to persevere in this endeavour. A platform for doing so is the fourth section of this book. It presents a view of recent trauma survivors as neither passively dependent nor submissive. Also, their behavioural, cognitive, affective and psychobiological reactions are best understood as typically adaptive and conducive to improved chances of survival. These perspectives carry clear implications for interventions applied in the early aftermath of traumatic events. For instance, to the extent evoked reactions serve adaptive ends, care should be taken not to interfere with processes that are conducive to natural recovery. Intervention should aspire to minimize negative influences exerted by the recovery environment and maximize those associated with favourable outcomes.

The fact that such processes are at work is demonstrated in the non-intervention follow-up study of accident victims reported by Schnyder and Moergeli. Some of its key findings are reproduced below in a line diagram plotting scores on the Clinician-Administered PTSD Scale for 106 subjects over a 1-year period. Assuming the subjects are representative of other accident victims, this study shows what happens if no specific post-incident psychological help and support is given. Based on the listed facts, it is possible, to make informed decisions about whether or not and for whom early intervention may be indicated, and what forms this may take.

As can be appreciated from Figure 24.1 the case for routine administration of early intervention for all recent accident victims is not supported by published evidence. Equally, some survivors report significant adjustment difficulties at various time intervals. These may be remedied by psychological first aid, but at current levels of evidence such declarations are speculative. Carefully designed, randomized, controlled intervention studies will have to be conducted to differentiate between natural resolution and specific intervention effects. Only at this juncture will the field have progressed to the point of having empirically demonstrated which effects and effect sizes can be achieved by new forms of early intervention. Based on recent experience some studies might well identify negative consequences from ill-advised help given at a phase inappropriate time.

Only upon this type of evidence base is it possible to reach informed decisions about whether or not to offer psychological first aid, to whom and when. Also to be addressed is the empirical question of when not to offer assistance. Many survivors report naturally occurring resolution of reactions evoked by trauma. This is a confounding phenomenon that, if not taken into consideration, may lead enthusiastic service providers to presume all positive effects are attributable to help given. In fact, changes may have occurred naturally over time. As long as this particular line of empirical evidence is poorly developed, the field should be alert to an even worse scenario. Namely, certain forms of early intervention administered to some survivor groups may produce worse outcomes. Embarrassingly, this as exactly the scenario suggested by some studies in the Cochrane Review.

Several chapters demonstrate risks inherent in assuming that early intervention invariably promotes resolution of trauma reactions. Particularly important in this regard are the Cochrane

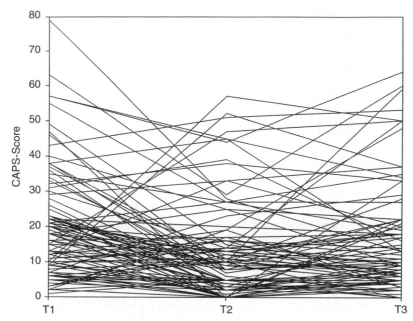

Figure 24.1   Individual total scores on the Clinician-administered PTSD Scale (CAPS-2) in 106 severely injured accident victims shortly after the accident (T1), at 6 (T2) and 12 months follow-up (T3).

Reviews undertaken by Rose and her colleagues. These have failed to demonstrate consistent and distinct beneficial effects from one-off early interventions administered to a variety of survivor groups. The need for continued caution with regard to presumptions made about early intervention is further reinforced by two long-term follow-up studies of road traffic accident and burn trauma victims. Some were taken through an early intervention protocol and others were not (Bisson *et al.*, 1997; Mayou *et al.* 2000). At follow-up the former groups endorsed more continuing symptoms indicative of poorer adjustment. Similar results are also reported in a follow-up study of police officers mobilized for disaster response in the Netherlands (Carlier *et al.*, 1998).

These particular results were obtained from specific groups of trauma survivors and, therefore, may not generalize to other populations. Trauma such as rape, displacement during war and torture may carry significantly worse prognoses than accidents. Also, some occupational groups, such as emergency services staff or soldiers on peacekeeping missions, typically make positive adjustments to work-related trauma. This is a point taken up in the Cochrane Review. Although cautious in its general conclusions, it acknowledges that some interventions were associated with more favourable group outcomes than reported by those allocated to non-intervention control conditions. By implication, therefore, future research should establish the exact parameters (nature of critical incident or trauma, initial reactions to event, demographic characteristics of survivor populations and availability of social support) under which psychological first aid engenders positive, neutral or negative post-trauma adjustment.

Schnyder and Moergeli's study prompts recognition of further factors that are important for early intervention. This is the tension between results reported for groups of survivors and the development of trauma reactions in particular individuals. Figure 24.1 is particularly illuminating on this respect. It plots marked individual variations between subjects over time and demonstrates how accident victims' scores fluctuate during the follow-up period. So, although tests of statistical significance for group differences are crucial for evidence-based early intervention, decisions about whether or not to offer psychological first aid should also be guided by considerations of the interests of particular individuals or even sub-groups of survivors. Recognition of tensions that exist between these approaches does not make these mutually exclusive. Despite apparent differences of emphasis, both approaches are important for reconstructing early intervention. Considerations raised by these approaches are sometimes complex, difficult and inconvenient, but little is gained by nurturing controversy about these matters. Instead, more considered approaches to psychological first aid can be achieved through creative integrating of separate strands of evidence.

One step towards integration is to encourage changes in the ways results from large group studies of early intervention are reported and interpreted. Current practice focuses on group differences. More consideration might be given to raising profiles of subjects whose characteristics do not conform to mean, median and modal values. Some investigators have started using this extended format for reporting findings relevant to sub-groups. Most notably they include long-term follow-up by Mayou *et al.* (2000) plus the study reported by Brewin and colleagues in this book.

Mayou's team did not only report findings of group differences observed between road traffic accident victims who had been taken through a standardized early intervention protocol and those who had not. More detailed examination of symptom endorsement patterns revealed the early intervention group comprised of subsets of individuals. Some had adjusted as well as subjects in the non-intervention group, but experimental subjects also comprised of a subset that had adjusted so poorly they raised group mean differences to a statistically significant level. So, on the basis of evidence presented in this expanded format, it would appear disappointing outcomes found for the early intervention group were not necessarily representative of the whole sample, but a product of a subset of subjects who had done particularly poorly. Further analysis revealed subjects with particularly high levels of agitation and distress soon after the accident to be over-represented in the poor outcome subgroup. Indications are, therefore, survivors who present in this manner should be given help to reduce levels of agitation before being taken through more complex early interventions.

The emergent body of evidence offers strong support for the principle of phased provision of psychological first aid. It is interesting to note these nuanced findings are consistent with the perspectives explicitly formulated by Gersons, Shalev and Ursano in this book. The former draws on crisis theory and accumulated experience with crisis intervention, while the latter two use recent evidence about the psychobiology of early reactions to trauma.

Screening

Brewin, Rose and Andrews present another example of what can be learned from studying sub-groups of large samples of trauma survivors. Their study was inspired by a recognition that long-term adjustment difficulties are experienced by a relatively small subgroup of all individuals exposed to trauma. Prevalences vary according to the nature of trauma, pre-incident adjustment and the quality of the recovery environment. Once service providers can identify sub-samples of survivors at greatest risk it is possible for resources to be mobilized to track symptom developments, assess emergent needs and address these in phase appropriate stages. The evidence base generated by this study engenders a simple screening technique to establish current diagnostic status and identify high-risk individuals or groups for systematic follow-up and study. A questionnaire devised to identify relevant predictors recommends itself for being simple to administer, easy to score with clear guidelines for how results are to be interpreted and can be used by non-specialists. The fact that highest predictive validity of later PTSD can be obtained by setting a cut-off point at three re-experiencing symptoms is an indication of the promise of this approach.

It is now important for practitioners to understand the principles governing the use of screening instruments. Their purpose is to correctly identify survivors whose early reactions indicate a risk of developing longer-term adjustment difficulties. Simplest is the notion of test sensitivity; the probability that a screening instrument will correctly identify individuals at risk if no help and support were given. In theory, all that is required to get a 100% sensitivity score is to positively identify all survivors implicated in a particular traumatic incident. Logic dictates that this strategy will be perfectly sensitive. However, such a strategy is useless because the selected population will also include many who will not develop adjustment difficulties. A screening instrument's sensitivity must therefore be complemented by considerations of its specificity; that is, the probability of those not at risk being correctly categorized as such. Once again, for obvious reasons, it is easy to devise tests with high sensitivity. All it takes is to include all subjects screened.

However, when these two criteria are jointly applied, an exacting requirement is set to help practitioners decide which screening method to use. To date, no test has been designed that achieves ideal sensitivity and specificity values for predicting longer-term trauma-related difficulties. Before a screening instrument is used, therefore, its actual performance characteristics should be explicitly stated. Describing positive predictive power and negative predictive power does this. The former is the probability of someone given a positive test will, in fact, develop longer-term problems and the latter is the probability of someone with a negative test not having these difficulties (Baldessarini *et al.*, 1983). Finally, the performance of a test can be expressed in terms of the percentage of cases correctly identified as belonging in these two groups. This is referred to as its overall efficiency.

Brewin and colleagues review the status of screening instruments published so far. Some practitioners rely on rather long and complicated interview schedules. These are impractical for mass screenings that call for brief, paper and pencil questionnaires. How this can be designed is meticulously documented by these authors. At current levels of knowledge longer-term difficulties are optimally predicted by endorsement of at least three moderately intensive re-experiencing symptoms taken from criterion B of the DSM-IV diagnosis of PTSD (sensitivity 0.71, specificity 0.85, positive predictive value 0.55, negative predictive value 0.92 and overall efficiency 0.83). As can be appreciated from the figures quoted above, there is considerable scope for using these screening criteria, but their limitations should also be recognized. An overall efficiency of 0.83 indicates that approximately 20 out of 100 assault victims will be incorrectly classified.

From a screening point of view practical problems also arise because the range of survivor populations (e.g. children, adults, war veterans and emergency responders) require different predictive tests. Furthermore, overall efficiency measures of screening tools are likely to vary according to the severity and duration of particular trauma. So, despite the optimism associated with this line of enquiry, the evidence cautions against practitioners and clinicians having unrealistically high expectations of its accuracy. As a consequence, service planners and providers should adopt flexible and phased strategies for identifying those who, in fact, develop difficulties over time.

Flexible and phased interventions for complex reactions

Protocol prescriptions for early intervention have enjoyed broad popularity for putatively being simple to implement to address trauma reactions said to conform to a narrow pattern of set responses the course of which are readily amenable to change. Recent controversies about the scope and limitations of early intervention have questioned the veracity of these assumptions.

The extent to which these presumptions and advocated techniques are misguided is explained in a chapter jointly authored by Shalev and Ursano. They help foster an informed appreciation of the complexities of early reactions to trauma and the theoretical frameworks that promote a more comprehensive understanding of these phenomena. However, diversity is not an impediment to a constructive and creative synthesis of evidence published to date. In fact, these two authors' endeavours demonstrate that commitment to evidence base practice engenders opportunities for creative speculation that promotes new insights and sensible innovation.

Shalev and Ursano present a new way of structuring observations of reactions evoked in the early aftermath of trauma. By mapping and detailing the multidimensional picture of survivors' reactions readers are helped to appreciate that unfolding situations are rarely simple. A pattern of phased and sequential reactions is described with the qualification that these may overlap in real life situations. Secondary stressors or individual survivors' strategies for coping and adjusting can also change these reactions. Of central importance to their emergent perspective is the notion that trauma evokes powerful adaptive mechanisms promoting survival. For these reasons there is no justification for continuing to view survivors as typically being rendered passive and dependent by unfolding events. It is therefore imperative that early interventions incorporate a recognition that interactions between survivors and their environment, including those who wish to offer help, remain active and dynamic at all times.

Shalev and Ursano explain how this may be achieved. In the early aftermath of trauma, natural forces operate in the service of physical and psychological survival. A basic requirement of psychological first aid is that it enhances or complements ongoing adjustment processes. If helpers keep this in mind, an appreciation may develop of survivors being well-informed guides, rather than dependent charges. To the extent that dialogues are premised by this recognition, early reactions to trauma can be construed as functional, since they enhance communication with others, mobilize support and set in place processes that promote reappraisal, staged readjustment and eventually formative learning. The catalyst for these processes to unfold is improved communication between survivors and helpers.

Also, it is essential for the process of reconstructing early intervention that reciprocal reactions evoked in helpers should mirror what survivors actually say they need and want. In the past, provision may have been unduly influenced by parallel processing and helpers' preconceived ideas about survivors' needs, rather than by the latter's expressed wishes.

To the extent that survivors' initial reactions are functional and adaptive they are likely to encompass elements not included in DSM-IV or ICD-10 symptom lists or diagnostic criteria. They will also be rapidly changing. Reactions that carry greatest personal significance are likely to be transient feelings of apprehension, anger, bewilderment, grief, regret, depression, agitation, stupor, numbing, irritability and yearnings. These will be paired with attempts to control emotions, find distractions and also re-appraisals to make sense of the event (Grinker and Spiegel, 1945; Yitzhaki *et al.*, 1991). Once survivors are listened to, an appreciation can develop that their narratives give expression to 'lived experiences' of, for example, loss, threats to established habits and routines, being uprooted, isolated and disconnected, feeling degraded by others, plus having to live with a new and keenly felt sense of uncertainty and doubt (Dasberg, 1976; Shalev and Munitz, 1989).

Given such inherent complexities, the question of appropriate timing of early interventions after trauma and the form this should take is unlikely ever to have one correct answer. A reasonable rule of thumb may therefore be to follow and respond to the progressive paths of individual development that occur after trauma. Helpers should take account of secondary stressors and ongoing trauma in the recovery environment, e.g. relocation, enduring injury, exposure to the media, painful medical examinations, surgery and other therapeutic procedures, juridical examinations, etc. Successive stressors evoke new sets of responses that further complicate survivors' preoccupations with basic survival. Thus, the purpose of early intervention can be redefined as a multidimensional process that seeks to identify and manage, in a staged and phase appropriate manner, obstacles to self-regulation and recovery. In so doing, it is important to recognize that impediments may be manifest at any level, ranging from the individual to that of the whole community.

This is not to argue that acute responses to trauma are always and invariably adaptive, or will necessarily promote problem resolution. Clearly, the evidence points to instances where individual characteristics (e.g. previous life trauma) and situational demands (e.g. intensity and duration of exposure, degree of continuing threat) militate against a favourable prognosis. It is under such circumstances that the case for early intervention is most clear and that it is not an end in itself, but a precursor for longer-term management involving family, social and clinical reconstruction.

Field experience indicates phased trauma reactions do not necessarily progress in a sequence through impact, rescue, recovery and return to life. Given the idiosyncratic demand characteristics of trauma, and their immediate aftermath reconstructed early intervention has to be flexibly tailored to each and every evolving situation. A key prerequisite is to consult with possible service users so as to be factually informed if help and support will be welcomed. To proceed on this basis makes good practical sense: it tempers helpers' inclinations to make unwarranted claims of expertise and militates against fostering passive dependencies on the part of survivors. This strategy for psychological first aid recommends itself for being consistent with Pearlin and Schooler's (1978) coping model of emitted behaviours, and the emergent evidence base about survivors resilience, coping and competency.

Table 24.1 is copied from Shalev and Ursano's chapter. It offers guidance on how to integrate the emergent evidence base within emergent approaches to early intervention. For each of the four stages the principal stressor is identified along with the presumed goals of emitted reactions and the forms of help that may be considered appropriate.

Once survivors have been rescued from primary stressors and are settled in a place of relative safety the emergent challenges for ongoing early interventions are to facilitate appropriate processing of confusion and bewilderment. At this stage, helpers may dampen the immediate impact

Table 24.1 Successive and overlapping stages of the response to traumatic events

	Impact phase	Rescue	Recovery	Return to life
Principal stressor	Threat, separation, exposure, incongruence etc.	New external and internal realities	Learning about the consequences of the event	Incongruence between inner experience or resources and external demands
Concrete goals of behaviour	Survival	Adjustment to new realities	Appraisal and planning	Re-integration
Psychological tasks	Primary stress responses	Accommodation	Assimilation	Practicing and implementing change
Salient behaviour pattern	Fight/flight, freezing; surrender, etc.	Resilience versus exhaustion	Grief, re-appraisal, intrusive memories, narrative formation	Adjustment versus phobias, avoidance, depression and PTSD
Role of all helpers	Rescue and protection	Orientation, provision for needs	Presence, responsiveness and sensitive interaction	Continuity of concrete and symbolic assistance
Role of professional helpers	Organizer	Holder	Interlocutor	Diagnostician and therapist

of the evolving situation by ensuring survivors are not abandoned with intensifying feelings of estrangement or alienation. Active psychological intervention may not be indicated at this stage. Instead, the 'holding' presence and warmth of helpers who model a capacity to endure and contain emotions may promote coping and adjustment.

During the recovery phase survivors distance themselves from the trauma and also re-evaluate what has happened. Intrusive re-experiencing might preclude the former from occurring, but this set of evoked reactions are powerful motivators for sharing with others what has happened and jointly assess its significance. In particular, this is a time for trying to understand the meaning and implications of trauma, examine key learning points, taking account of previous life experiences and amend expectations about the future. Whilst this is ongoing helpers should be available as facilitators for talking about what happened and helping make sense of the often surprising or unfamiliar reactions provoked by trauma. Intervention to block or eliminate trauma reactions is not usually indicated at this stage. However, much benefit can be derived from educating survivors about the typical course of these reactions over time.

Pearlin and Schooler (1978) suggested progress can be monitored by assessing the extent to which survivors actively engage in interactions that foster relief of distress, maintain a sense of personal worth involving rewarding interpersonal contacts and a capacity for sustained task performance. Note should also be made of signs that give rise to concerns about obstructions to the unfolding of a natural healing path. Particularly important in this regard are persisting inability to modulate emotions, impaired task performance, self-blame or worthlessness, and being unable to enjoy the company of others.

Making early intervention complementary to survivors' coping strategies

By presuming some degree of survivor coping and competence early intervention can be transformed into a service that aspires to validate and complement preferred adjustment strategies. Ørner's chapter about adjustment strategies used by experienced emergency services officers illustrates the promise of this approach. This establishes an entirely new empirical baseline of self-help strategies that can be taught in training programmes or post-qualification workshops. It also provides a foundation for assessing whether non-routine early intervention strategies are indicated, and assessing if the preference for naturally emergent, largely informal self and peer support can be reconciled with recommendations for formal early intervention.

Early self-identification of distress appears to be a skill that emergency services staff acquire in the course of their careers. At critical times, a majority turn to colleagues for support. Thereafter, and with minimal delay, help and support is sought from others with whom they feel close. While these generalizations apply to the samples surveyed findings also indicate many exceptions at individual or subgroup levels. Of particular interest to those who are committed to delivering evidence-based early interventions is the finding that approximately 20% of emergency responders did not typically wish to talk about what had happened immediately after the event. Clearly, presumptions of uniformity and the notion that one form of early intervention can address the needs of all are ill advised.

It is interesting to note that emergency services staff develop idiosyncratic patterns of preferred coping and adjustment strategies that are flexibly applied. A principal component analysis of deliberate adjustment strategies produced the following categories; 'wait and monitor the nature and course of reactions', 'rest and relaxation', 're-establish control and routines', 'confront what has happened' and 'find release from somatosensory sequelae'. A guiding principle that underpins these coping strategies is to reduce levels of arousal and re-establish a sense of control. These objectives turn out to be entirely consistent with arguments put forward by other chapter authors, most especially Gersons, Shalev and Ursano. Further concurrent research is called for to monitor the ongoing impact of each strategy on unfolding reactions to service related trauma. This reformulation highlights differences between new guidelines and past protocol prescriptions for early intervention. For instance, an emergent imperative is to foster informed leadership practices that encourage peer support during and in the immediate aftermath of major or unusual events. Here, the challenge is one of staff education, rather than clinical intervention. The value of educational, rather than prescriptive practices is further demonstrated during the post-incident phase. At this stage, the process of monitoring officers' coping and adjustment, and seeking their advice about additional help and support can only be achieved through dialogue with possible service users. The process is therefore didactic and educational, and marks the end of an era in which experts insisted on mandatory attendance for meetings facilitated by mental health professionals.

Emergency services officers have helped identify some practical strategies, the principles of which may prove highly relevant to other survivor populations. Research will establish if these principles offer more refined guidance for general provision of early intervention. This will be a step towards ensuring that help and support is both rooted in evidence and delivered in a manner that complements survivors' preferred practices. With these considerations in mind, reconstructed early intervention can be promoted as a means of effecting agreed and operationalized improvements in the quality of survivors' recovery environment.

25 Progress made towards reconstructing early intervention after trauma: principles of evidence based practice

R.J. Ørner and U. Schnyder

For the last decade or so, a self-perpetuating debate has raged about the scope and limitations of early intervention (Gist and Woodhall, 1998; Mitchell, 1998; Avery *et al.* 1999). While controversies were endlessly rehearsed some service providers continued to address the practical imperative of mobilizing systematic help and support for survivors of recent and ongoing trauma. All chapters in the penultimate section of this book add substance to the view that evidence-based early psychosocial intervention is a crucial dimension of comprehensive post-incident care. Format and techniques vary according to the actualities of complex, unfolding situations and the many survivor populations being served. All the same, it is instructive to review the new guiding principles of early intervention as they emerge, from these chapters. With these in mind, it becomes possible to speculate constructively about future developments and priorities.

Formulation, diagnosis, objectives and aims

The search for a unifying diagnosis for early reactions to trauma continues under difficult circumstances. McFarlane and other authors caution against presuming a precise clinical diagnosis can be formulated to serve as a definitive marker. In this regard, the multi-factorial nature of initial reactions to trauma is a mitigating factor and preoccupations with diagnosis run the risk of bringing psychopathological perspectives to natural human distress.

Shalev and Ursano promote a view of initial reactions to trauma having adaptive functions promoting survival. Diagnostic fervour should therefore be contained and early intervention should not be made contingent on survivors' diagnoses. Decisions about whether or not a particular form of psychological first aid is indicated should, at least initially, be informed by a resolve to address practical needs. However, for the purposes of systematic service evaluation it is essential to carry out assessment and screening of evoked reactions, and their development over time.

Initially, a common sense pragmatism will inspire a recognition that survivors may need help and support after recent exposure to trauma. However, Shalev and Ursano warn against assuming survivors' needs are so marked and immediate that any forms of early intervention will be welcomed. These authors point to the adaptive characteristics of initial reactions serving the biological imperative of survival. Primitive reactions of distress and despair can help bring into closer physical and psychological proximity those in danger, and those who can provide safety, security and other basic needs. This interactive perspective clarifies, to some extent, the basis for mental health professionals' preoccupations with extending their complex or sophisticated interventions into the field of acute post-trauma care. Within the advocated framework of early intervention such help and support is considered appropriate only during later phases of post-trauma reactions.

These considerations have several important implications. For instance, de Jong and Kleber, as well as Ajduković and Ajduković, describe early interventions premised by considerations of the status of community resources and social networks. They recognize extreme circumstances, such as war and mass violence, will engender nightmares, fears, shock reactions and despair in virtually all survivors. However, even in the absence of formalized access to mental health services, 60–90% do not go on to develop diagnosable mental disorders (Kleber and Brom, 1992). According to these authors, the objective of some forms of reconstructed early intervention is therefore to promote social reconstruction with a view to strengthening survivors' resilience and capacities for coping. An early objective is for service users to resume more complex adaptive roles and, once again, be functioning community members. Exact details about how this may be achieved will vary according to the contexts within which early intervention is provided. Clearly, pertinent factors conducive to adaptive coping and mastery reside both beyond and within individual survivors. This broad-based supra-individual perspective advocated by de Jong and Kleber marks a significant development in the range of complementary rationales available to inform service providers.

In their chapters about early intervention for soldiers with combat stress reactions (CSR) Weisæth and Mehlum give examples of how adjustment is a function of both contextual and personal considerations. Through preparation and training soldiers know they function in settings where the predominant presumption is of individual coping and mastery. This is made explicit in their 'operational orders' that specify how prompt help is to be given near or in the battle zone under expectations of rapidly resuming active combat roles. However, early intervention relies both implicitly and explicitly on recognition of important restorative group processes. The same principles of balancing considerations pertinent to the individual and the group inform the staged interventions advocated by Avery and King, and Ørner for emergency services staff. Their approach also illustrates how service planning should incorporate options to access counselling or brief therapy.

As happens after disclosed sexual violence, some countries have health and judicial procedures in place for activation in the aftermath of trauma. Similarly, hospitals provide a specific organizational context for those patients who may be in psychological crisis and several authors have demonstrated the scope for effecting significant hospital service improvements by incorporating early intervention in care planning. These examples illustrate the underlying principle of evidence based early intervention. Namely, a preoccupation with achieving an optimal balance between social and contextual influences that facilitate coping through appropriately phased assistance.

A recurrent theme of this book is the sheer scale of the challenges presented to practitioners. As pointed out by Gersons, trauma takes a multitude of forms and will, if a lifetime perspective is taken, be the norm, rather than an exception. So, even under conditions of relative social stability, over 50% of inhabitants in western countries will in the course of their lives experience at least one critical event that fulfils the DSM-IV stressor criteria for PTSD (Breslau *et al.*, 1991; Kessler *et al.*, 1995). Accidents and assaults are the most commonly experienced trauma, but within 3 months approximately 80% will have adjusted and do not endure persistent event-related sequelae (Rothbaum *et al.*, 1992; Riggs *et al.*, 1995). The non-intervention study reported by Schnyder and Moergeli in this book found even lower prevalence rates at 6 and 12 months follow-up.

Such generalizations mask massive variations in the course and developments of post-trauma reactions. For instance, Kessler and colleagues (1995) found PTSD after rape in 65% of the men and 46% of the women interviewed. An additional complicating consideration is the growing body of evidence about prognosis not being exclusively linked to level and intensity of acute reactions. Their course and development are subject to a multitude of influences. Only some of these can be changed by psychological first aid. Vigilance beyond the short term is therefore of the essence.

To systematically confront the challenge of delivering evidence-based early intervention it is useful to construe it as consisting of the broad base of services that Beverley Raphael refers to as psychological first aid (Raphael, 1986):

First attend to basic needs

- Safety, security and survival
- Food and shelter
- Orientation
- Communication with family, friends and community
- Assess the environment for ongoing threats

First level of reconstructed early intervention

- Protect survivors from further harm
- Reduce physiological arousal
- Mobilize support for those in greatest distress
- Keep families together, facilitate reunion with chosen friends and loved ones
- Provide information, encourage communication and education
- Use effective risk communication techniques

Needs assessment and screening

- Assess current status.
- Are immediate needs being addressed?
- Improve immediate recovery environment.
- Consider if additional interventions are needed for whole groups or communities, particular sub-populations or individual survivors.

Monitor the rescue and recovery environment

- Observe, listen to and consult with those most affected.
- Monitor the environment for additional threats and stressors.
- Monitor past and ongoing threats.
- Monitor services being provided.
- Monitor media coverage and rumours.

Outreach and information dissemination

- Use established community structures, information leaflets for general distribution, set up new websites, prepare and distribute media releases, participate in media interviews and public information programmes.

Technical assistance, consultation and training

- Improve capacity of organizations and caregivers to provide what is needed to re-establish community structures, support family recovery to foster cohesion plus resilience and safeguard community infrastructures.

- Technical assistance, consultation and training should be prioritized for relevant organizations involved in trauma and disaster response; professional responder groups, other caregivers and volunteers; leaders and incident commanders.

Foster resilience, coping and recovery

- Facilitate social interaction at family, group and community levels.
- Offer structured modules for coping skills awareness training and ways of conducting risk assessments.
- Provide education about stress response, traumatic reminders, ways of reducing impact of recent trauma, differentiating normal and abnormal functioning, draw attention to risk factors, inform survivors of available services and how to access these. They may comprise of;

    individual, group and family interventions
    fostering natural social support
    looking after the bereaved

- Restore organizations to operational readiness through staff support.

Assessing different levels of immediate need: triage

- Clinical assessment by professional health care staff.
- Referral when indicated.
- Identify vulnerable, high-risk individuals and groups.
- Arrange emergency hospitalization if necessary.

Treatment

- Reduce or ameliorate symptoms to improve functioning using individual, family and group psychotherapies.
- Consider pharmacotherapy.
- Offer and provide spiritual support.
- Short- or long-term hospitalization.

Such a broad-based perspective is useful when planning and delivering comprehensive early intervention. Eventually, independent strands of evidence should document the impact of each constituent part of psychological first aid. In this regard, it is encouraging to note a new realization of the case in favour of one-off, very early, single problem-focused interventions. As described by Mehlum and Weisæth, forward combat psychiatry can effect recovery from CSR in 80–90% of uninjured battle casualties and resumption of combat ability within 72 hours (Solomon and Benbenishty, 1986). This focus on single, specific trauma-related reactions is also being used with recent survivors of rape and sexual assault (Resnick et al., 1999). Practice is inspired by evidence demonstrating the remedial impact over the longer term of promoting improved functioning during the immediate post-trauma phase. In this book, Resnick and her colleagues describe specific elements of early rape survivor care that focus on circumscribed, but significant distress reaction. By using techniques known to reduce victims' acute post-rape distress and taking steps to minimize risks of further traumatization by invasive forensic examinations, targeted early interventions for rape survivors can facilitate improved coping in the short term and positive adjustment in the longer term. In keeping with the above are recent innovations that specifically target known risk factors to mitigate their detrimental impact (Dansky et al., 1994; Najavits et al., 1996).

Targeted early interventions offer opportunities to initiate or plan more specialist forms of therapy. For instance, Falsetti and Resnick (2000) advocate a 12-session treatment package called Multiple Channel Exposure Therapy (M-CET) for survivors with civilian trauma-related PTSD and co-morbid panic attacks. It incorporates elements from cognitive processing therapy (Resick and Schnicke, 1993), stress inoculation training (Kilpatrick et al., 1982) and the 'Mastery of Your Anxiety and Panic' approach advocated by Barlow and Craske (1988). Preliminary outcome results for M-CET are encouraging (Falsetti and Resnick, 2000). Furthermore, strong indications exist for treating acute stress disorder (ASD) following road traffic accidents with cognitive behaviour therapy (Bryant *et al.*, 1999). As reported by Bisson, CBT techniques have been adapted, with encouraging results, in an early intervention programme for recently hospitalized survivors of accidents and violent assault.

It is in relation to these more complex, phase appropriate interventions that systematic diagnoses demonstrate both their value and limitations for early intervention. Pitfalls inherent in confining descriptions of early reactions to trauma to accepted diagnoses are highlighted in Harvey and Bryant's (1998) prospective treatment study of acute stress disorder. They found 78% of motor vehicle accident survivors initially identified as presenting with ASD were given a PTSD diagnosis 6 months post-trauma. However, 60% of those with subsyndromal ASD, which does not include dissociative reactions, were also diagnosed with PTSD at this follow-up. Two years later, 63% of those initially diagnosed with ASD and 70% of those with its subsyndromal condition still qualified for a PTSD diagnosis (Harvey and Bryant, 1999). On its own, therefore, the ASD diagnosis may not be a reliable marker for event-related adjustment problems experienced in the longer term.

In hospitals, uniformed services and other similar settings the organizational climate tends to favour set routines with guaranteed outcomes. Those who champion psychological first aid cannot offer such assurances. Therefore, promoting the introduction of early psychosocial interventions within organizations where this has not been standard practice is difficult. A strategic view of the need to educate leaders and managers increases the chances of accepting service developments. As pointed out by Buus-Jensen and Baron in their chapter on training programmes this may involve actively campaigning for human rights.

Screening

Reconstructed early intervention is informed by the presumption that survivors' resourcefulness can promote coping and positive adaptations to trauma. Although appropriate in most instances, the expectation will not apply for all individuals. An immediate practical challenge is therefore to develop screening techniques that accurately identify individuals most at risk of experiencing longer-term psychosocial adjustment difficulties.

Several authors have advocated the use of screening in support of early intervention. Although the screening methods to be used will vary according to circumstances, the case for focusing on individuals or groups most at risk, or in greatest need is compelling. In a study of hospitalized patients carried out by Ruzek and Zatzick (2000), a majority reported welcoming opportunities to undergo comprehensive psychosocial assessments because it prompted recognition of previously ignored factors that might promote recovery. Techniques are available to gauge levels of immediate psychological distress such as depressive and dissociative symptoms (Harvey and Bryant, 1998; Freedman *et al.*, 1999) or intrusive memories (Brewin *et al.*, 1998). Symptom screening can also help identify other clinically significant conditions, such as co-morbid alcohol and substance abuse, acute stress disorder, post-traumatic stress disorder, situational and social phobias, plus other stress-related impairments (Green *et al.*, 1993) that might not otherwise have been disclosed or identified. All the same, the extent to which screening is indicated varies according to type of trauma (mass violence, disasters, individual accidents or assaults) and the ways phased early intervention is implemented.

Several chapters list screening instruments used to gauge reactions evoked by recent trauma. None are perfect, but four measures are singled out to identify adults with acute stress disorder. They are the Stanford Acute Stress Reaction Questionnaire (SASRQ; Cardeña *et al.* 2000), the Acute Stress Disorder Interview (ASDI; Bryant *et al.*, 1998), the Acute Stress Disorder Scale (ASDS; Bryant *et al.*, 2000) and the Brief Screening Instruments for PTSD (Brewin *et al.*, 2002).

For more general screening of trauma reactions, Bisson used the Trauma Distress Scale (Brewin *et al.*, 1998).

If screening is indicated under circumstances where the number of survivors is very large, it is advisable to use standardized questionnaires. As reported by Brewin and colleagues, current evidence suggests that measures of intrusive memories have good predictive power. They have developed a 10-item screening instrument for general use with recent trauma survivors (Brewin *et al.*, 2002). However, practitioners should also recognize that improved identification rates are achieved if screening encompasses considerations of pre-trauma levels of psychosocial stress (Schnyder *et al.*, 2001a,b), anxiety and depression (McFarlane, 1988; Breslau *et al.*, 191; Resnick and Newton, 1992) and family history of psychiatric disorder (Breslau *et al.*, 1991; Davidson *et al.*, 1991). Other important indicators include measures of cortisol immediately post-trauma (Yehuda *et al.*, 1998) and current availability of social support (Davidson *et al.*, 1991).

Field experience and clinical practice has led Yule to conclude the criteria for screening very young children probably differ from those that may be indicated with older, more mature and articulate children. Working within communities disrupted by war, early intervention involved calling meetings to advise young survivors and their families about stress reactions plus elementary strategies conducive to coping. Once assembled it proved possible to carry out informal triage to ensure those with greatest immediate need were given priority help (Yule and Unwin, 1991).

Recent enthusiasm about early screening should not distract from possible misuses of the information so gathered. Practitioners who are inclined to provide psychological therapy at the moment of identifying a need should temper their therapeutic fervour. This is especially so in the early aftermath of trauma. Evidence indicates there is a phase during which many survivors resolve initial crises without professional involvement. Responding to 'presumed need' can have aversive consequences if survivors are mistakenly led to believe they are functioning in maladaptive or pathological ways, or are deficient in the personal or social resources conducive to coping and adjusting to difficult situations.

Despite these contextual limitations survivor screening will continue to generate streams of evidence to inform the process of reconstructing early intervention. The fact that scales and techniques advocated in this book typically focus on psychosocial reactions manifest at later stages of the post-trauma response should not distract from the initial imperative of addressing survivors' primary needs for safety and security.

Timing and consultation with service users

This book confirms an important historical shift in respect of when to deliver early intervention after trauma. Past protocol prescriptions gave high prominence to this aspect of service provision. So much so, it seemingly constituted one of the defining characteristics of early intervention. This emphasis on chronological time goes some way towards explaining Yule's comment about a propensity amongst providers to overlook the primacy of physical needs in the early aftermath of trauma. Similarly, a focus on time has fostered a presumption of survivors necessarily needing professional help even when studies demonstrated their resilience and capacity for coping. Within emergency services, for instance, an organizational climate has evolved in which peers and friends support one another after work-related critical incidents and trauma. As pointed out by Ørner, routine imposition of precipitate and mandatory early intervention is therefore strongly contraindicated on several counts. Clearly, for some high risk populations provision of comprehensive early intervention is rooted in anticipation of trauma and should be education based.

Assessment and screening of recent survivors of trauma may establish they are in no state to benefit from complex psychological interventions requiring recall, reflection or developing trauma narratives. For this reason, reconstructed early intervention places less emphasis on timing than on observation, assessment and consultation that establishes which forms of phased help and support are required. Based on accumulated field experience, some chapter authors advocate making survivors aware that help with emotional reactions will be offered at some point, but not immediately after a particular event. The evidence base reviewed by Shalev and Ursano in Table 24.1 informs this guidance. Early intervention after trauma should therefore be appropriately phased and flexibly applied, since survivors' needs are not a given in the complex aftermath of trauma. Needs evolve, increase and decrease. In some instances, adjustment takes place against a background of new or ongoing threat to life. These are some of the reasons why timing of interventions should not be prescribed by 'the clock'. Furthermore, there are circumstances that may warrant a return to earlier stages of phased interventions to be followed through with help and support programmes that extend into the intermediate or long-term future.

This emergent perspective on early intervention has several implications. For instance, service providers should be cautious about making mandatory recommendations unless unequivocal evidence can be quoted in their support. Avery and King describe how this recognition helped establish a systematic approach to consultation with service users. It also resulted in radical re-definitions of aims and objectives of a staff care initiative for emergency services personnel. When asked about their post-incident care preferences, officers tend to prioritize education and awareness raising, fostering good leadership practices, reinforcing their capacity for coping and making sensible adjustments to work-related trauma. Low priority was given to focusing on specific symptoms evoked by trauma.

As if to reinforce the above, formal therapeutic interventions such as cognitive behaviour therapy for ASD or other brief trauma focused therapies are typically not indicated within 2 weeks of the precipitating event (Brom et al., 1989; Foa et al., 1995). In general, therefore, the theory and practice of psychological therapies relevant to general clinical practice informs only some of the more specialist aspects of psychological first aid. Some delay in administering therapy after recent trauma decreases the likelihood of reported symptoms being transient reactions. It also allows survivors additional time to consolidate their coping resources, increases opportunities for addressing, and resolving many practical or contextual problems that typically emerge in the aftermath of trauma.

Education and prevention

Beyond the initial aims of providing safety and security for survivors early intervention can engender change through psycho-education. Being well informed about reactions evoked by trauma, and being aware of how to use personal and social resources to control these are prerequisites for coping and eventually making positive adaptations to unfolding events. Broadly speaking, the key challenges of early intervention are to educate, rather than treat and to optimize conditions for imparting relevant knowledge about coping and mastery. This tends to occur after trauma have impacted, but early intervention is, more than most specialist fields, explicit about its preoccupations with prevention.

As pointed out by Buus-Jensen and Baron, a psycho-educational perspective positively emphasizes the importance of being explicit about the content of training curricula for different groups of survivors and helpers. In respect of the latter, training towards competence should be followed by ongoing supervision, on the job coaching and peer review. Not only are these natural extensions of training objectives, but they also become essential components for monitoring and improving service quality standards. As such, they are important adjuncts for research activities to engender the evidence base that informs providers of early intervention.

Providers will do well to anticipate that some types of trauma generate their own educational needs; the nature of which survivors may not be fully aware. For instance, accident survivors may experience distress because they are uncertain about the extent or implications of their injuries. Equally, they may be uninformed about the scope, limitations and side effects from psychotropic medication. Resnick, for instance, has recommended that concerns about negative health outcomes associated with assault and rape be addressed soon after the trauma. Matters for consideration include worries about injuries, risks of developing sexually-transmitted diseases, future medical care requirements plus options for testing and preventing unwanted pregnancy. Early intervention also offers opportunities to engage survivors in a series of follow-up consultations to monitor adjustment and health status over the longer term.

Competence to provide reconstructed early intervention

The great majority of chapter authors do not recommend that provision of early intervention be an exclusive prerogative of a particular professional group. Given that most survivors cope and adjust positively without access to professional helpers there is strong reason to be cautious about prescriptions of competency or who is suitable for training. In its emergent manifestations early intervention should encourage practices unburdened by doctrinaire orthodoxy, or the promotion of personal and professional self-interest. Nonetheless, it is important to develop an informed perspective on who is to be formally sanctioned to provide the various forms of psychological first aid. Given that provision covers a very broad range of services the crucial question to address is who is best placed to do what and at what stage? A starting point for answering this question is to examine who is actually involved in service provision. Given the many and varied traumas to which survivor populations are exposed the realization dawns that competence is not an exclusive prerogative of professional carers. Flexible and phased interventions inevitably involve a broad spectrum of service providers. In some instances, practical help and emotional support is provided by front line emergency services personnel and at a later stage services may be provided by experienced psychotherapists.

In the former instance, basic psychological help is provided as an adjunct to addressing survivors' primary needs. Emergency services responders, soldiers on peacekeeping missions, nurses on medical wards and some volunteer helpers are typically deployed to attend to the physical safety and security of survivors. Their manner of doing so is crucially important for creating circumstances conducive to achieving improved psychological adjustment in the short, intermediate and long term. Over time, experienced officers accumulate extensive hands on experience in attending to survivors' immediate distress and needs. It is contrary to common sense, therefore, to presume front line responders are not competent to provide early intervention even though they may not be specifically trained to provide psychosocial care.

Looking to the future

We hope reconstructed early intervention will be a practically orientated specialist field with a multidisciplinary ethos that is firmly rooted in sensible theory and enriched by a developing evidence base. With this aspiration in mind it becomes possible to speculate about its future directions and engender informed public debates about appropriate provision for survivors of recent trauma.

The need for a reconstruction of early intervention is not in doubt. Rather, the pervasiveness of trauma in the lives of most people warrants greater recognition. More nuanced perspectives should be promoted about survivors' needs, and how these can be systematically addressed by flexible, practical, phased and evidence-based measures.

Each constituent element of early intervention seeks, in its own particular way, to promote particular aims and objectives. Given the phased nature of early intervention each initiative is not necessarily an end in itself, but a stepping-stone towards improved coping and positive adjustment.

Depending on the circumstances, early intervention may comprise of measures to promote social reconstruction. At other times it seeks to address immediate emotional needs of sub-groups of survivors or individuals traumatized by violence, rape, serious accidents, assaults and any number of personal misfortunes.

Significant too is the recognition that early intervention is not necessarily defined by considerations of time relative to a particular trauma. Under some circumstances 'early' precedes trauma as in the case of educational initiatives for high-risk groups in uniformed and emergency services or public information campaigns. At other times, early intervention extends into the longer term as part of comprehensive care provision. Early intervention is likely to become increasingly preoccupied with delivery of preventive public health programmes to educate the general public about sensible adjustment strategies to be used. This will also raise awareness about indications for seeking specialist care and how this can be done for a broad range of survivor groups. Along with the above a greater understanding will evolve of specific sub-population needs. In view of the complexities inherent in providing early intervention a core element of expertise is to recognize the importance of consultation with possible service users. This emerges as an essential precondition for promoting aims and objectives consistent with service users priorities in the short, intermediate and long term.

All the same, reconstructed early intervention should aspire to be brief and informed by the evidence that post-trauma distress typically remits naturally without access to specialist care. Outcome studies carried out by Resnick and colleagues with survivors of rape demonstrate that very brief focused interventions can, at critical times, help improve adjustment in the longer term (Resnick and Newton, 1992). Such approaches present a particularly interesting challenge for early intervention because they combine elements of specialist care with a recognition of survivors' capacity for coping and mastery. All of the above should, of course, be the subject of further systematic research.

Bryant draws attention to the difficult and rarely discussed matter of professional responsibilities owed by service providers to those who do not seek help or fail to complete an agreed programme of early intervention. Amongst road traffic accident survivors a dropout rate of approximately 20% has been recorded. Indications are that the individuals concerned may be survivors with high morbidity and severe adjustment problems for whom additional, flexibly administered and individually tailored early intervention is strongly indicated. Weisæth (1989, 2001) has laid the foundations for an informed debate on these matters.

Trauma survivors are increasingly taking legal action to secure compensation for the effects of trauma (e.g. after road traffic accidents, military and emergency services staff). Legal arguments often centre on questions of negligence or failure to satisfy duty of care responsibilities. It is therefore reasonable to anticipate more attention will be given to agreeing minimum standards for duty of care in respect of early intervention. Even at present levels of knowledge, it is strongly advisable for organizations to have contingency arrangements in place that anticipates trauma and screen survivors for the course and development of their evoked reactions.

Given the large numbers of individuals who are implicated and affected by trauma there is a requirement for screening techniques to be further improved. Current practice of defining 'caseness' and planning provision from self-report symptom questionnaires should be refined to take fuller account of the high numbers of survivors whose reactions remit naturally.

Future advances within the field will also facilitate an explicit recognition of the extent to which 'natural remission' is a function of individual, group or whole community processes. This book describes a range of approaches that draw on these processes to different degrees. It also sets the stage for an appreciation of the fact that the constituent parts of psychological first aid are complementary and not mutually exclusive. An ongoing challenge, therefore, is to develop practices and guidelines based on the relative merits of these approaches. In these regards, contextual factors are going to be seen to be increasingly important, as are the hitherto largely neglected influences of cultural variations in survivors expressed preferences.

Liaison with non-clinical service managers and planners is likely to become an increasingly important aspect of the psycho-educational initiatives embraced by those who advocate early intervention. A starting point for doing so is to counteract the unfortunate effects of recent doctrinaire controversies about early intervention. More informed public and professional debate about trauma care should be fostered. Liaison is also crucial for ensuring that innovative practices are made acceptable to institutions and organizations that have so far not incorporated early intervention into routine service provision. This applies as much to international humanitarian aid organizations as to local hospitals and providers of specialist community care schemes.

To its credit the field of early intervention has established a sound reputation for engendering research and systematic evaluation. In years to come a shift is likely to occur away from an almost exclusive preoccupation with evoked symptoms and clinical outcomes. In part, this change will reflect the realization that early intervention has aims and objectives extending far beyond those commonly addressed in clinical trials and symptom focused research. Examples of such extended aims and objectives may be the facilitation of a return to work, less time lost through illness, improvement of general and health-related quality of life, etc. Reconstructed early intervention is a continuum of provision that encompasses a broad range of phased services. An aspiration is for these to be synchronized with the staged nature of human reactions to trauma so as to improve the quality of the recovery environment. Research should therefore engender conclusions that inform practitioners about what can realistically be achieved by early intervention, whilst also being relevant to actual 'field' practice. Therapies should also be developed to address the full range of chronic and co-morbid conditions experienced by some trauma survivors.

In the final count, this book delivers early intervention from an inauspicious start. Ill-informed controversy increases risks of discrediting endeavours to recognize the evidence-based imperative of offering some help and support to survivors. On the strength of contributions made by chapter authors much progress has been made to advance the process of reconstructing early intervention. For instance, all practice should now be related to sound theory, as well as empirical evidence. However, the process of reconstruction has not reached a final end point. Rather, reconstructed early intervention eschews orthodoxy and doctrinaire dogmatism. It favours approaches that tolerate uncertainty, but makes prompt action an imperative on the basis of consultation with possible service users.

The process of reconstruction fostered by this book is about new beginnings for early intervention. However, it also raises the possibility that the radical shifts in current conceptualizations of human reactions to adversity may also prompt other specialist fields, within and outside psychotraumatology, to consider if their areas of interest are in need of reconstruction.

References

Allen, J.G. (1995) *Coping with Trauma*. Washington DC: American Psychiatric Press.

APA (1952) *Diagnostic and Statistical Manual of Mental Disorders*, 1st edn. Washington DC: American Psychiatric Press.

APA (1968) *Diagnostic and Statistical Manual of Mental Disorders*, 2nd edn. Washington DC: American Psychiatric Press.

APA (1980) *Diagnostic and Statistical Manual of Mental Disorders*, 3rd edn. Washington DC: American Psychiatric Press.

APA (1994) *Diagnostic and Statistical Manual of Mental Disorders*, 4th edn. Washington DC: American Psychiatric Press.

Avery, A., King, S., Bretherton, R. and Orner, R. (1999) Deconstructing psychological debriefing and the emergence of calls for evidence-based practice. *Traum Stress Points* **13**, 6–8.

Ayalon, O. (1998) Community healing for children traumatized by war. *Int Rev Psychiat* **10**, 224–33.

Baldessarini, R.J., Finklestein, S. and Arana, G.W. (1983) The predictive power of diagnostic tests and the effect of prevalence of illness. *Arch Gen Psychiat* **40**, 569–73.

Barlow, D.H. and Craske, M.G. (1988) The phenomenology of panic. In Rachman, S. and Maser, J.D. (eds) *Panic; Psychological Perspectives*. Hilldale: Lawrence Erlbaum Associates, pp.11–35.

Beck, A.T. and Emery, G. (1985) *Anxiety Disorders and Phobias: a cognitive perspective*. New York: Basic Books.

Bisson J.I., Jenkins P., Alexander J. and Bannister, C. (1997) Randomised controlled trial of psychological debriefing for victims of acute burn trauma. *Br J Psychiat* **171**, 78–81.

Breslau, N., Davis, G.C., Andreski, P. and Petersen, E. (1991) Traumatic events and posttraumatic stress disorder in an urban population of young adults. *Arch Gen Psychiat* **48**, 216–22.

Breslau, N., Kessler, R.C., Chilcoat, H.D., Schultz, L.R., Davis, G.C. and Andreski, P. (1998) Trauma and posttraumatic stress disorder in the community—the 1996 Detroit Area Survey of Trauma. *Arch Gen Psychiat* **55**, 626–32.

Brewin, C.R., Andrews, B., Rose, S. and Kirk, M. (1998) Acute stress disorder and post-traumatic stress disorder in victims of violent crime. *Am J Psychiat* **156**, 360–6.

Brewin, C.R., Andrews B. and Valentine, J.D. (2000) Meta-analysis of risk factors for posttraumatic stress disorder in trauma-exposed adults. *J Consult Clin Psychol* **68**, 748–66.

Brewin, C.R., Rose, S., Andrews, B., Green, J., Tata, P., McEuedy, C., Turner, S. and Foa, E. (2002). Brief screening instrument for post-traumatic stress disorder. *British Journal of Psychiatry* **181**, 158–62.

Briole, C, Lebigot, F., Lafont, B., Faure, J.D. and Vallet, D. (1996) Le Traumatisme Psychique: rencontre et devenir, Masson Pb, Paris.

Brom, D., Kleber, R.J. and Defares, P.B. (1989) Brief psychotherapy for posttraumatic stress disorders. *J Consult Clin Psychol* **57**, 607–12.

Bryant, R.A., Harvey, A.G., Dang, S. and Sackville, T. (1998) Assessing acute stress disorder: psychometric properties of a structured clinical interview. *Psycholog Assess* **10**, 215–20.

Bryant, R.A., Sackville, T., Dang, S.T., Moulds, M. and Guthrie, R. (1999) Treating acute stress disorder: an evaluation of cognitive behavior therapy and counseling techniques. *Am J Psychiat* **156**, 1780–6.

Bryant, R.A., Moulds, M. and Guthrie, R. (2000) Acute stress disorder scale: a self-report measure of acute stress disorder. *Psycholog Assess* **12**, 61–8.

Cannon, W.B. (1932) *The Wisdom of the Body*. New York: Norton.

Caplan, G. (1964) *Principles of Preventive Psychiatry*. New York: Basic Books.

Caplan, G. and Killilea, M. (1976) *Support Systems and Mutual Help; Multidisciplinary Exploitations*. New York: Grune & Stratton.

Caplan, G. (1981) Mastery of stress: psychosocial aspects. *Am J Psychiat* **138**, 413–20.

Cardeña, E., Koopman, C., Classen, C., Waelde, L.C. and Spiegel, D. (2000) Psychometric properties of the Stanford Acute Stress reaction Questionnaire (SASRQ): a valid and reliable measure of acute stress. *J Traum Stress* **13**, 719–34.

Carlier, I.V.E., Lamberts, R.D., van Uchelen, A.J. and Gersons, B.P.R. (1998) Disaster-related post-traumatic stress in police officers: a field study of the impact of debriefing. *Stress Med* **14**, 143–8.

Daligand, L. (1997) Analyse critique du debriefing. *Rev Franc Psychiat Psycholog Med* **10**, 46–7.

Dansky, B.D., Brady, K.T. and Roberts, J.T. (1994) Post-traumatic stress disorder and substance abuse: empirical findings and clinical issues. *Subst Abuse* **15**, 247–57.

Dasberg, H. (1976) Belonging and loneliness in relation to mental breakdown in battle. *Isr Ann Psychiat Relate Sci* **14**, 307–21.

Datillio, F. and Freeman, M. (2000) *Cognitive-behavioral Strategies in Crisis Intervention*, 2nd edn. New York: Guilford.

Davidson, J.R., Hughes, D., Blazer, D.G. and George, L.K. (1991) Post-traumatic stress disorder in the community. *Psycholog Med* **21**, 713–21.

Dohrenwend, B.S. and Dohrenwend, B.P. (1981) *Stressful Life Events & their Contexts*. New Brunswick: Rutgers University Press.

Falsetti, S.A. and Resnick, H.S. (2000) Treatment of PTSD using cognitive and cognitive behavioral therapies. *J Cognit Psychother* **14**, 261–85.

Foa, E.B., Hearst-Ikeda, D. and Perry, K.J. (1995) Evaluation of a Grief cognitive-behavioural program for the prevention of chronic PTSD in recent assault victims. *Annual Review of Psychology* **48**, 449–80.

Freedman, S.A., Peri, T., Brandes, D. and Shalev, A.Y. (1999) Predictors of chronic PTSD—a prospective study. *Br J Psychiat* **174**, 353–9.

Freud, S. and Breuer, J. (1893) *On the Psychical Mechanism of Hysterical Phenomena: preliminary communication*, Vol. 2. London: Hogarth Press.

Gist, R. and Woodall, S.J. (1998) Social Science versus social movements: the origins and natural history of debriefing. *Aust J Disaster Trauma Stud*, electronic journal. Available at: http:/www.massey.ac.nz/~trauma/issues/1998–1/gist1.htm.

Green, M.M., McFarlane, A.C., Hunter, C.E. and Griggs, W.M. (1993) Undiagnosed post-traumatic stress disorder following motor vehicle accidents. *Med J Aust* **159**, 529–34.

Grinker, R.R and Spiegel, J.P (1945) *Men Under Stress*. Philadelphia: Blakistan.

Harvey, A.G. and Bryant, R.A. (1998) The relationship between acute stress disorder and post-traumatic stress disorder: a prospective evaluation of motor vehicle accident survivors. *J Consult Clin Psychol* **66**, 507–12.

Harvey, A.G. and Bryant, R.A. (1999) Relationship of acute stress disorder and posttraumatic stress disorder: a two-year prospective study. *J Consult Clin Psychol* **67**, 985–8.

Holmes, T.H. and Rahe, R.H. (1964) The social readjustment rating scale. *Am J Psychiat* **121**, 141–8.

Janoff-Bulman, R. (1985) The aftermath of victimization: rebuilding shattered assumptions (pp. 15–34). In Figley, C.R. (ed.) *Trauma and Its Wake: the study and treatment of post-traumatic stress disorder*. New York: Brunner/Mazel.

Kessler, R.C., Sonnega, A., Bromet, E. and Nelson, C.B. (1995) Posttraumatic stress disorder in the National comorbidity survey. *Arch Gen Psychiat* **52**, 1058–60.

Kilpatrick, D.G., Veronen, L.J. and Resick, P.A. (1982) Psychological sequelae to rape: assessment and treatment strategies. In Doleys, D.M., Meredith, R.L. and Ciminero, A.R. (eds) *Behavioral Medicine: assessment and treatment strategies*. New York: Plenum Publishing Corporation, pp. 473–97.

Kleber, R.J. (2000) Psychosocial acute care: current state of research on coping with trauma and acute stress interventions. *Psycho-social Acute Care in the Event of a Crisis Workshop*, 14–22 May 2000, Vienna.

Kleber, R.J. and Brom, D. (1992) *Coping with Trauma: theory, prevention and treatment*. Amsterdam: Swets and Zeitlinger International.

Klein, D.C. and Lindemann, E. (1961) Preventive intervention in individual and family crisis situations. In G. Caplan (ed.) *Prevention of Mental Disorder in Children*. New York: Basic Books.

Lacan J. (1966) *Ecrits*. Paris: Seuil.

Lindemann, E. (1944) Symptomatology and management of acute grief. *Am J Psychiat* **101**, 141–8.

Mayou, R., Ehlers, A. and Hobbs, M. (2000) Psychological debriefing for road traffic accident victims. *Br J Psychiat* **176**, 589–93.

McFarlane, A.C. (1988) The longitudinal course of post-traumatic morbidity: the range of outcomes and their predictors. *J Nerv Ment Dis* **176**, 30–9.

Mitchell, J. (1983) When disaster strikes: the critical incident stress debriefing process. *J Emerg Med Serv* **8**, 36–9.

Mitchell, J. (1998) Critical incident stress management: a new era in crisis intervention. *Traum Stress Pts*, **12**, 9–11.

Mowrer, O.H. (1960) *Learning Theory and Behavior*. New York: John Wiley and Sons.

Najavits, L.M., Weiss, R.D. and Liese, B.S. (1996) Group cognitive-behavioral therapy for women with PTSD and substance use disorder. *J Subst Abuse Treat* **13**, 13–22.

Paykel, E.S. (1969) Life events and depression: a controlled study. *Arch Gen Psychiat* **21**, 753–60.

Pearlin, L.I. and Schooler, C. (1978) The structure of coping. *J Hlth Soc Behav* **22**, 337–56.

Peddle, N., Monteirlo, C., Guluma, V. and Macauley, T.E.A. (1999) Trauma, loss and resilience in Africa: a psychosocial community based approach to culturally sensitive healing. In Nader, K., Dubrow, N. and Stamm, B.H. (eds) *Honoring Differences: issues in the treatment of trauma and loss*. Philadelphia: Brunner/Mazel, pp. 121–49.

Pilgrim, H. (1999) Cognitive aspects of PTSD. PhD Thesis. University of Manchester, England.

Post, R.M. (1992) Transduction of psychosocial stress into the neurobiology of recurrent affective disorder. *Am J Psychiat* **149**, 999–1010.

Raphael, B. (1986) *When Disaster Strikes; a Handbook for the Caring Professionals*. Boston: Unwin Hyman.

Reichenberg, D. and Friedman, S. (1996) Traumatized children. In Danieli, Y., Rodely, N. and Weisaeth, L. (eds) *International Response to Traumatic Stress*. New York: Baywood, pp. 307–26.

Resick, P.A. and Schnicke, M.K. (1993) *Cognitive Processing Therapy for Rape Victims: a treatment manual*. Newbury Park: Sage Publications.

Resnick, H., Acierno, R., Holmes, M., Kilpatrick, D. and Jager, N. (1999) Prevention of post-rape psychopathology: preliminary evaluation of an acute rape treatment. *J Anx Disord* **13**, 359–70.

Resnick, H.S. and Newton, T. (1992) Assessment and treatment of posttraumatic stress disorder in adult survivors of sexual assault. In Foy, D.W. (ed.) *Treating PTSD*. New York: Guilford Press, pp. 99–126.

Riggs, D.S., Rothbaum, B.O. and Foa, E.B. (1995) A prospective examination of symptoms of posttraumatic stress disorder in victims of non-sexual assault. *J Interpers Violence* **10**, 201–13.

Rothbaum, B.O., Foa, E.B., Riggs, D.S., Murdock, T. and Walsh, W. (1992) A prospective examination of post-traumatic stress disorder in rape victims. *J Traum Stress* **5**, 455–75.

Ruzek, J.I. and Zatzick, D.F. (2000) Ethical considerations in research participation among acutely injured trauma survivors: An empirical investigation. *Gen Hosp Psychiat* **22**, 27–36.

Schnyder, U. (1997) Crisis intervention in psychiatric outpatients. *Int Med J* **4**, 11–17.

Schnyder, U., Moergeli, H., Klaghofer, R. and Buddeberg, C. (2001a) Incidence and prediction of PTSD symptoms in severely injured accident victims. *Am J Psychiat* **158**, 594–9.

Schnyder, U., Moergeli, H., Trentz, O., Klaghofer, R. and Buddeberg, C. (2001b) Prediction of psychiatric morbidity in severely injured accident victims at one-year follow-up. *Am J Resp Crit Care Med* **164**, 653–6.

Selye, H. (1956) *The Stress of Life*. London: Longmans.

Shalev, A.Y. and Munitz, H. (1989) Combat stress reaction in Ries N.D. In Dolcv, E. (ed.) *Manual of Disaster Medicine*. Berlin: Springer Verlag, pp. 169–82.

Solomon, Z. and Benbenishty, R. (1986) The role of proximity, immediacy and expectancy in frontline treatment of combat stress reaction among Israelis in the Lebanon War. *Am J Psychiat* **143**, 613–17.

Solomon, Z, Laror, N. and McFarlane, A.C. (1996) Acute posttraumatic reactions in soldiers and civilians. In van der Kolk, B.A., McFarlane, A.C. and Weisaeth, L. (eds) *Traumatic Stress: the overwhelming experience on mind, body and society*. New York: Guilford Press, pp. 102–14.

Terr, L. (1990) *Too Scare to Cry*. New York: Harper Collins.

Terr, L. (1991) Childhood traumas: an outline and overview. *Am J Psychiat* **148**, 10–20.

Tyhurst, J.S. (1957) The role of transition states—including disasters—in mental illness. In *Symposium on Preventive and Social Psychiatry*. Washington DC: Walter Reed Army Medical Centre.

Weisæth, L. (1989) The importance of high response rates in traumatic stress research. *Acta Psychiat Scand* Suppl. 355, **80**, 131–7.

Weisæth, L. (2001) Acute posttraumatic stress: non acceptance of early intervention. *J Clin Psychiat* **62**, 35–40.

Wessells, M.G. (1999) Culture, power and community: Intercultural approaches to psychosocial assistance and healing. In Nader, K., Dubrow, N. and Stamm, B.H. (eds) *Honoring Differences: issues in the treatment of trauma and loss*. Philadelphia: Brunner/Mazel, pp. 267–82.

World Health Organization (1992) *The ICD-10 Classification of Mental and Behavioural Disorders. Clinical Descriptions and Diagnostic Guidelines*. Geneva: WHO.

World Health Organization (1993) *The ICD-10 Classification of Mental and Behavioural Disorders. Diagnostic Criteria for Research*. Geneva: WHO.

Yehuda, R., McFarlane, A.C. and Shalev, A.Y. (1998) Predicting the development of post-traumatic stress disorder from the acute response to a traumatic event. *Biolog Psychiat* **44**, 1305–13.

Yitzhaki, T., Solomon, Z. and Kotler, M. (1991) The clinical picture of acute combat stress reaction among Israeli soldiers in the 1982 Lebanon War. *Mil Med* **156**, 193–7.

Yule, W. and Unwin, O. (1991) Screening child survivors for posttraumatic stress disorders: experiences from the 'Jupiter' sinking. *Br J Clin Psychol* **30**, 131–8.

Index